Concise
Osteology

Muscles, Clinical Orientation and Viva Voce

Concise
Osteology

Muscles, Clinical Orientation and Viva Voce

BD Ghosh DMS, Dip. NIH, MD (Hom)

Professor and Head
Department of Anatomy
KS Homoeopathic Medical College and Hospital
Lashkar, Gwalior, MP

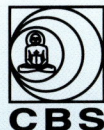

CBS

CBS Publishers & Distributors Pvt Ltd

New Delhi • Bengaluru • Chennai • Kochi • Kolkata • Mumbai

Bhopal • Bhubaneswar • Hyderabad • Jharkhand • Nagpur • Patna • Pune • Uttarakhand • Dhaka (Bangladesh)

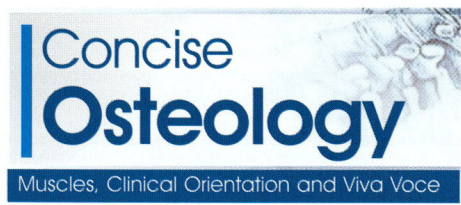

ISBN: 978-93-88178-85-3

Copyright © Author and Publisher

First Edition: 2019

Published by Satish Kumar Jain and produced by Varun Jain for

CBS Publishers & Distributors Pvt Ltd

4819/XI Prahlad Street, 24 Ansari Road, Daryaganj, New Delhi 110 002, India.
Ph: 23289259, 23266861, 23266867   Fax: 011-23243014   Website: www.cbspd.com
e-mail: delhi@cbspd.com; cbspubs@airtelmail.in.
Corporate Office: 204 FIE, Industrial Area, Patparganj, Delhi 110 092
Ph: 4934 4934   Fax: 4934 4935   e-mail: publishing@cbspd.com; publicity@cbspd.com

Branches

- **Bengaluru:** Seema House 2975, 17th Cross, K.R. Road,
  Banasankari 2nd Stage, Bengaluru 560 070, Karnataka
  Ph: +91-80-26771678/79   Fax: +91-80-26771680   e-mail: bangalore@cbspd.com
- **Chennai:** 7, Subbaraya Street, Shenoy Nagar, Chennai 600 030, Tamil Nadu
  Ph: +91-44-26680620, 26681266   Fax: +91-44-42032115   e-mail: chennai@cbspd.com
- **Kochi:** 42/1325, 1326, Power House Road, Opposite KSEB Power House,
  Ernakulam 682 018, Kochi, Kerala
  Ph: +91-484-4059061-65   Fax: +91-484-4059065   e-mail: kochi@cbspd.com
- **Kolkata:** 6/B, Ground Floor, Rameswar Shaw Road, Kolkata-700 014, West Bengal
  Ph: +91-33-22891126, 22891127, 22891128   e-mail: kolkata@cbspd.com
- **Mumbai:** 83-C, Dr E Moses Road, Worli, Mumbai-400018, Maharashtra
  Ph: +91-22-24902340/41   Fax: +91-22-24902342   e-mail: mumbai@cbspd.com

Representatives

- **Bhopal** 0-8319310552
- **Bhubaneswar** 0-9911037372
- **Hyderabad** 0-9885175004
- **Jharkhand** 0-9811541605
- **Nagpur** 0-9021734563
- **Patna** 0-9334159340
- **Pune** 0-9623451994
- **Uttarakhand** 0-9716462459
- **Dhaka (Bangladesh)** 01912-003485

Printed at Magic International, Greater Noida, UP, India

_to_

my daughter Payel Ghosh

Forewords

It is a great pleasure for me to introduce the book *Concise Osteology* written by Dr BD Ghosh. Nowadays original bones are not easily available. This book contains original pictures of bones which are explained clearly.

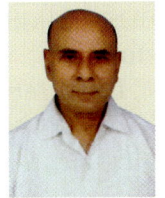

This book reveals the effort and long experience of the author. I hope this book will create interest about the osteology among the students.

Ravindra Kumar
Principal
Dr Ram Balak Singh Homoeopathic
Medical College and Hospital
Amwan, Gaya, Bihar

Concise Osteology written by Dr BD Ghosh, Professor of Anatomy, is hands down, one of the best osteological textbooks I have ever come across. Its value lies mainly in the systematic way, it guides you through a detailed study of bones. The information is concise, accurate and as comprehensive as I imagine it could be.

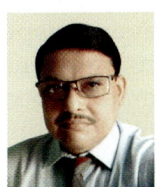

I have gone through this book thoroughly and acquired valuable information on bones. I am pretty sure that this book will be inevitable for medical students and aspirants for achieving better marks in written as well as oral examinations.

Champak Chattopadhyay
Reader and Head
Department of Anatomy
Birbhum Vivekananda Homoeopathic
Medical College and Hospital
Sainthia, Birbhum, West Bengal

I am glad to know that Professor Dr BD Ghosh has written the book *Concise Osteology*. Nowadays original bones are scarcely available to students. So, the illustrations of original bones in this book will be treasure for all medical students.

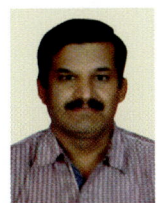

I congratulate Dr Ghosh for this amazing work in the field of anatomy and wish him good luck.

Atul Kumar Singh
Principal
Dr MPK Homoeopathic Medical College,
Hospital and Research Centre
Jaipur, Rajasthan

I convey my warm greetings for the book *Concise Osteology* written by Dr BD Ghosh. This book is concentrated on the problems faced by the students during the *viva voce* and practical examinations. In this book, minute features of every bone are explained by giving illustrations. It will surely help students to have the clear idea about bones.

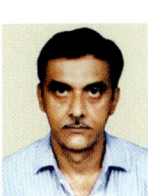

I wish Dr BD Ghosh all the success for this book.

Mrinal Mukherjee
Assistant Professor/Reader
Netai Charan Chakraborty
Homoeopathic Medical College and Hospital
45 F Road, Belgachia, Howrah, West Bengal

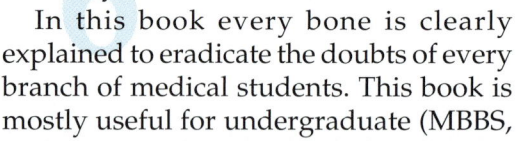

I am very happy to recommend the book *Concise Osteology* authored by Dr BD Ghosh Professor and Head, Department of Anatomy, KS Homoeopathic Medical College and Hospital, Gwalior, MP. I have gone through the book and I found that author has covered 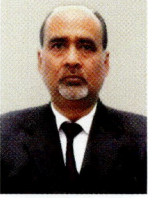 every aspect of subject which represents the comprehensive study of osteology. The author has made a beautiful effort in presenting the original photographs of bones. The book will be a testimony to his experience and with clearly justify his untiring efforts and his versatility. Dr BD Ghosh has been an excellent academician.

I extend my blessings and wish him great success for his future life.

Narendra Singh Sengar
Principal
Homoeopathic Medical College
Piproli, Chirwai Naka, Lashkar Gwalior, MP

The book *Concise Osteology* by Dr BD Ghosh is very good for preparation of theory and *viva voce* examinations.

In this book every bone is clearly explained to eradicate the doubts of every branch of medical students. This book is mostly useful for undergraduate (MBBS, 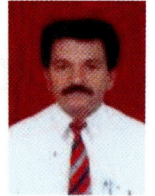 BDS, BHMS, BAMS, physiotherapy and BSc nursing) students.

I congratulate Dr BD Ghosh for bringing this book. May God bless him in every walk of his professional life.

Jadi Rajamallu
Professor and Head
Department of Anatomy
Merchant Homoeopathic Medical College
Ahmedabad, Gujrat

Preface

After a long teaching experience in anatomy, I observed that there is need of knowledge and proper conception of osteology as it is the backbone of anatomy.

The medical students in India are increasing day by day. On the other hand, the number of skeleton and bones is decreasing proportionately. The bone sets are less available and costly. So students cannot easily collect these.

So I have given original photographs of each and every bone for proper understanding and clear knowledge of each and every feature of the bones, hoping that it will be helpful for students to understand osteology properly.

BD Ghosh

Acknowledgements

This book *Concise Osteology* is enriched with Dr Manatosh Pahari's great knowledge in anatomy, which I have extracted from him and applied from beginning to end of this book.

Dr Manotosh Pahari, Dr Tapas Kumar Modak, Dr Mrinal Mukherjee and Dr Champak Chatterjee have also contributed their valuable knowledge and advice for editing of this book.

I am lucky enough to work with Desarda family Dr SM Desarda, Dr KS Desarda and Dr Yogesh Desarda whose support have encouraged me to my best outcome in anatomy writing.

My hearty respect to Dr Ramjee Singh, Dr Rabindra Kumar for introducing me in nation for anatomy.

I am also very thankful to Dr BB Jana, Dr Goutam Ash, Dr Srimanta Saha, Dr Swapan Kumar Halder, Dr Paromita Goswami, Dr Alpana Ghosh, Dr Netai Chandra Ghosh, Dr KR Pal, Dr Deb Kumar Das, Dr Jaya Bhattacharya, Dr Upendra Singh, Dr Tapaur Hausain, Dr BC Ghosh, Dr Tanmoy Mitra, Dr Anil Kumar Mishra, Dr Birendra Prasad Srivastava, Dr Somen Kundu, Dr Pritam Gupta, Dr Bharat Kumar Singh, Dr Narendra Singh Sengar, Dr Rajvardhan Singh Bhadoria, Dr BB Hati, Dr Balachandran, Dr Sujit Kumar Pal, Dr Jagdish Darak, Dr BL Dudhmal, Dr Toofan Chakravorty, Dr Usha Garge, Dr Minal Vinayak Rachalwar, Dr Arvinda Kumar Verma, Dr Pravin Kumar, Dr Pradip Das, Dr Ujjal Bhowmick, Dr TK Saha, Dr Biswajit Biswas, Dr Vikrant Tripathi, Dr Ankita Acharya Tripathi, Dr Timir Baran Datta, Dr Somnath Ganguli, Dr Atul Kumar Singh, Dr UK Jawahar, Dr Jadi Rajamallu, Dr Sudip Ditti, Dr Sk Hasina, Dr Raghunath Kumar, Dr Shankar Sagar, Dr Vishal Kumar, Dr Raj Bondre, Dr Sanap Pandurang Sachin, Dr Sudhir Ashokrao Hatnoorkar, Dr Rameswar Patil, Dinesh kumar Maurya, Hafiz Quazi Ateek ur Rahaman, Mr Sudhir Kumar Singh, Vishesh Singhal, Dr Chandan Yadav, Pooja Sawaleram Wagh, Manish Bamb, Pravat Kumar Sinha, Arjun Kamble, Prasad Deshmukh, Anunka Sil, Samir Kumar Kar, Dibyendu Sarkar, Subham Sengupta, Sayyed Saim Anique, Sohail Ahmed, Zuber Mirza, Maksud Patel, Mujahed Pathan, Vijay Hiwale, Indrayni Londhe, SPhradha Chavan, Shivani Kadam, Bhagyashree Shindhe, Varsha Gvali, Zoya Khan, Anjali Verma, Aqsa Anam, Sana Begum, Saniya Saudagar, Pranjal Mahajan, Vaibhav Palve, Ashwini Bhosle, Kathwade Ashwini, Saherish Fatema for their support.

I am also thankful to Dibyendu Sarkar who with his expert artistic skill in computer technology has edited all the figures of this book.

I am grateful to Samir Kumar Kar for helping me in DTP and in every aspect he can.

I have been influenced and encouraged by the members of CBS team, Mr SK Jain (CMD), Mr YN Arjuna (Sr Vice President—Publishing, Editorial and Publicity), Mrs Ritu Chawla (AGM of Publishing), Mr PG Bandhu, Mr CB Bhattacharjee, and Mr Prasun Bhattacharya.

My beloved daughter Payel Ghosh and my wife Dr Sucheta Ghosh have supported me all the time during writing this book and also have encouraged me to devote for anatomy.

BD Ghosh

Contents

General Consideration

INTRODUCTION

The science, which deals with the bones, called osteology.

i. Known that all vertebrate animals have their inside the bodies made up of hard tissue called bone.

ii. The bones form the general framework of the body.

iii. Bones form important landmarks for determining position of internal visceras.

iv. Bones afford leverage to the muscle.

v. Careful study of bones is possible to estimate the age, sex, and cause of death of any individuals for medicolegal point of view.

vi. The characteristic features of bones vary with the race, occupation and customs of the individual.

vii. The skull of Europeans differs from that of Japanese in shape and size.

viii. The Mohammedans kneel down during prayer so that impressions on their patellae vary from those of Europeans who stand during prayer.

ix. Impression on the ischial tuberosities of Indians are different from those of the other races as Indians adopt their sitting position very often.

IMPORTANT TERMS USED IN OSTEOLOGY

- **Ala:** Wing in appearance.
- **Canal:** A bony tunnel.
- **Condyle:** This is a large rounded partly articular portion at the end of a long bone.
- **Cornu:** A horn-like bony projection.
- **Crest:** A ridge of some wide.
- **Epicondyle:** Non-articular bony projections lie above the condyles.

- **Facet:** The smooth articular surfaces between the two bones.
- **Foramen:** An opening in the bone.
- **Fossa:** Depression on the surface of the bone.
- **Groove:** A long narrow channel.
- **Hamulus:** A hook-like bony projection.
- **Hiatus:** A gap in the bone.
- **Incisura:** A notch or a cut on the general outline in the bone.
- **Lamina:** A flat piece of bone.
- **Lingula:** A tongue-shaped projection.
- **Meatus:** A narrow passage.
- **Notch:** An indentation on the edge of a bone.
- **Ossicle:** Any small bone especially bones of the ear.
- **Process:** Any localized elevation or projection.
- **Ridge:** A linear elevation.
- **Spine:** A pointed bony process.
- **Squama:** A large lamina.
- **Sulcus:** A groove or furrow.
- **Suture:** The line of union between the skull bones.
- **Trochanter:** Large non-articular projections, only in case of femur.
- **Trochlea:** A pulley-shaped articular surface.
- **Tubercle and tuberosity:** These are localized rounded thickenings on the surface of the bones with varying sizes. The smaller ones are known as tubercles whereas larger ones are known as tuberosities.
- **Uncus:** A hook-like projection.

OSSEOUS SYSTEM OR SKELETAL SYSTEM

Skeleton: It is the bony framework of the body also cartilages and membranous parts.

HISTOLOGY OF BONES

i. Bones consists of two kinds of tissues, the compact tissue and spongy tissue.

ii. The bone is covered externally by the tight vascular membrane—the periosteum, except the part covered by articular cartilages.

iii. From this highly vascular membrane the periosteal blood vessels enter the substance of the bone and supply it.

iv. In long bones there is a central cavity called medullary cavity filled with bone marrow.

v. This cavity is also lined by highly vascular membrane the endosteum or medullary membrane.

vi. When a thin transverse section of a bone is examined under microscope, it shows a large number of circular areas known as haversian canal surrounded by several concentric bony lamina.

vii. The haversian canal transmits an artery, vein, some lymphatics and nerve filaments.

CLASSIFICATION OF BONES

A. According to Shape

i. *Long bones:* Each long bone has an elongated shaft (diaphysis) and two expanded ends (epiphysis). The long bones are further following types.

  a. Typical long bones: These are most of the long bones of the limbs.
  Examples: Humerus, ulna, radius, femur, tibia and fibula.

  b. Miniature or short long bones: Here only one single epiphysis at one end only (epiphysis of medial four metacarpals at their distal ends whereas in the first metacarpal epiphysis at its base or proximal end).
  Examples: Metacarpals, metatarsals, phalangeal bones of fingers and toes.

  c. Modified long bones: The clavicle is a modified long bone, although it has no medullary cavity and ossified mostly in membrane.

ii. *Short bones:* Their shape is usually cuboid.
Examples: Carpals and tarsals.

iii. *Flat bones:* Flat bones consist of two plates of compact bones with intervening spongy bone and marrow.
Examples: Most of the bones of the vault of the skull.

iv. *Irregular bones:* These bones present irregular morphology.
Examples: Most of the bones of the base of the skull, vertebrae and hip bones.

v. *Pneumatic bones:* These bones contain air spaces which are lined by mucous membrane.
Examples: Maxillae, sphenoid, ethmoid, etc.

Functions of pneumatic bone

a. It makes the skull light in weight.

b. Helps in resonance of voice.

c. Acts as an air conditioning chamber by adding humidity and temperature for the inspired air.

vi. *Sesamoid bones:* These bones develop in the tendons of some muscles.

Sites where sesamoid bones are develop:

a. In the tendon of quadriceps femoris—patella develops.

b. In the tendon of lateral head of gastrocnemius—fabella.

c. In the tendon of flexor carpi ulnaris—pisiform.

d. In the tendon of adductor pollicis.

e. In the tendon of flexor pollicis brevis.

f. In the tendon of peroneus longus.

g. In the tendon of flexor hallucis brevis.

Functions of sesamoid bones

a. Reduce friction of tendons against bone.

b. To alter the direction of pull of the muscle (act as pulley for muscular contraction).

c. To maintain the local circulation.

Peculiarities of sesamoid bones

a. Bone develops within the tendon of muscle.

b. It has no periosteum.

c. Ossify after birth.

d. It has no Haversian system.

vii. *Accessory or supernumerary bones:* These bones may appear as ununited epiphysis developed from extracentres of ossification.
Example: Sutural bones, os trigonum (lateral tubercle of talus), os vesalianum (tuberosity of 5th metatarsal), etc.
Medicolegal importance: In X-ray films they may be mistaken for fracture.

viii. *Heterotopic bones:* Bones may develop in soft tissues.
Example: Bone may develop in the adductor longus muscle which is termed as rider's bone.

B. According to Development (Ossification)

i. **Membranous bones:** Ossify in membrane (derived from mesenchymal condensations).
Examples: Bones of the vault of the skull and facial bones.

ii. **Cartilaginous bones:** Ossify in cartilage.
Example: Bones of the limbs, thoracic cage and vertebral column.

iii. **Membrano-cartilaginous bones:** Ossify partly in membrane and partly in cartilage.
Examples: Clavicle, mandible, occipital, temporal and sphenoid bones.

C. According to Position

i. Axial bones: Examples are bones of the skull, ribs, sternum and vertebrae.

ii. Appendicular bones: Examples are bones of the limbs.

D. According to Structure

i. Macroscopically

a. Compact bone: Dense in texture like ivory, but extremely porous.

Examples: Cortex of long bones.

b. Cancellous or spongy or trabecular bone: It is made with of meshwork of trabeculae (rods and plates) with marrow containing spaces. These are of three types:

- Meshwork of rods.
- Meshwork of rods and plates.
- Meshwork of plates.

ii. Microscopically: There are again five types:

a. Lamellar bone: Most of the mature bones are composed of thin plates of bony tissue, called lamellae.

b. Woven bone: These are seen in fetal bone, fracture repair and in cancer of bone.

c. Fibrous bone: These are seen in young fetal bones.

Example: Dentine and cement in teeth.

FUNCTIONS OF BONES

i. To give shape, support and forms the rigid framework of the body.

ii. Bones act as levers for muscles therefore help in movements.

iii. To provide for the attachments of muscles, tendons and ligaments.

iv. Production of blood cells from the bone marrow.

v. Bones are store houses of calcium and phosphorus, which form two-thirds of the bone by weight. The mineral salts responsible for rigidity of bones and radiopaque in X-ray films.

vi. The reticuloendothelial cells of the bone marrow are phagocytic in nature and take part in immune responses of the body.

vii. The paranasal air sinuses affect the timbre (quality of sound) of the voice.

viii. The skull, vertebral canal and thoracic cage protect brain, spinal cord and thoracic visceras, respectively.

BONES OF SKELETON

The total number of bones in a human body are 206.

i. Bones of the axial skeleton: 80 bones

a. Vertebrae—26.

b. Bones of the skull and face—22

c. Hyoid bone—1

d. Sternum—1

e. Ribs (12 pairs)—24

f. Auditory ossicles—6

ii. Bones of appendicular skeleton: 126

a. Bones of the upper limbs—total 64 (32 in each side).

b. Bones of the lower limbs—total 62 (31 in each side).

FORMATION OF BONES

i. Bones are developed from the mesodermal tissue of the embryo.

ii. Some from fibrous membrane, called membranous ossification.

iii. Others from cartilaginous masses, called cartilaginous ossification.

iv. The process by which a bone is formed called ossification.

CENTERS OF OSSIFICATION

i. The place from which bone formation takes place called center of ossification.

ii. Centers of ossification may be primary or secondary.

iii. Those centers are appear in fetal life are known as primary center except carpal bones cuneiform and navicular of foot.

iv. Those centers that appear after birth known as secondary center except lower end of femur.

LAW OF UNION OF OSSIFICATION

i. During the process of development the center of ossification appears first in the body and later in the ends.

ii. The growth of bone is regulated by the mode of ramification of its blood vessels.

iii. In long bones which have got diaphysis and epiphysis. Epiphysis, which gets more blood supply, unites with the diaphysis first.

iv. In the arm and forearm, the nutrient artery being directed towards the elbow joint, the lower epiphysis of the humerus and upper epiphysis of radius and ulna unite with their respective diaphysis before their fellows on the other end.

v. Where there is only one epiphysis, the nutrient artery runs towards that side,

vi. The epiphysis, which begins to ossify, first unites with the diaphysis last and vice versa (in fibula law of union of epiphysis is violated).

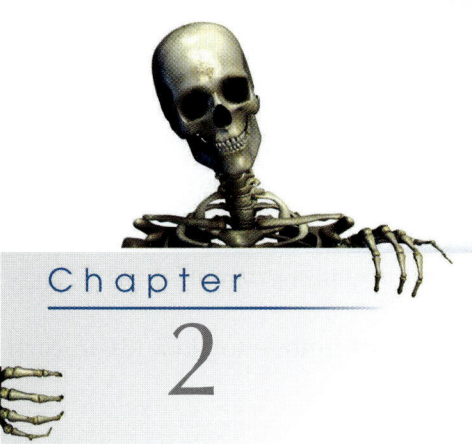

Bones of Upper Limb

CLAVICLE

▌ INTRODUCTION

The clavicle is a subcutaneous long bone extends laterally and horizontally across the front of the root of the neck and connects the sternum with the scapula.

Clavicle is a modified long bone: Clavicle is a modified long bone because it transmits forces or weight from the upper limb to the axial skeleton (specially its medial two-thirds). This is however an exception violating the following principles of a long bone.

Following are the peculiarities

  i. Clavicle has no medullary cavity.
  ii. Ossifies mostly by membrane.
  iii. Two primary centers of ossification in the shaft.
  iv. It is the first bone in the body to start ossification, and also last bone to complete ossification..
  v. It is wholly subcutaneous.
  vi. It is placed horizontally.
  vii. Sometimes, it is pierced by supraclavicular nerves.

▌ ANATOMICAL POSITION

  i. Bone should be held horizontally.
  ii. The enlarged sternal end directed medially.
  iii. The flattened acromial end directed laterally.
  iv. The medial two-thirds of the shaft convex forward.
  v. The lateral one-third of the shaft concave forward.
  vi. Presence of a groove on its inferior aspect of the intermediate part.
  vii. The conoid tubercle will be directed postero-inferiorly.

SIDE DETERMINATION

After holding the bone in anatomical position, the flattened lateral end on which side belongs will determine the side of the bone.

FUNCTIONS OF CLAVICLE

  i. Clavicle helps to place the scapula laterally, so the upper limb can swing from the side of the trunk.
  ii. It receives the weight of the upper limb through the coracoclavicular ligament and medial two-thirds of the bone to the axial skeleton.
  iii. The posterior surface of the medial two-thirds of the clavicle protects the neurovascular bundles of the root of the neck, apex of the lung and its covering pleura.
  iv. It helps in various scapular movements.
  v. Clavicle prevents the dropping of the point of the shoulder.

GENERAL FEATURES OF THE CLAVICLE

As it is a long bone, it has a shaft and two ends (medial and lateral).

Shaft

It is divided into medial two-thirds and lateral one-third.

Medial Two-thirds

It is roughly cylindrical with four surfaces but no borders.

Anterior surface: It is curved and rough but laterally smooth.

Superior surface: It is rough medially but smooth laterally (Fig. 2.1).

Posterior surface: The surface is smooth and concave posteriorly except close to its sternal end where it is rough.

Relations: From medial to lateral—
i. Lower end of internal jugular, subclavian and beginning of the brachiocephalic veins.
ii. Trunks of brachial plexus and third part of subclavian artery.
iii. Suprascapular vessels.

Inferior surface
i. On the middle one-third of this surface a groove for the subclavius muscle, called subclavian groove.
ii. Close to sternal end a rough costal impression
iii. Nutrient foramen present on the lateral end of the subclavian groove transmits nutrient vessels (Fig. 2.2).

Lateral One-third

It is flat and contains following features.

Surfaces
Superior surface: This surface is smooth and subcutaneous in the center but near the margins, it is rough due to muscular attachments.

Inferior surface: It is rough and present conoid tubercle at the junction of medial three-fourths and lateral one-fourth of the bone and trapezoid ridge runs forwards and laterally from the conoid tubercle to the acromial end.

Borders
Anterior: It is rough concave and may present deltoid tubercle.

Posterior: It is thick and convex.

Tubercles
Conoid tubercle: It is present on the inferior surface near to the posterior border at the junction of medial three-fourth of the bone.

Deltoid tubercle: Anterior border of the lateral one-third may show a small tubercle, called deltoid tubercle.

Ends
Sternal or medial end: This end is enlarged and presents a convex rough articular surface to articulate with the clavicular notch of the manubrium to form the sternoclavicular joint.

Acromial or lateral end: It is flat and presents an oval facet to articulate with a similar facet on the medial border of the acromion process to form the acromioclavicular joint.

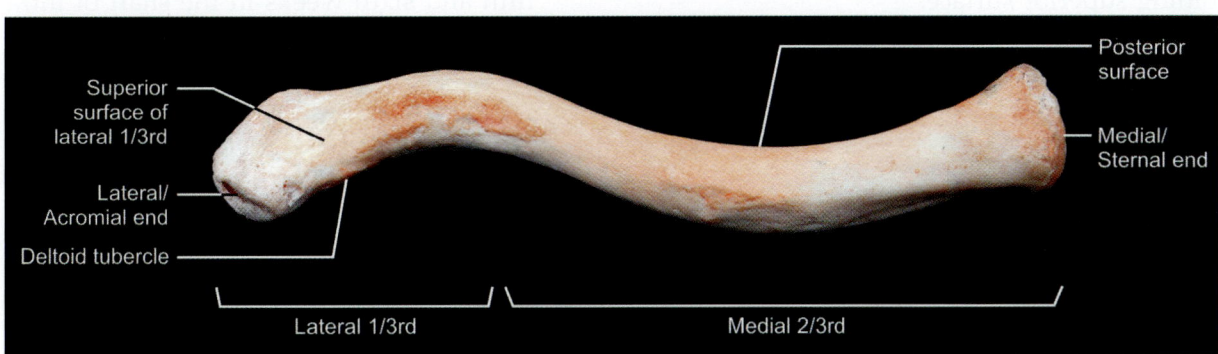

Fig. 2.1: General features of right clavicle (superior view)

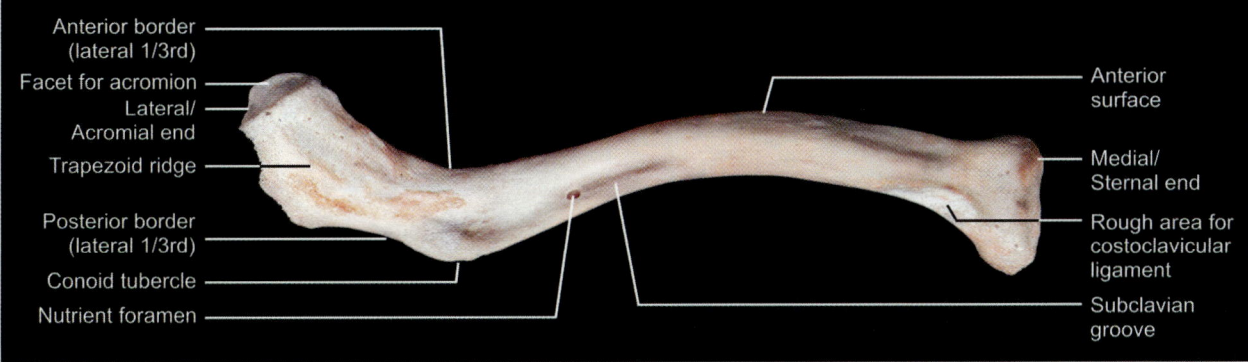

Fig. 2.2: General features of right clavicle (inferior view)

ATTACHMENTS OF CLAVICLE

Medial Two-thirds of the Shaft

i. **Origin of** (Fig. 2.3)

    a. **Pectoralis major:** from the medial half of the anterior surface.

    b. **Clavicular head of the sternocleidomastoid:** Medial part of the superior surface.

    c. **Sternohyoid:** close to the medial end of the posterior surface.

ii. **Insertion of** (Fig. 2.4)

    Subclavius: In the floor of the subclavian groove of inferior surface.

iii. **Fascia and ligament**

    a. **Clavipectoral fascia:** Lips of the groove give attachment of the two layers of clavipectoral fascia.

    b. **Costoclavicular ligament:** to the rough costal impression of the inferior surface (Fig. 2.3).

Lateral One-third of the Shaft

i. **Origin of** (Fig. 2.3)

    Deltoid: To the anterior border, including deltoid tubercle and also the adjoining superior surface.

ii. **Insertion of**

    Trapezius: To the posterior border and also adjoining superior surface.

iii. **Ligaments**

    a. **Conoid part of the coracoclavicular ligament:** To the conoid tubercle.

    b. **Trapezoid part of the coracoclavicular ligament:** To the trapezoid ridge (Fig. 2.4).

Ends

Sternal or medial end

i. **Capsular ligament:** Around the margin of the articular surface of the sternal end.

ii. **Articular disc and interclavicular ligament:** Rough upper part of the sternal end.

iii. **Sternoclavicular ligaments:** To the corresponding margins of sternal end.

Acromial or lateral end

i. **Capsular ligament:** Along the margin of the articular facet.

ii. **Acromioclavicular ligament:** At the upper margin of the articular facet.

iii. **Coracoclavicular ligament:** This ligament connects the clavicle and coracoid process of scapula.

OSSIFICATION

Ossification begins from the membrane.

i. **Two primary centers** of ossification between the fifth and sixth weeks in the shaft of intrauterine life.

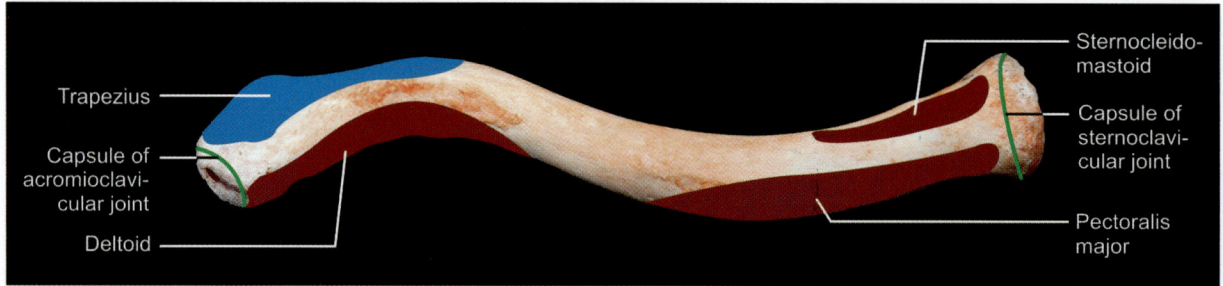

Fig. 2.3: Attachment of right clavicle (superior view)

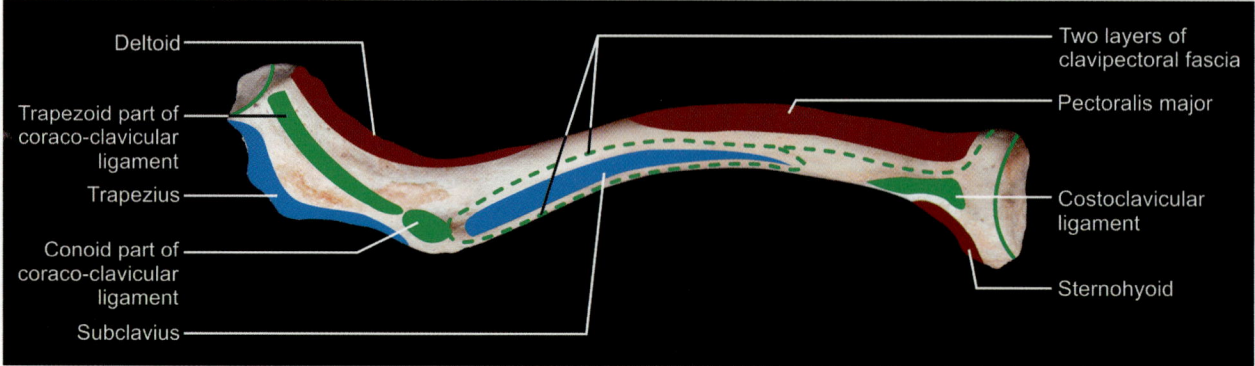

Fig. 2.4: Attachment of right clavicle (inferior view)

ii. **One secondary center** appears in the sternal end about 18 years, which fused with the shaft starts about 20 years and completed the fusion about 31 years.

iii. Occasionally, a secondary center may appear at the acromial end between 18 and 20 years.

The above helps in age determination

Deference between male and female clavicles as shown in Table 2.1.

CLINICAL ANATOMY

i. Fracture of the clavicle

a. Clavicle is one of the most frequently fractured bones as a result of indirect violence due to fall on the outstretched hand or on the shoulder or by direct violence on the shoulder.

b. Fracture usually takes place at the junction of medial two-thirds with the lateral one-third which is the weakest part of the bone because two curvatures meet, the transmission of forces from the clavicle to scapula occur at this site through coracoclavicular ligament and presence nutrient foramen on the lateral end of the subclavian groove.

c. Lateral segment is displaced downwards by the weight of the upper limb as a result drooping of the shoulder. The medial segment displaced upwards by the pull of the sternocleidomastoid muscle.

ii. Greenstick pattern fracture

a. This type of fracture is usually seen in young children where clavicle often breaks in a "greenstick" pattern.

b. The bones in children, are so elastic that when twisting or angulating force is applied the whole thickness of bone does not break. Instead, one cortex breaks while the other cortex is simply moulded.

c. This fracture requires no operative treatment, usually a sling support or by immobilization with figure 8 bandages is sufficient for stability of the bone within three to four weeks.

iii. **Cleidocranial dysostosis:** Clavicle may be congenitally absent one or both. This patient can bring the soulders close to each other in front of chest.

SCAPULA

▌ INTRODUCTION

The scapula is a large flat, triangular bone situated on the posterolateral aspect of the chest wall, extends from second to seventh ribs, and forms the part of the shoulder girdle.

Type: Flat bone.

ANATOMICAL POSITION

i. The dorsal surface carrying the spine looks backwards.

ii. The inferior angle looks downwards.

iii. The glenoid cavity directed forwards, laterally and slightly upwards.

iv. Tip of the coracoid process directed anteriorly.

SIDE DETERMINATION

After holding the bone in anatomical position the glenoid cavity will determine the side to which the bone belongs.

GENERAL FEATURES OF THE SCAPULA

Surfaces

i. Costal

ii. Dorsal.

Borders

i. Superior

ii. Medial or vertebral

iii. Lateral or axillary.

Angles

i. Superior

ii. Inferior

iii. Lateral.

Processes

i. Spinous

ii. Acromion

iii. Coracoid.

Table 2.1	Difference between male and female clavicles	
Male	**Female**
Clavicle is longer, thicker and more curved	Clavicle is shorter, thinner and less curved
Musclular impressions are more marked in male than female	Musclular impressions are less marked in male than female
Lateral end is either at the same level or slightly higher than medial end	Lateal end is slightly lower than the medial end.

Notches
i. Suprascapular
ii. Spinoglenoidal.

Neck
i. Anatomical
ii. Surgical.

Fossa
i. Supraspinous
ii. Infraspinous.

Tubercles
i. Supraglenoid tubercle
ii. Infraglenoid tubercle.

Costal surface
i. It is directed anteromedially.
ii. It is slightly hollow especially above.
iii. Near the lateral border a rounded ridge.
iv. Three or more oblique ridges run upwards and laterally from the medial border produced by the origin of intermuscular tendon of subscapularis muscle (Fig. 2.5).

Dorsal surface
i. The dorsal surface presents a triangular self-like projection, called spinous process.
ii. By the spinous process the dorsal surface is divided in to upper smaller area, called supraspinous fossa and lower larger area, called infraspinous fossa.
iii. Spinoglenoid notch, presents between lateral border of the spinous process and the dorsal aspect of the neck, transmits the suprascapular vessels and nerves (Fig. 2.6).

Superior border
i. It is thinnest and shortest of all borders.
ii. It extends from the superior angle to the root of the coracoid process.
iii. Marked by the suprascapular notch.

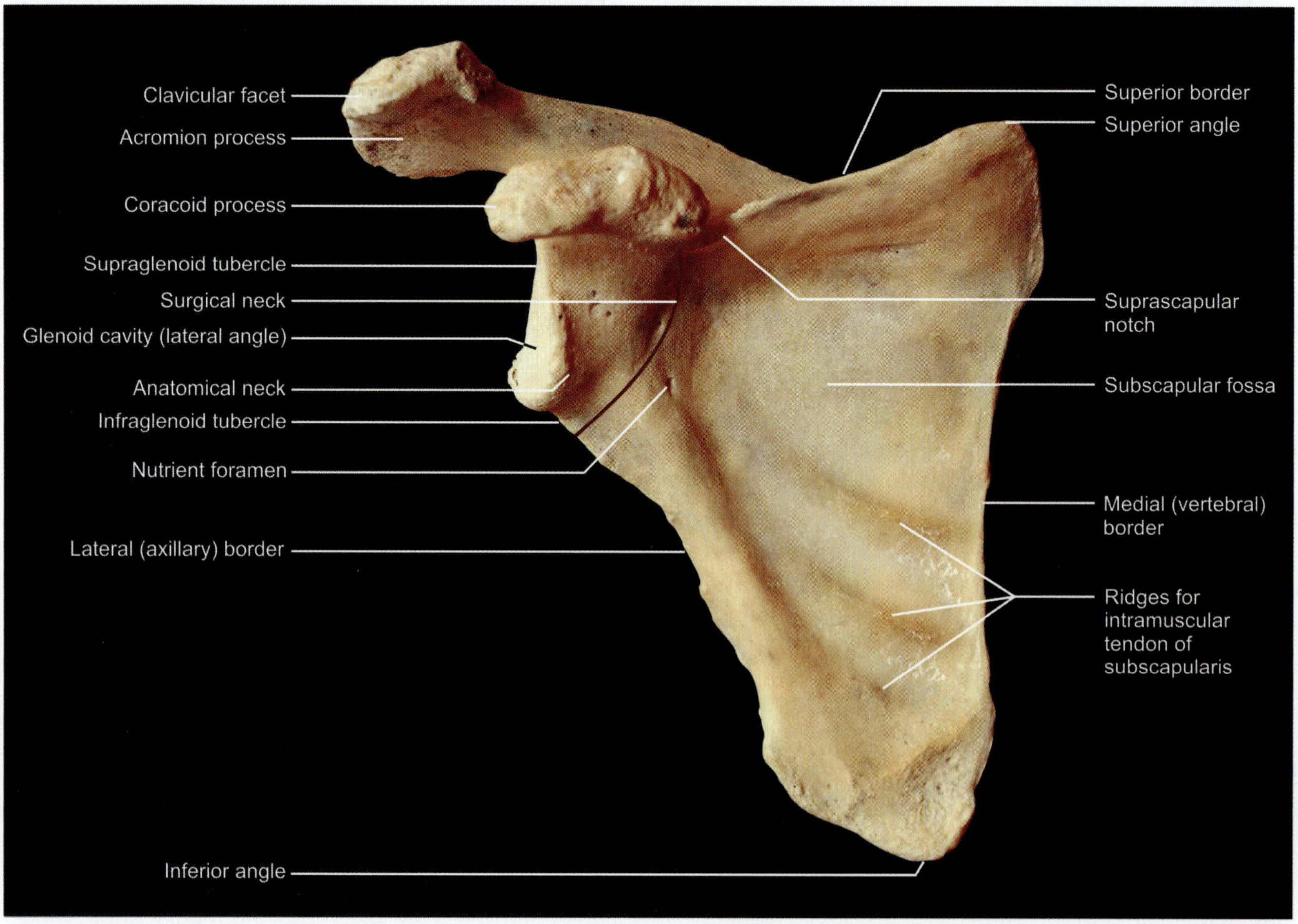

Clavicular facet

Acromion process

Coracoid process

Supraglenoid tubercle

Surgical neck

Glenoid cavity (lateral angle)

Anatomical neck

Infraglenoid tubercle

Nutrient foramen

Lateral (axillary) border

Inferior angle

Superior border

Superior angle

Suprascapular notch

Subscapular fossa

Medial (vertebral) border

Ridges for intramuscular tendon of subscapularis

Fig. 2.5: General features of right scapula (costal surface)

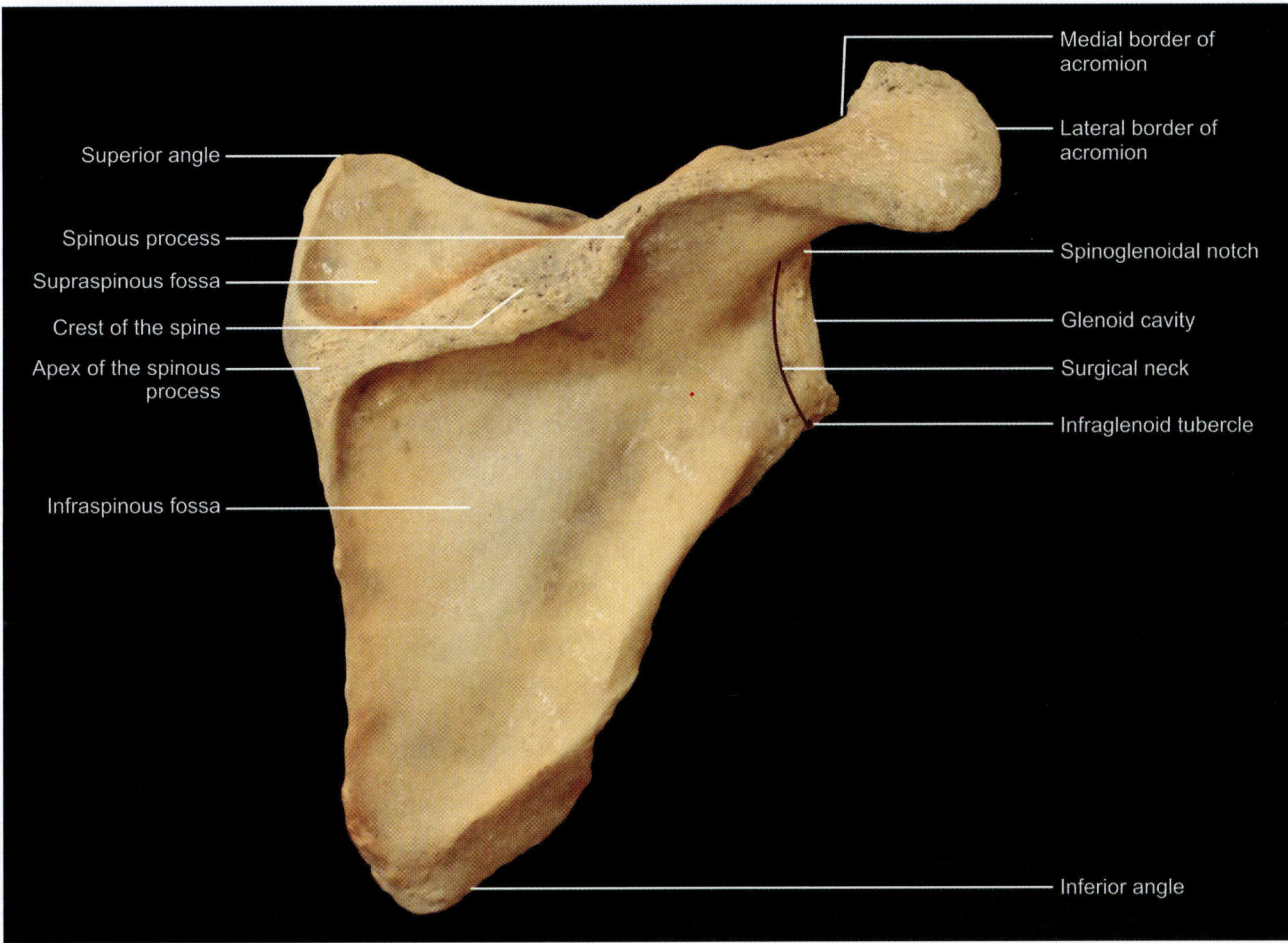

Fig. 2.6: General features of right scapula (dorsal surface)

Medial or vertebral border

   i. Longest of all borders

  ii. Extends from superior to inferior angles.

Lateral or axillary border

   i. Thickest of all borders.

  ii. Extends from the lower end of the glenoid cavity to the inferior angle.

 iii. Below the glenoid cavity lies the infraglenoid tubercle.

Superior angle: Formed by the junction of the superior and medial borders.

Inferior angle

   i. Formed by the junction of the lateral and medial borders.

  ii. Lies opposite the seventh rib or intercostal space.

Lateral angle

   i. Having the glenoid cavity and forms the head of the scapula.

  ii. Having the supraglenoid tubercle lies above the glenoid cavity and at the root of the coracoid process.

 iii. **Anatomical neck** is the constricted part of the bone beyond the glenoidal margin.

 iv. **Surgical neck** is represented by a line passing from the anterior margin of the suprascapular notch to the infraglenoid tubercle, and posteriorly line passes through the spinoglenoid notch.

Spinous process

   i. It is a self-like triangular projection from the upper part of the dorsal surface.

  ii. It divides the dorsal surface in to supra- and infraspinous fossae.

 iii. Spine consists of base, apex, anterior, posterior and lateral borders and upper and lower surfaces.

    a. **Apex:** It is smooth triangular area, lies at the medial border of the scapula at the level of TV3 spine.

b. **Anterior border:** Fused with the dorsal surface of the scapula obliquely upwards and laterally.

c. **Posterior border**
   - This border thick, subcutaneous and forms the crest of the spine
   - Crest presents upper and lower lips
   - The upper lip laterally continuous with the medial border of the acromion process
   - The lower lip continuous with the lateral border of acromion process at the lateral angle.

d. **Lateral border:** It is thick and free, forms the medial boundary of the spinoglenoidal notch.

e. **Upper surface:** It is gently concave, continuous with the supraspinous fossa.

f. **Lower surface:** It is slightly convex, continuous with the infraspinous fossa.

Acromion process

i. It is the expanded plate of bone.

ii. It consists of superior and inferior surfaces and medial and lateral borders.

iii. Its superior surface is subcutaneous.

iv. The lateral border of the acromion meets the lower lip of the spine to form a subcutaneous bony prominence.

v. Its medially having a small articular facet for articulation with the clavicle to form the acromioclavicular joint.

Coracoid process

i. It arises from the upper part of the glenoid cavity.

ii. Its tip directed forwards, lies 1 inch below the junction of medial three-fourths and lateral one-fourth of the clavicle.

iii. It has ascending and horizontal parts.
   a. Ascending part having anterior and dorsal surfaces,
   b. Horizontal part directed forwards, having lateral and medial borders and upper and lower surfaces and a conical tip.

Supraglenoid tubercle: It lies just above the glenoid cavity, a rough elevation.

Infraglenoid tubercle: It lies just below the glenoid cavity, a rough elevation.

ATTACHMENTS OF SCAPULA

A. Costal Surface

Origin of

Subscapularis (Fig. 2.7): From the most of the costal surface (except the region of the neck) and the oblique ridges.

Insertion of

Serratus anterior: Along the costal surface of the medial border

i. First and second digitations from superior angle to the point opposite the spinous process of scapula.

ii. Third and fourth digitations from opposite the apex of the process of the scapula to the superior part of the inferior angle of the scapula.

iii. Fifth to eight digitations from the opposite the inferior angle of the scapula (Fig. 2.7).

B. Dorsal Surface

Origin of

i. **Supraspinatus:** From the medial two-thirds of the supraspinous fossa.

ii. **Infraspinatus:** From the infraspinous fossa (except near the neck).

iii. **Teres minor:** From the upper two-thirds of the rough strip on the dorsal surface near the lateral border.

iv. **Teres major:** From the lower one-third of the rough strip along the lateral border of the dorsal surface.

v. **Latissimus dorsi:** From the dorsal surface near the inferior angle (Fig. 2.8).

C. Superior Border

Origin of

Inferior belly of omohyoid: From the suprascapular notch.

Others: The suprascapular notch is converted into suprascapular foramen by the suprascapular ligament, which transmits the suprascapular nerve, but suprascapular vessels pass above the ligament.

D. Medial or Vertebral Border

Insertion of

On the dorsal aspect

i. **Levator scapulae:** From superior angle to the upper part of the apex of the spine.

ii. **Rhomboideus minor:** Opposite the apex of the spine.

iii. **Rhomboideus major:** Below the apex of the spine up to the inferior angle.

On the ventral aspect

iv. **Serratus anterior:** From whole of the medial border of the costal surface, which extends to:

   a. **The first and second digitations:** From the superior angle to a point opposite the apex of the spine.

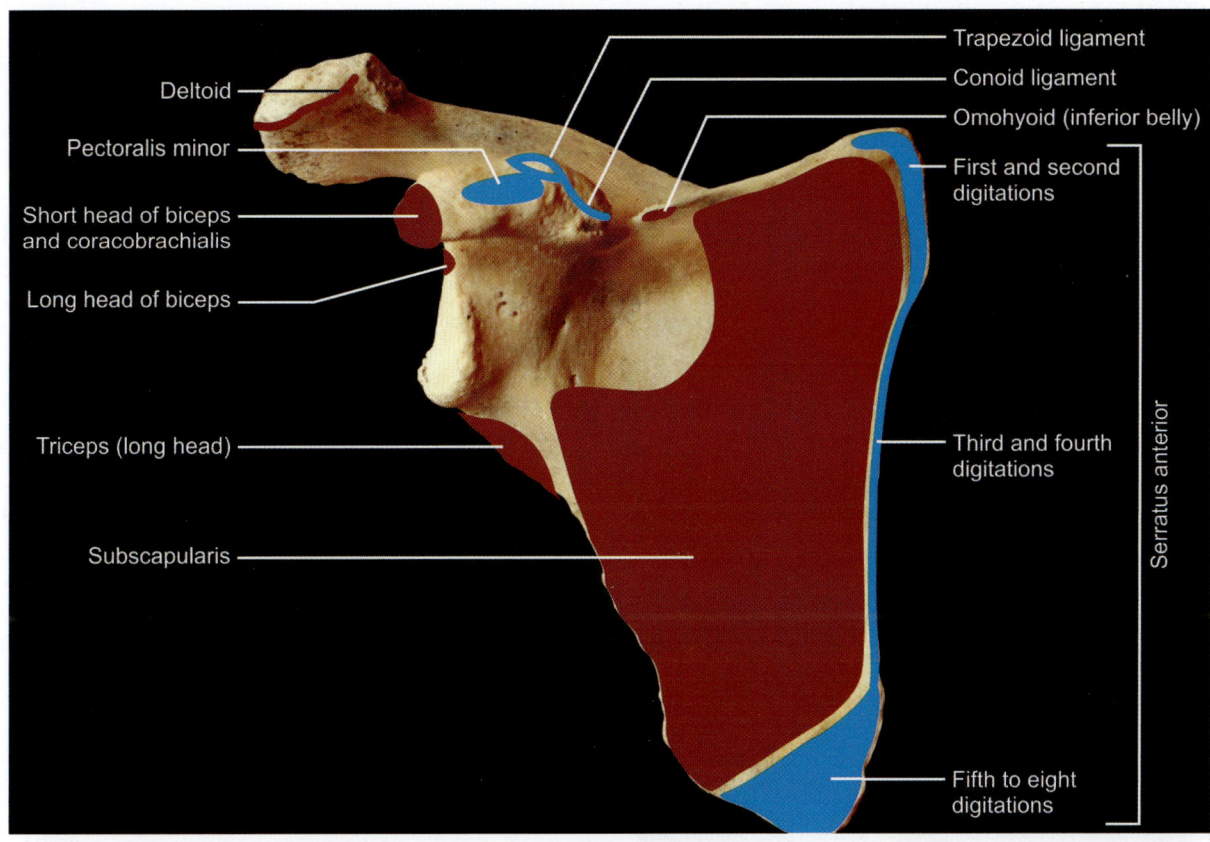

Fig. 2.7: Attachments of right scapula (costal surface)

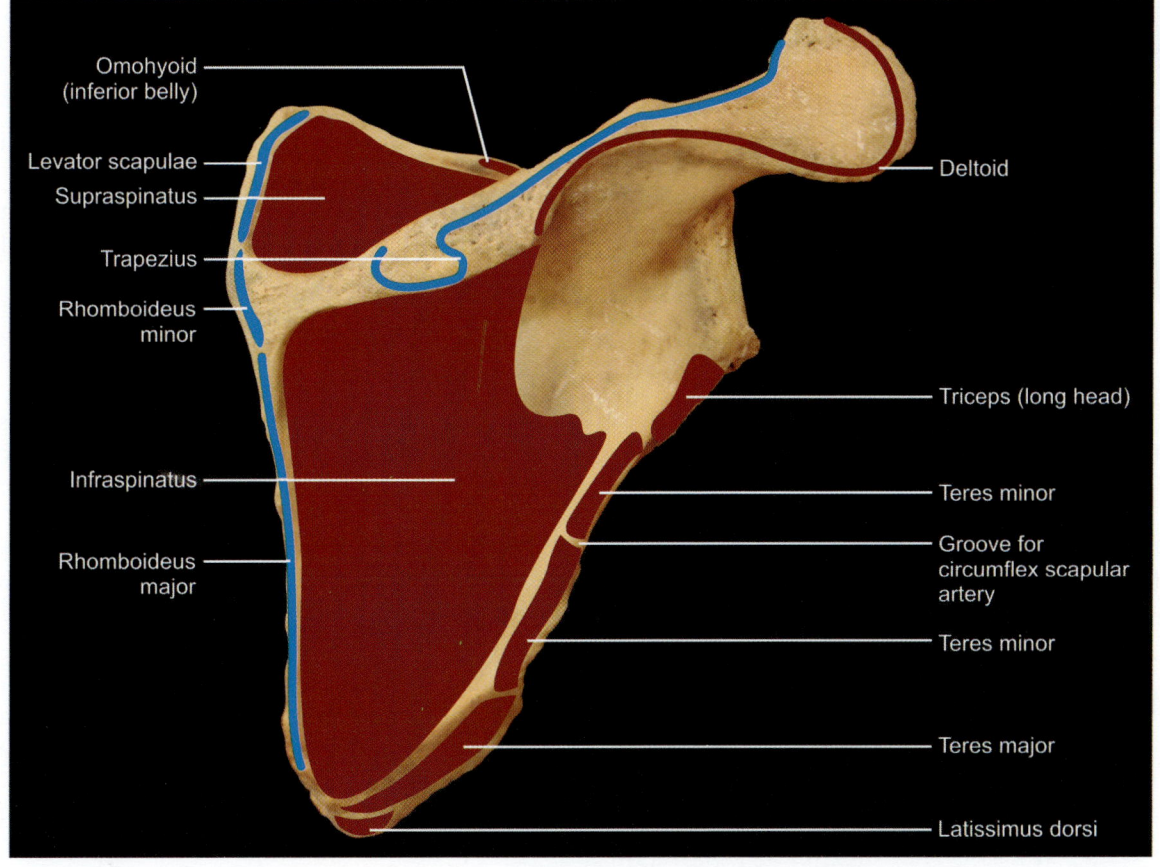

Fig. 2.8: Attachments of right scapula (dorsal surface)

b. The third and fourth digitations: From below the apex of the spine to the up to the upper part of the inferior angle.

c. The fifth to eighth digitations: From opposite the inferior angle.

E. Lateral or Axillary Border

Origin of (Fig. 2.9)

i. **Long head of triceps brachii:** From the infraglenoid tubercle.

ii. **Subscapularis:** Along the costal surface.

iii. **Teres minor and major:** Along the dorsal surface (Fig. 2.9).

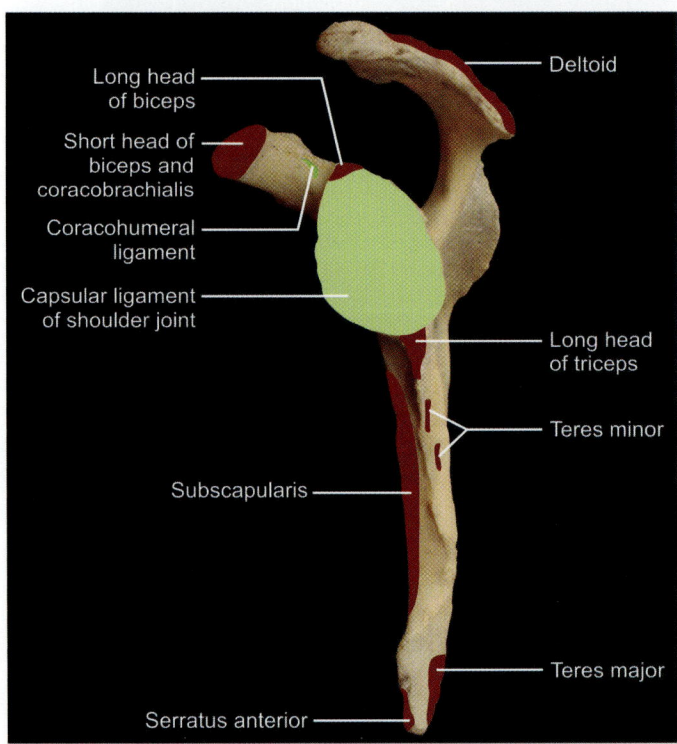

Fig. 2.9: Attachments of left scapula (lateral view)

Inferior angle

On the dorsal aspect

Origin of

i. Teres major

ii. Few fibers of the latissimus dorsi.

On the ventral surface:

Insertion of

iii. Serratus anterior (fifth to eight digitations).

Lateral angle

Origin of

Long head of biceps brachii: From the supraglenoid tubercle.

Ligaments and others

i. **Articular hyaline cartilage:** It covers the floor of the glenoid cavity.

ii. **Glenoidal labrum:** Attached to the margins of the glenoid cavity.

iii. **Capsular ligament of the shoulder joint:** Attached to the peripheral margins of the glenoid cavity outside the glenoidal labrum, except superiorly where it extends to root of the coracoid process.

Spinous process

Origin of

i. **Deltoid:** From the lower lip of the crest of the spine (posterior fibers).

ii. **Supraspinatus:** From the upper surface of the spinous process.

iii. **Infraspinatus:** From the lower surface of the spinous process.

Insertion of

Trapezius: Into the upper lip of crest.

Acromion process

Origin of

Deltoid: From the lateral border (middle fibers).

Insertion of

Trapezius: From the medial border (middle fibers).

Ligaments

i. **Coracoacromial ligament:** At the tip of the acromion process.

ii. **Capsular ligament of the acromioclavicular joint:** At the margins of the articular facet on the medial border.

Coracoid process

Origin of

Coracobrachialis and short head of biceps brachii: From the tip of the coracoid process of which coracobrachialis is medially and biceps laterally.

Insertion of

Pectoralis minor: From the medial border of the horizontal part and adjoining upper surface.

Ligaments

i. **Conoid part of the coracoclavicular ligament:** To the rough impression at the junction of ascending and horizontal parts.

ii. **Trapezoid part of the coracoclavicular ligament:** Attached to the ridge on the upper surface of the horizontal part.

iii. **Supraclavicular ligament:** To the ascending part, this forms the upper margin of the suprascapular notch.

iv. **Coracoacromial ligament:** To the lateral border of the horizontal part both in front and behind.

v. **Coracohumeral ligament:** To the middle of the lateral border of the horizontal part.

Supraglenoid tubercle

Origin of: Long head of biceps brachii.

Infraglenoid tubercle

Origin of: Long head of triceps brachii.

OSSIFICATION

Scapula has eight centers of ossification of which one primary and seven are secondary.

i. **Primary center:** Appears in the body during eighth week of intrauterine life.

ii. **Secondary centers**

a. The coracoid process having two centers, one appears in the first year and second center appears about the age of puberty at the root of the coracoid process called subcoracoid center, which fused with the body by age of fifteenth years.

b. By the age of puberty two centers for the acromion process.

c. One center for the medial border.

d. One center for the inferior angle.

e. One for the lower margin of the glenoid cavity.

f. These centers fused with the body of the scapula at about the age of 20 year.

CLINICAL ANATOMY

i. **Winging of the scapula:** It is a deformity of the scapula characterized by the inferior angle and medial border of scapula become unduely prominent and difficulty of abduction of arm above 90°. It is due to paralysis of serratus anterior muscle in case of injury of the long thoracic nerve.

ii. **Fracture of the blade of the scapula** producing haematoma deep to infraspinatus fascia, Which is a strong fascia covers the infraspinatus and teres minor muscles.

iii. **Sprengel's deformity (congenital high scapula):** The scapula develops in the cervical region during intrauterine life then it normally migrates from cervical to thoracic position at about fifth week of intrauterine life. Failure of descent results in scapula situated in neck region.

HUMERUS

INTRODUCTION

The humerus is the longest and strongest bone of the upper limb having upper and lower ends and an intervening portion, called shaft or body.

ANATOMICAL POSITION

i. Spheroidal head looks upwards, medially and backwards.

ii. Prominent lesser tubercle projected forwards from the anterior part of the upper end.

iii. The olecranon fossa looks backwards of the lower end.

SIDE DETERMINATION

After holding the bone in anatomical position the head of the humerus or medial epicondyle will determine the opposite side of the bone.

GENERAL FEATURES

Upper or Proximal End

It consists of head, neck, lesser tubercle, greater tubercle and intertubercular sulcus.

Head

i. It is less than half a sphere

ii. Directed upwards, medially and backwards.

Neck: Humerus having the anatomical, surgical and morphological neck.

Anatomical neck: It is the constriction just succeeding the head.

Surgical neck: It is a constriction between the expanded upper end and the cylindrical shaft.

Morphological neck

i. It is line of fusion between upper epiphysis and diaphysis that passes across the lower parts of greater and lesser tubercles or about 0.5 cm above the surgical neck of the humerus

ii. Morphological neck disappears in adult.

Lesser tubercle

i. It projects forwards from the anterior part of the upper end of the humerus

ii. On its superior part there is a smooth muscular impression

iii. It is separated from the greater tubercle by the intertubercular sulcus.

Greater tubercle

i. It is most lateral of the upper end

ii. Its convex lateral part projects beyond the acromion process with many vascular foramina

iii. Its medial margin forms the lateral lip of the intertubercular sulcus

iv. On its posterosuperior aspect presents three impressions for muscular attachments.

Intertubercular sulcus/bicipital groove

i. It is a vertical deep groove between the lesser and greater tubercles

ii. It has lateral and medial lips and a floor (Fig. 2.10).

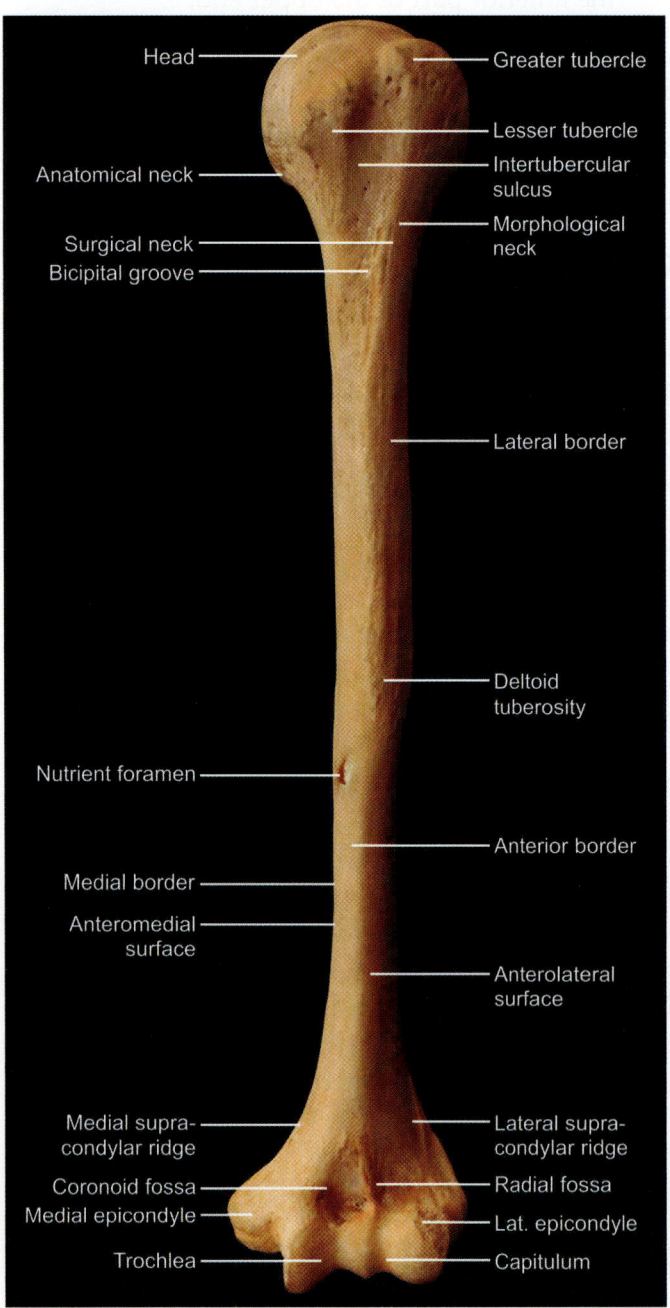

Fig. 2.10: Anterior aspect of the left humerus showing general features

Shaft

i. Upper half is cylindrical and lower half is triangular on cross-section

ii. Three borders—anterior, lateral and medial

iii. Three surfaces—anterolateral, anteromedial and posterior.

Anterior border

i. It extends from the front of the greater tubercle to the lower end of the humerus

ii. Opposite of middle forms the anterior edge of V-shaped deltoid tuberosity on the anterolateral surface of the bone.

Lateral border

i. It extends from the lower and posterior part of the greater tubercle and ends below above the lateral epicondyle

ii. Its upper part is indistinct

iii. Its lower part is very prominent called lateral supracondylar line or ridge.

Medial border

i. It extends from the medial lip of bicipital groove to the medial epicondyle

ii. Lower part is very prominent called medial supracondylar line or ridge.

Anterolateral surface

i. It lies between the anterior and lateral borders

ii. Near the middle a V-shaped muscular elevation called deltoid tuberosity.

Anteromedial surface

i. It lies between the anterior and medial borders

ii. Opposite the middle a rough area for muscular attachment

iii. Immediately below the midpoint of the shaft close to the medial border presents nutrient foramen directed downwards transmits nutrient artery.

Posterior surface

i. It lies between the medial and lateral borders

ii. In its upper one-third a rough oblique line descends laterally

iii. In the middle one-third crossed by a shallow groove passes downwards and laterally, called spiral or radial groove

iv. Lower one-third is flat, smooth and widens (Fig. 2.11).

Lower end

i. It is flattened anteroposteriorly and broader transversely.

ii. It consists of articular and non-articular parts.

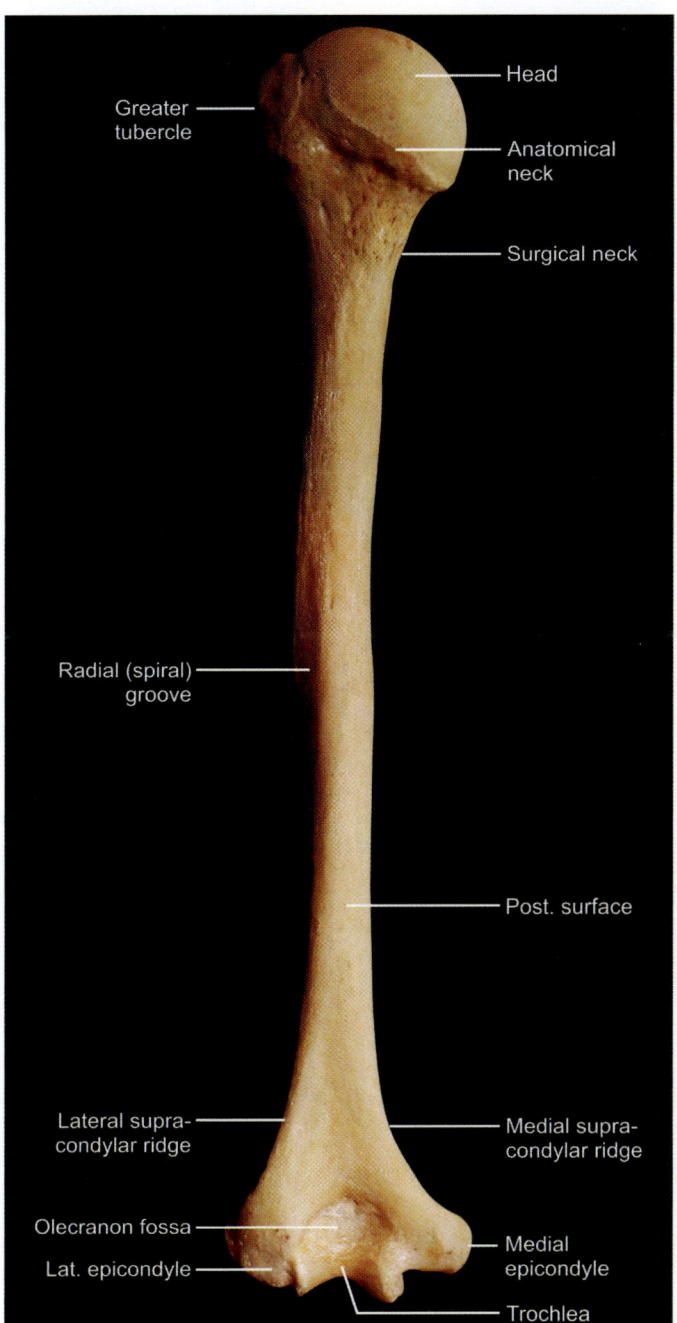

Fig. 2.11: Posterior aspect of the left humerus showing general features

Articular part (forms the elbow joint)

Capitulum

i. It is convex and less than half a sphere lies laterally
ii. Between the capitulum and trochlea there is a faint groove.

Trochlea

i. It is like a asymmetrical pulley
ii. It has anterior, posterior and inferior surfaces
iii. Its medial margin is prominent and projects downwards about 6 mm below the lateral margin

Non-articular part

Medial epicondyle

i. It is blunt, more prominent and subcutaneous
ii. Its anterior part is rough
iii. Posterior part is smooth
iv. On its anteroinferior surface presents a impression for muscular attachments
v. Immediately above the medial epicondyle forms a prominent margin called medial supracondylar ridge or line.

Lateral epicondyle

i. It is less prominent projection on the lateral part of the lower end of humerus.
ii. Its anterolateral aspect presents an impression for muscular attachments.
iii. Its posterior surface is convex.
iv. Immediately above the lateral epicondyle forms a prominent margin called lateral supracondylar ridge or line.

Olecranon fossa: It is deep depression on the lower part of the posterior surface of the humerus lodges the olecranon process of ulna in fully extended elbow.

Radial fossa: It is situated just above the capitulum on the anterior surface of the lower end, it lodges head of the radius in full flexion of elbow.

Coronoid fossa: Situated above the trochlea medial to the radial fossa, it lodges the coronoid process of ulna in full flexion of elbow.

ATTACHMENTS OF HUMERUS

Upper or Proximal End

Head

i. It is covered by the hyaline cartilage, which is thicker centrally and thinner peripherally.
ii. Head articulates with the glenoid cavity to form the shoulder (ball and socket) joint.

Neck: Capsular ligament of the shoulder joint—along the anatomical neck except the following areas:

i. At the upper end of the intertubercular sulcus.
ii. Medially, descends 1 cm more on the shaft.

Surgical neck: Relations—posteriorly related with axillary nerve and posterior circumflex humeral vessels.

Lesser tubercle

Insertion of: Subscapularis—on the superior part, it extends 12 mm below on the shaft.

Ligament: Transverse humeral ligament—on its lateral margin.

Greater tubercle
Insertion of
i. **Supraspinatus:** To the upper impression
ii. **Infraspinatus:** To the middle impression
iii. **Teres minor:** To the lowest impression.

Ligament: Transverse humeral ligament—to the medial margin of the tubercle.

Intertubercular sulcus/bicipital groove
Insertion of: From lateral to medial
i. **Pectoralis major:** To the lateral lip
ii. **Latissimus dorsi:** To the floor
iii. **Teres major:** To the medial lip (Fig. 2.12).

Contents
i. Long head of biceps brachii with synovial sheath
ii. Ascending branch of the anterior circumflex humeral artery.

Shaft

Anterolateral surface

Insertion of: Deltoid—at the deltoid tuberosity.

Origin of
i. **Brachialis:** Rest of the surface below the insertion of deltoid
ii. **Brachioradialis:** From the upper two-thirds of the lateral supracondylar ridge and adjoining anterolateral surface
iii. **Extensor carpi radialis longus:** From lower one-third of the lateral supracondylar ridge.

Other
Lateral intermuscular septum: In the lateral supracondylar ridge and lateral border of the humerus as far as the insertion of deltoid.

Anteromedial surface
Insertion of
Coracobrachialis—rough area on the middle.

Origin of
i. **Brachialis:** Lower half of the surface
ii. **Humeral head of pronator teres:** Lower part of the medial supracondylar ridge.

Other
Medial intermuscular septum: In the medial supracondylar line and medial border of the humerus as far as the insertion of coracobrachialis.

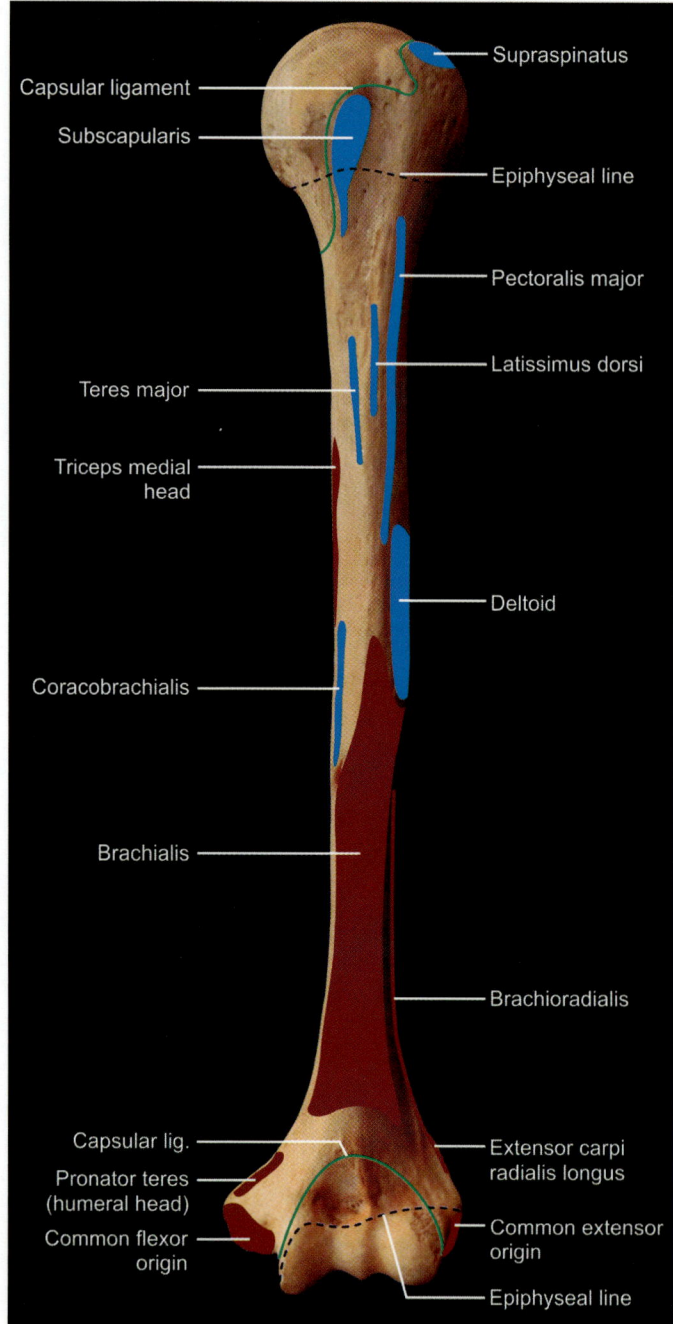

Fig. 2.12: Anterior aspect of the left humerus showing attachments

Posterior surface
Origin of (Fig. 2.13)
i. **Lateral head of triceps brachii:** From the oblique line on the upper one-third
ii. **Medial head of triceps brachii:** Rest of the surface below the radial groove.

Relations
Radial or spiral groove: This groove transmits radial nerve and profunda brachii vessels.

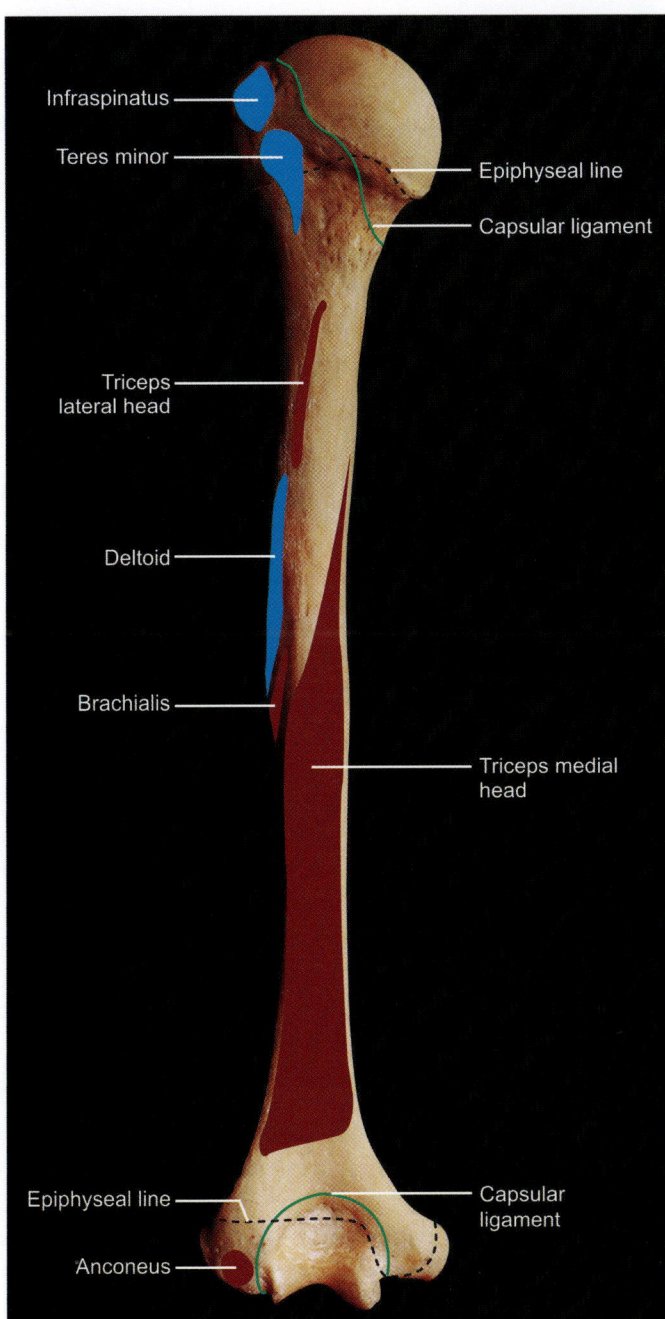

Labels on figure:
Infraspinatus
Teres minor
Epiphyseal line
Capsular ligament
Triceps lateral head
Deltoid
Brachialis
Triceps medial head
Epiphyseal line
Capsular ligament
Anconeus

Fig. 2.13: Posterior aspect of the left humerus showing attachements

Lower End

Capitulum

Articulations: It articulates with the upper surface of the head of the radius.

Trochlea

Articulations: It articulates with the trochlear notch of ulna.

Medial epicondyle

Origin of

Common origin of the superficial group of flexor muscles of forearm: From anterior part of the medial epicondyle.

Ligament

Anterior and posterior bands of ulnar collateral ligament: At the tip of the medial epicondyle.
Relation: Ulnar nerve (lodges in the sulcus nervi ulnaris present on the posterior surface of the medial epicondyle).

Lateral epicondyle

Origin of

i. **Common origin of the superficial group of extensor muscles of forearm:** From the impression present on its anterolateral aspect
ii. **Anconeus:** From the posterior surface.

Ligament

Radial collateral ligament: From the tip.
Olecranon fossa: It is deep depression on the lower part of the posterior surface of the shaft of the humerus.

Lodges: the olecranon process of ulna in fully extended elbow.

Radial fossa: It is situated just above the capitulum on the anterior surface of the lower end of the humerus.

Lodges: The head of the radius in full flexion of elbow.

Coronoid fossa: Situated above the trochlea medial to the radial fossa.

Lodges: the coronoid process of ulna in full flexion of elbow.

OSSIFICATION

Humerus ossified from one primary center and seven secondary centers of which three for the upper end and four for the lower end.

i. **Primary center:** It appears in the shaft during eighth week of embryonic life.
ii. **Secondary centers:**

For upper end

a. For the head—first year
b. For the greater tubercle—third year
c. For the lesser tubercle—fifth year
   The three secondary centers unite in the sixth year and upper end fused with the shaft about the twentieth year.

For lower end

a. For the medial epicondyle—about fifth year

b. For the medial part of trochlea—tenth year

c. For the lateral part of trochlea with capitulum—second year

d. For the lateral epicondyle—twelfth year.

The medial epicondyle fuses with the shaft by a separate epiphyseal line about sixteenth year or seventeenth year and rest three centers unite to form single epiphysis, which fuses with the shaft about eighteenth year.

The formers help in age determination.

CLINICAL ANATOMY

i. Fracture of humerus may occur by muscular action or by direct or indirect trauma.

ii. Commonly fracture occurs at the surgical neck, middle one-third of the shaft or supracondylar region

iii. Fracture of the surgical neck may injure the axillary nerve because of their close relationship, as a result paralysis of deltoid muscle

iv. Fracture of the mid-shaft may injure the radial nerve

v. Fracture of the medial epicondyle may injure the ulnar nerve

vi. Fracture of the middle one-third may cause delayed or non-union due to poor blood supply

vii. In supracondylar fracture (commonest) the proximal fragment may compress or tear the brachial artery.

viii. **Positive Duga's sign:** In shoulder dislocation patient is unable to touch the shoulder of the normal side with the palm of the affected side.

RADIUS

INTRODUCTION

The radius is the lateral bone of the forearm having upper and lower ends, and an intervening portion called shaft.

ANATOMICAL POSITION

i. Broader lower end looks downwards

ii. Concave surface looks forwards

iii. The dorsal tubercle on the back of the lower end looks backwards.

SIDE DETERMINATION

After holding the bone in anatomical position the styloid process on which side belongs will determine the side of the bone.

GENERAL FEATURES

Upper End

It consists of head, neck and a tubercle.

Head

i. It is rounded

ii. It overhangs all sides except medially where it articulates with the radial notch of the ulna

iii. Upper surface of the head is concave and articulates with the capitulum of the humerus.

Neck and radial tuberosity

i. Neck is the constricted part succeeding the head

ii. Below the medial part of the neck there is an elevation called radial tuberosity (Fig. 2.14).

Shaft

It is narrow above and broader below, with lateral convexity

Borders: Anterior, posterior and interosseous.

Anterior border

i. This border begins from the anterolateral part of the radial tuberosity and ends where it continuous with with the anterior border of the styloid process.

ii. At first this border descends obliquely downwards and laterally indistinctly, round in its middle one-third, then vertically downwards like a ridge at the distal one-fourth of the shaft,

Posterior border

i. This border is well-defined in its middle one-third but upper and lower parts are ill-defined

iii. It begins from the posteroinferior part of the radial tuberosity, then descends obliquely downwards and laterally, then descends vertically to end in the dorsal (Lister) tubercle of the lower end.

Interosseous border

i. It is most distinct and sharp border

ii. It begins from the posteroinferior part of the radial tuberosity then vertically downwards, bifurcates below to enclose a triangular area above the ulnar notch of radius.

Surfaces: Anterior, posterior and lateral.

Anterior surface

i. Between anterior and interosseous borders

ii. Broader below and narrow above

iii. Presence of nutrient foramen directed upwards lies near the midpoint.

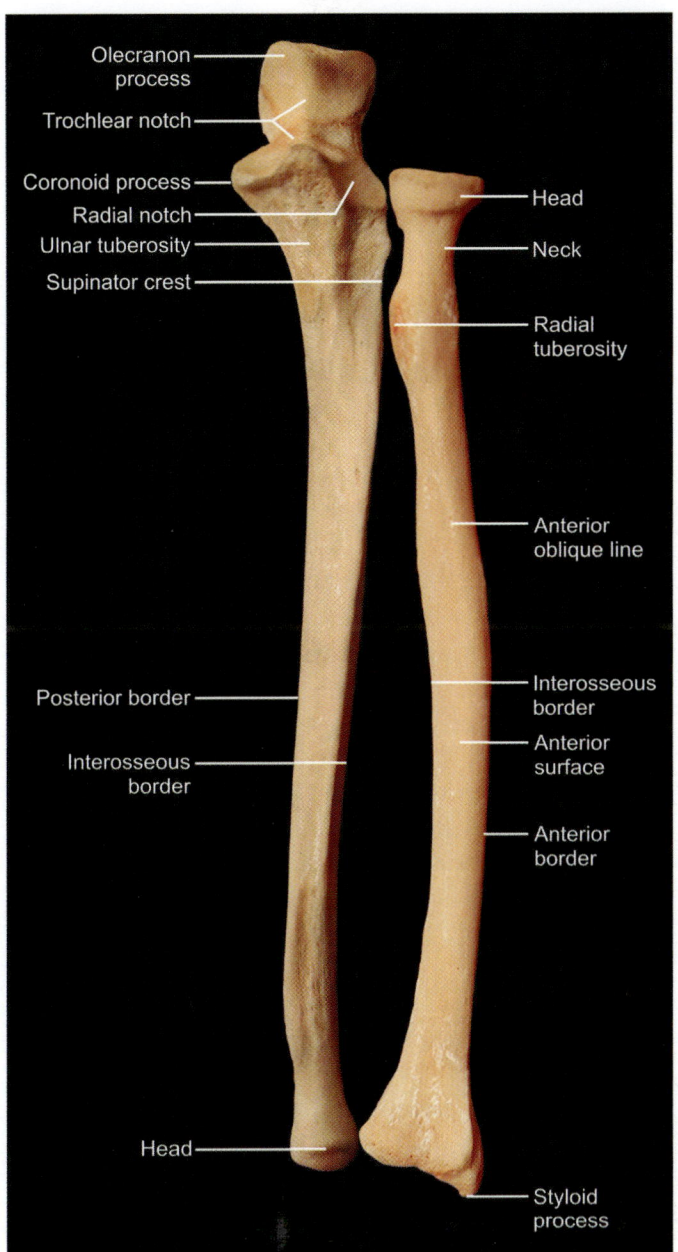

Fig. 2.14: Right radius and ulna general features (anterior view)

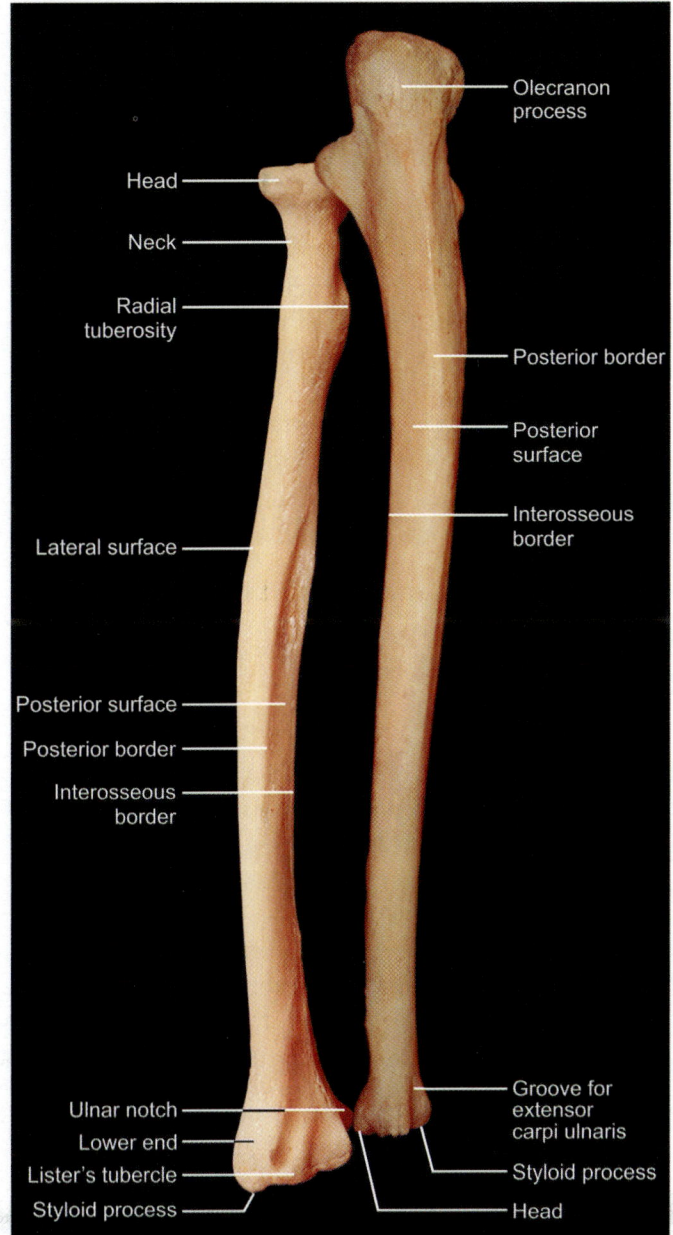

Fig. 2.15: Right radius and ulna general features (posterior view)

Posterior surface: It lies between posterior and interosseous borders (Fig. 2.15).

Lateral surface
i. Between the anterior and posterior borders
ii. This surface is convex
iii. A rough oblique ridge is present at the middle (Fig. 2.15).

Lower End
i. It is the widest part of the bone

ii. It has anterior, posterior, lateral, medial and inferior surfaces.

Anterior surface
i. It is narrow
ii. Represented by a thick prominent ridge.

Posterior surface
i. Broad and irregular
ii. Presents a palpable dorsal tubercle (Lister's tubercle)
iii. Presents three longitudinal grooves one lateral to the tubercle and two medial to the tubercle.

Lateral surface

   i. It is rough
   ii. A conical process projects downwards called styloid process.
   iiii. Lateral surface of the styloid process has two faint grooves.

Medial surface

   i. It presents a smooth articular notch at its lower part, called ulnar notch of radius articulates with the head of the ulna to form the distal radioulnar joint
   ii. This surface separates from the inferior surface by a smooth ridge.

Inferior surface: It is concave, which is divided by a ridge into lateral triangular and medial quadrilateral areas.

ATTACHMENTS OF RADIUS

Upper End

Head

Ligament: Annular ligament—it encircles margin of the head except medially where it forms the superior or proximal radioulnar joint.

Neck and radial tuberosity

Insertion of

Biceps brachii: On posterior rough part of the radial tuberosity.

Ligaments

   i. Annular ligament: In the upper part of the neck
   ii. Oblique cord: Lower end of the tuberosity.

Shaft

Anterior border

Origin of (Fig. 2.16)

Flexor digitorum superficialis: From the oblique part of the anterior border with adjoining surface.

Other

Extensor retinaculum (lateral end): At the lower sharp part of the border.

Interosseous border

Interosseous membrane: It begins from the 25 mm below the radial tuberosity between the radius and ulna.

Insertion of: Pronator quadratus—from the triangular area and its anterior border.

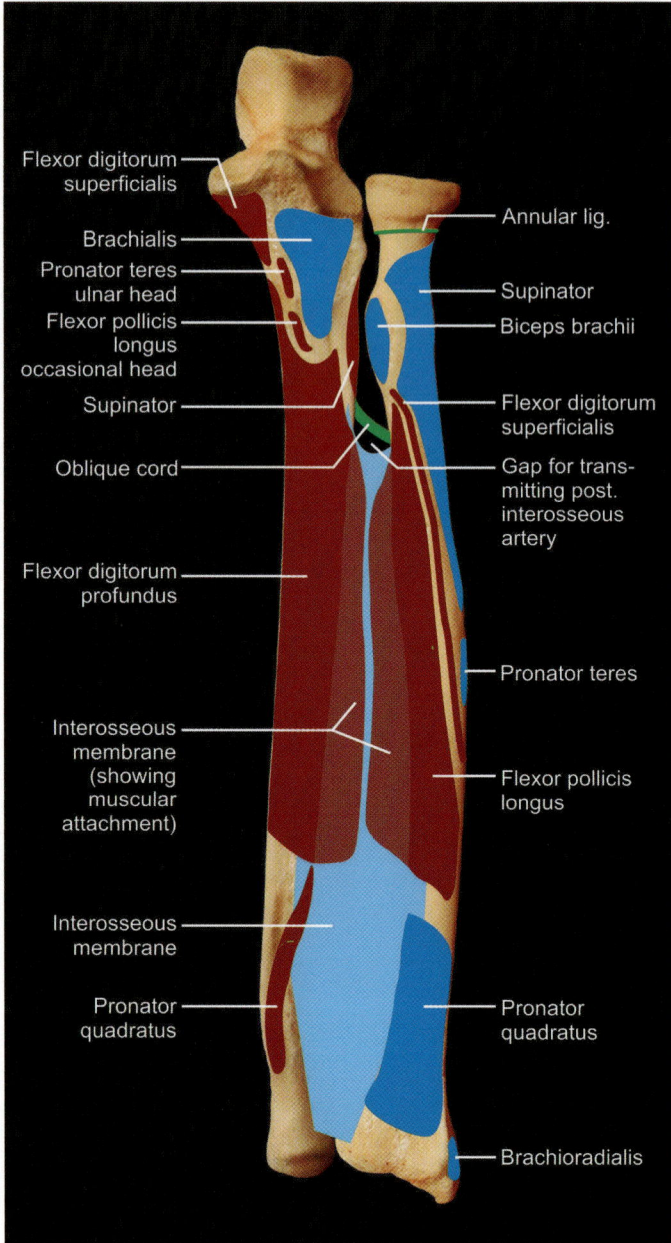

Fig. 2.16: Right radius and ulna attachments (anterior view)

Anterior surface

Origin of

Flexor pollicis longus: From the upper two-thirds.

Insertion of

Pronator quadratus: Lower one-fourth with triangular area and its anterior border.

Posterior surface

Origin of (Fig. 2.17)

   i. Abductor pollicis longus: From the upper part
   ii. Extensor pollicis brevis: From the lower part

Lateral surface

Insertion of (Fig. 2.17)

  i. **Pronator teres:** Rough impression on the middle
  ii. **Supinator:** Above the rough impression on the lateral surface.

Relations: Below the insertion of pronator teres the rest part of the surface is covered by the tendons of extensor carpi radialis longus and brevis.

Lower End

Anterior surface

Ligaments

  i. Palmar radiocarpal ligament.
  ii. **Capsular ligament of wrist joint:** Immediately below the ridge in a faint groove.

Importance: Radial pulse is felt against this surface.

Posterior surface

Ligaments

  i. **Capsular ligament and dorsal radiocarpal ligament:** At the lower margin of the posterior surface
  i. **Extensor retinaculum:** At the dorsal tubercle.

Relations of tendons: Lateral to medial (Fig. 2.18)

  i. Extensor carpi radialis longus
  ii. Extensor carpi radialis brevis
  iii. Extensor pollicis longus
  iv. Extensor digitorum
  v. Extensor indicis.

Lateral surface

Insertion of

Brachioradialis: On the lateral surface proximal to the styloid process.

Ligament

Lateral carpal ligament: at the tip of the styloid process.
Relations: Abductor pollicis longus and extensor pollicis brevis (Fig. 2.18).

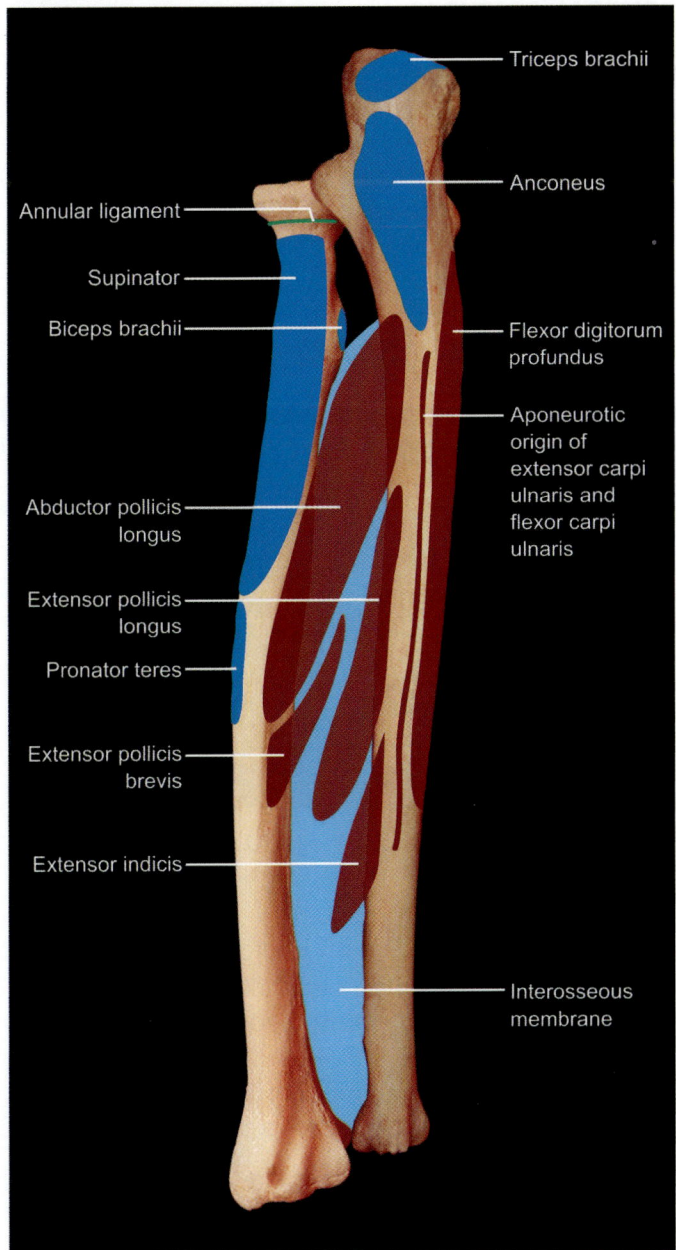

Fig. 2.17: Right radius and ulna attachments (posterior view)

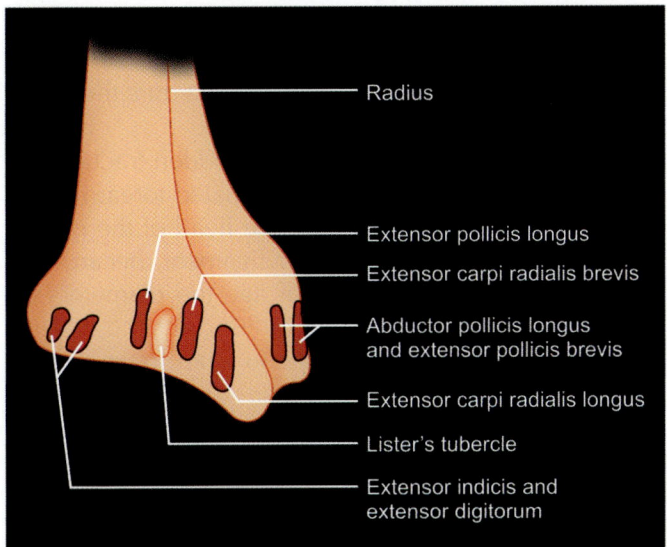

Fig. 2.18: Tendons related to posterior and lateral surfaces of lower end of right radius

Medial surface

Triangular articular disk: To the smooth ridge between the ulnar notch and inferior surface of the lower end of the radius.

Inferior Surface

Articulations

i. Lateral triangular area: With the scaphoid
ii. Medial quadrilateral area: With the lunate.

Ligament: Capsular ligament—attached along the periphery of the inferior surface and at the ulnar notch of radius.

OSSIFICATION

It has one primary center and two secondary centers of ossification.

i. **Primary center:** It appears in the shaft in the eighth week of intrauterine life.
ii. **Secondary centers:**
   a. For the lower end in the one year which unite with the shaft in the 20th year
   b. For the head of the radius in the fourth or fifth year which unite with the shaft in the 18 th year helps in age determination.

CLINICAL ANATOMY

i. **Colles' fracture with dinner fork deformity:** The most common site of fracture of radius occurred, which is about 2 cm above its lower end due to fall on the outstretched hand in which the distal segment is displaced upward, backward and laterally caused by the pull of brachioradialis producing a shape known as dinner-fork deformity.
ii. **Smith's fracture:** It is the reverse of Colles' fracture due to fall with flexed wrist. In this fracture the distal segment is displaced anteriorly.
iii. **Sub-luxation or pulled elbow:** Sudden traction on the hand of a child in semi-pronated forearm may cause partial dislocation of the head of the radius from the grip of the annular ligament, because in children below six years of age the diameters of the head and neck of the radius are similar. This condition is corrected by the forcible supination of the forearm.

ULNA

INTRODUCTION

Ulna is the medial bone of the forearm having upper and lower ends, and an intervening portion called shaft or body.

ANATOMICAL POSITION

i. Hook like olecranon process looks upwards
ii. Concave articular surface (trochlear notch) looks forward
iii. Head looks downward
iv. The sharp interosseous border laterally.

SIDE DETERMINATION

After holding the bone in anatomical position the interosseous border on which side belongs it will determine the side of the bone.

GENERAL FEATURES

Upper End

i. It is hook-like expanded part of bone with concavity forwards:
ii. It has two processes
   a. Olecranon process
   b. Coronoid process.
iii. It also has two articular areas
   a. Trochlear notch
   b. Radial notch (Fig. 2.19).

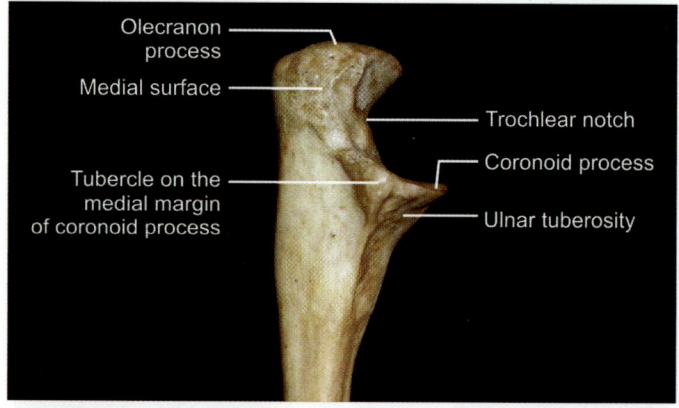

Fig. 2.19: Proximal end of the left ulna (medial view)

Olecranon process

i. It projects upwards with bent forward
ii. Its upper end forms a beak-like projection which occupies in the olecranon fossa of humerus in extended elbow
iii. It consists of—upper, medial, lateral, posterior and anterior surfaces.

Upper surface

i. It is rough
ii. In flexed elbow the three bony points, olecranon process, medial and lateral epicondyles forms a triangle known as triangle of isoscele.

Medial surface: Continuous with the medial surface of the body.

Lateral surface: It is continuous with the posterior surface of the body of the ulna.

Posterior surface: It is smooth, subcutaneous and triangular in shape with apex directed downward.

Anterior surface

i. Deeply concave
ii. It forms the upper part of the trochlear notch
iii. Continuous with the superior surface of the coronoid process to form the trochlear articular surface
iv. This anterior articular surface is divided into three parts (medial, intermediate and lateral) by vertical lines.

Coronoid process

i. It is a self-like process
ii. It projects forwards from the upper and anterior part of the shaft
iii. Medial margin is sharp and bears a tubercle.
iv. It consists of superior, anteroinferior and lateral surfaces.

Superior surface: Forms the lower part of the trochlear notch.

Anteroinferior surface: It presents a rough triangular elevation called ulnar tuberosity.

Lateral surface

i. Presents an oval concave articular area called radial notch of ulna, articulates with the head of the radius.
ii. Below the notch presents a triangular depression with raised on its behind called supinator crest.

Trochlear notch

i. It is formed by the anterior surface of the olecranon process and superior surface of the coronoid process
ii. It articulates with the trochlea of the humerus.

Shaft

i. It gradually narrows from above downwards
ii. Upper part is triangular
iii. Lower part is rounded
iv. Dorsally it is convex

Features of the shaft

Borders—anterior, posterior and interosseous.

Anterior border (Fig. 2.14)

i. It is ill-defined rounded border
ii. Begins from the lower end of the ulnar tuberosity to the front of the styloid process of the ulna.

Posterior border: It begins from the apex of the triangular area on the posterior surface of the olecranon process of ulna to the back of the styloid process of ulna. This border is entirely subcutaneous.

Interosseous border (lateral border): It begins from the apex of the grooved triangular area below the radial notch of ulna.

Surfaces—anterior, posterior and medial.

Anterior surface: It lies between the anterior and interosseous borders.

Posterior surface (*Fig. 2.15*)

i. It lies between the posterior and interosseous borders.
ii. An oblique ridge divides the posterior surface into upper small and lower large areas.
iii. A vertical ridge further subdivides the lower area into lateral and medial areas.

Medial surface: It lies between the anterior and posterior borders.

Lower End

i. Slightly expanded
ii. Consists of head and styloid process.

Head

i. On the lateral part presents a smooth articular area for articulation with the ulnar notch of radius.
ii. Inferiorly a semilunar articular area lies laterally articulates with the upper surface of the base of the triangular articular disk and rough and groove area lies medially attached with the apex of the triangular articular disk.

Styloid process

i. It projects downwards from posteromedial aspect of the lower end.
ii. Presents a groove between the styloid process and posterior surface of the head.
iii. The radial styloid process about 2 cm below than the ulnar styloid process.

ATTACHMENTS OF ULNA

Upper End

Olecranon process

Upper surface

Insertion of

Triceps brachii: On the rough part of the superior surface.

Ligament

Capsular ligament: Attached to the groove on the superior surface.
Other: A bursa present between the above two attachments.
Medial surface: From anterior to posterior.
Ligament: Capsular ligament of the elbow joint.

Origin of

   i. Flexor carpi ulnaris
   ii. Flexor digitorum profundus.

Lateral surface

From anterior to posterior.

Ligaments

   i. Capsular ligament of the elbow joint
   ii. Radial collateral ligament of the elbow joint.
Insertion of: Anconeus.

Coronoid process

On its medial margin and the tubercle: Anterior and oblique bands of the ulnar collateral ligament of the elbow joint.

Anteroinferior surface

Insertion of: Brachialis: On the ulnar tuberosity.
Origin of: From above downwards.
   i. Part of the flexor digitorum superficialis
   ii. Ulnar head of pronator teres
   iii. Occasional head of the flexor pollicis longus.

Ligament

Oblique cord: At the lower part of the lateral border of the ulnar tuberosity.

Lateral surface

Origin of

Supinator: From supinator crest.

Trochlear notch

Articulation: It articulates with the trochlea of the humerus.

Shaft

Anterior border

Origin of

Flexor digitorum profundus: From the upper three-fourths.

Posterior border

Origin of

   i. Flexor digitorum profundus: From the proximal three-fourths.
   ii. Flexor carpi ulnaris: From the proximal half.
   iii. Extensor carpi ulnaris: From the middle one-third.
Other: Common aponeurosis derived from the deep fascia of forearm.

Interosseous border

Attachment

Interosseous membrane: It presents a gap between its upper part and oblique cord passing the posterior interosseous vessels.

Anterior surface

Origin of (Fig. 2.16)

   i. Flexor digitorum profundus: From the upper three-fourths
   ii. Pronator quadratus: Form the ridge in the lower one-fourth part.

Posterior surface

Insertion of (Fig. 2.17)

Anconeus: On the upper area.

Origin of

Lower lateral area—from above downwards.
   i. Abductor pollicis longus
   ii. Extensor pollicis longus
   iii. Extensor indicis.

Medial surface

Origin of

Flexor digitorum profundus: From the upper three-fourths.

Lower End

Styloid process

Ligament

Ulnar collateral ligament of the wrist joint: At the tip of the styloid process.
Structure lodged: Tendon of the extensor carpi ulnaris.

OSSIFICATION

It has one primary center and two secondary centers of ossification.

i. **Primary center:** It appears in the eighth week in the shaft during intrauterine life.

ii. **Secondary centers**

a. For the lower end—in the fifth year and unites the shaft in the eighteenth year.

b. For the proximal part of the olecranon process—in the tenth year and unites with the shaft in fifteenth or sixteenth year.

The aboves help in age determination.

CLINICAL ANATOMY

i. Alteration of positions of the three bony points—medial and lateral epicondyles and olecranon process in same horizontal line in fully extended elbow indicates the dislocation of elbow joint.

ii. Fracture of the shaft of the ulna easily detected because its posterior border is subcutaneous.

SKELETON OF THE HAND

i. Skeleton of the hand is composed of three segments.

ii. The proximal segment composed of carpus or wrist consisting of eight small carpal bones arranged in two rows.

iii. The intermediate segment consists of five metacarpal bones.

iv. Distal segment consists of phalanges arranged in three rows excepting the thumb in which one phalanx is absent (Fig. 2.20).

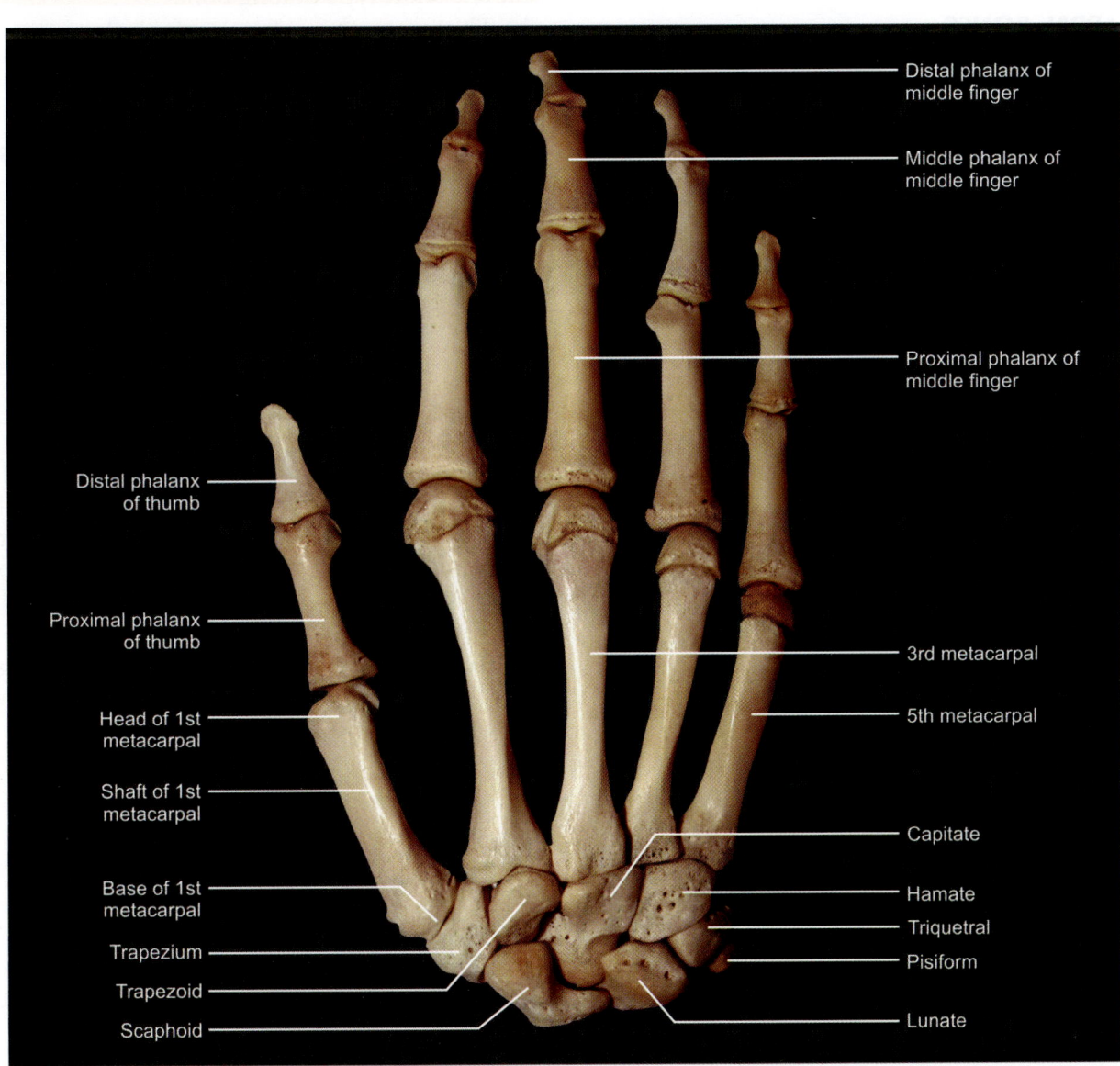

Fig. 2.20: Bones of the right hand (dorsal surface)

CARPAL BONES

▌ INTRODUCTION

The carpal bones are eight in number. They arranged in two rows, proximal and distal.

  i. **Proximal row**—from lateral to medial side
    a. Scaphoid
    b. The lunate
    c. The triquetral
    d. The pisiform.
  ii. **The distal row**—from lateral to medial side
    a. The trapezium
    b. The trapezoid
    c. The capitate
    d. The hamate.

METACARPAL BONES

Identifying Characters

  i. The metacarpal bones are five in number
  ii. They are named numerically from lateral to medial side
  iii. Each of them has a head or distal end, a base or proximal end and a shaft or body
  iv. The body is concave forwards and convex backwards
  v. The head is larger than the base
  vi. The body becomes thicker gradually from above downwards
  vii. The dorsal surface of the body presents a flattened triangular area (Fig. 2.21).

PHALANGES OF HAND

▌ INTRODUCTION

  i. Phalanges are fourteen (14) in number. Two for the thumb and three for the other fingers
  ii. Each of them consists of a base or proximal end, the shaft and the head or distal end

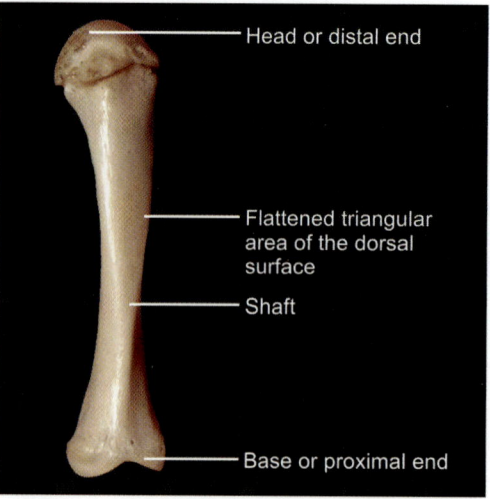

Fig. 2.21: Metacarpal bone dorsal view

  iii. It is short type of long bone
  iv. There are three types of phalanges such as proximal phalanx, middle phalanx and the distal phalanx.

GENERAL CHARACTERISTICS OF PHALANGES

  i. Tapers from proximal to distal end
  ii. Dorsal surface of the shaft is smooth and convex
  ii. The volar surface of shaft is flattened from side to side and gently concave from above downwards.

CLINICAL ANATOMY

  i. **Polydactyly:** It is an abnormality of fingers or toes where presence of extra fingers or toes. Often the extra digit is incompletely formed and lacks proper muscular development; it is thus useless. It is mostly bilateral, extra digit is most commonly medial or lateral rather than central. In the foot the extra toe is usually on the lateral side. Polydactyly is inherited as a dominant characteristic.
  ii. **Brachydactyly:** Shortness of the digits of fingers or toes. It is uncommon and is the result of reduction in the length of the phalanges.

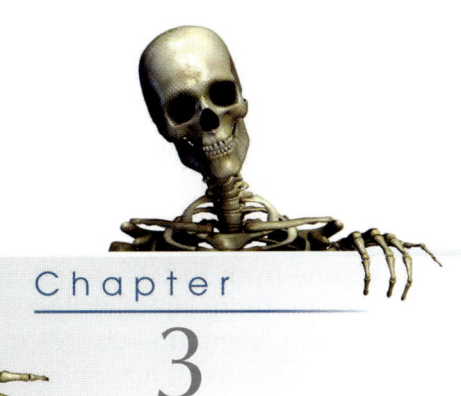

Chapter 3

Bones of Lower Limb

HIP BONE

INTRODUCTION

i. The hip or innominate bone is large irregular bone, constricted in the middle, presents a cup-shaped socket, acetabulum on its outer surface which articulates with the head of the femur to form the hip joint.
ii. The bone is expanded above and below the acetabulum.

ANATOMICAL POSITION

i. Expanded part ilium directed upwards
ii. Pubis is directed forwards and medially above the obturator foramen
iii. The acetabulum directed downwards, forwards and laterally
iv. Acetabular notch looks vertically downwards
v. Anterior superior iliac spine and pubic crest lie in the same vertical plane.

SIDE DETERMINATION

After holding the bone in anatomical position the acetabulum on which side belongs will determine the side of the bone.

GENERAL FEATURES

Parts

i. Ilium
ii. Ischium
iii. Pubis.

Ilium

i. Upper part flat and expanded
ii. Ends—upper and lower
iii. Borders—anterior, posterior and medial
iv. Surfaces—gluteal or external and internal
v. Internal surface further subdivided into anterior hollow part, called iliac fossa and posterior part, called sacropelvic surface.

Upper end (iliac crest)

i. It is thick called iliac crest extends from anterior superior iliac spine to posterior superior iliac spine
ii. Anteriorly a bony projection called anterior superior iliac spine
iii. Posteriorly also a bony projection called posterior superior iliac spine
iv. Anterior two-thirds of the iliac crest convexity outward known as ventral segment
v. Posterior one-third of the iliac crest concavity outward known as dorsal segment.
vi. Ventral segment—consists of:
   a. Outer lip
   b. Intermediate area
   c. Inner lip.
vii. On the outer lip, 5 cm behind the anterior superior iliac spine presents a tubercle called tubercle of the iliac crest, at the level of LV5 (to draw the transtubercular plane).
viii. Dorsal segment—it consists of:
   a. Outer sloping area
   b. Inner sloping area.

Lower end

i. At the beginning the ilium connected with the ischium and pubis by a Y-shaped cartilage, but at the time of puberty the three parts are fused together
ii. Upper two-fifths of the acetabulum is formed by the ilium.

Borders

Anterior border

i. Begins from the anterior superior iliac spine and ends into the anterior margin of the acetabulum
ii. Presents a notch below the anterior superior iliac spine
iii. Presents anterior inferior iliac spine below the notch.

Posterior border

i. Begins from the posterior superior iliac spine, then forming a deeply concave greater sciatic notch, then continuous with the posterior border of the ischium.
ii. Below the posterior superior iliac spine there is posterior inferior iliac spine.

Medial border

i. It passes downwards, forwards and medially
ii. Posterior one-third is rough
iii. Middle one-third is sharp
iv. Anterior one-third forms arcuate line and continuous anteriorly with the pectineal line of pubis (pecten pubis).

Surfaces

Internal surface: This surface is divided into iliac fossa and sacropelvic surface by the medial border.

Iliac fossa (Fig. 3.1)

It is shallow, concave and smooth surface situated on the anterior part of the internal surface.

Sacropelvic surface

It is divided into:
i. Upper rough sacral area
ii. Lower smooth pelvic area.
i. Sacral area further subdivided into:
   a. Upper non-articular tuberosity called iliac tuberosity
   b. Lower articular area called auricular surface (looks like pinna of ear).
ii. Pelvic area is further subdivided into:
   a. Upper pelvic area—just below the auricular surface presents a rough groove, called preauricular sulcus (more prominent in female)

   b. Lower pelvic area—smooth and continuous with the pelvic surface of the body of the ischium.

Gluteal surface: It is divided into four areas by three-gluteal lines (Fig. 3.3).

Posterior gluteal line

i. It is shortest, begins from the iliac crest about 5 cm in front of the posterior superior iliac spine
ii. Then curving backwards and downwards to end in front of the posterior inferior iliac spine.

Anterior gluteal line

i. It is largest, begins from the middle of the greater sciatic notch
ii. Then ascends upwards and forwards to end just in front of the tubercle of the crest of the ilium of the outer lip.

Inferior gluteal line

i. It begins from the upper part of the anterior inferior iliac spine
ii. Then turns backwards to end opposite the lower part of the greater sciatic notch
iii. Between the inferior gluteal line and acetabular margin presents a rough grooved area.

Ischium

i. It consists of body and a ramus
ii. Lower part of the acetabulum is formed by the ischium.

Body: It consists of
i. **Surfaces**—femoral, dorsal and pelvic
ii. **Ends**—upper and lower
iii. **Borders**—anterior, posterior and lateral.

Surfaces

Femoral surface: Situated between the lateral and anterior borders.

Dorsal surface

i. It lies between the posterior and lateral borders.
ii. This surface is divided by a groove into:
   a. Upper area, smooth and convex
   b. Lower area, rough called ischial tuberosity
   c. The ischial tuberosity is further subdivided by a transverse ridge into—
     • Upper quadrilateral area
     • Lower triangular area.
   d. Again upper quadrilateral area subdivided into upper lateral area and lower medial area by an oblique ridge
   e. The lower triangular area further subdivided into lateral and medial areas by a ridge.

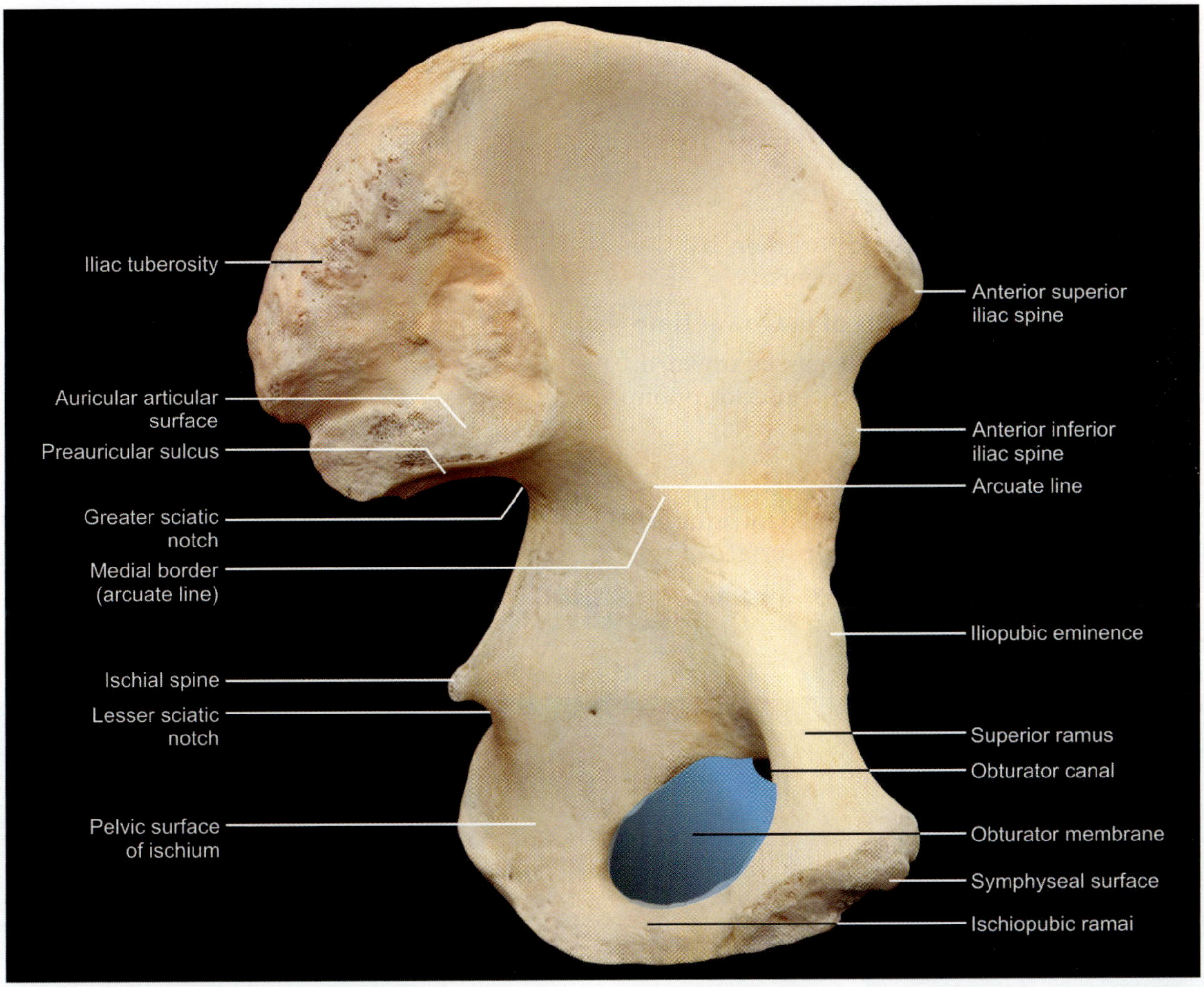

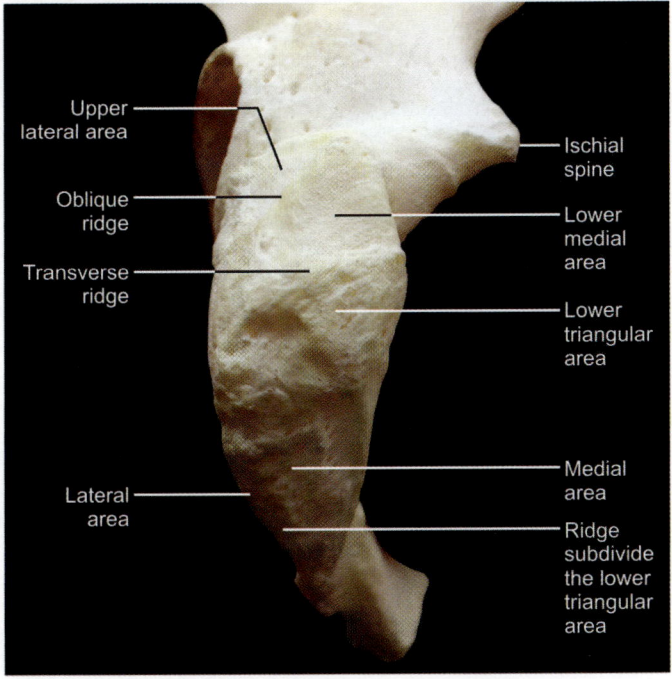

Fig. 3.1: Left hip bone (medial view)

Iliac tuberosity

Auricular articular surface

Preauricular sulcus

Greater sciatic notch

Medial border (arcuate line)

Ischial spine

Lesser sciatic notch

Pelvic surface of ischium

Anterior superior iliac spine

Anterior inferior iliac spine

Arcuate line

Iliopubic eminence

Superior ramus

Obturator canal

Obturator membrane

Symphyseal surface

Ischiopubic ramai

Pelvic surface: It lies between the anterior and posterior borders

Ends

Upper end: It is fused with the ilium and pubis at the acetabulum (along the floor).

Lower end: It is the most dependent part of the ischial tuberosity (Fig. 3.2).

Borders

Anterior border: It forms the posterior margin of obturator foramen.

Posterior border

i. It is continuous above with the posterior border of the ilium

ii. Below the greater sciatic notch the bony projection is called ischial spine

iii. Further below the ischial spine there is lesser sciatic notch.

Upper lateral area

Oblique ridge

Transverse ridge

Lateral area

Ischial spine

Lower medial area

Lower triangular area

Medial area

Ridge subdivide the lower triangular area

Fig. 3.2: Dorsal aspect of left ischial tuberosity

Lateral border

i. Upper part is indistinct

ii. Lower part is prominent

iii. It separates the femoral surface from the dorsal surface.

Lesser sciatic notch

It is converted into lesser sciatic foramen by the sacrotuberous and sacrospinous ligaments.

Structures transmit: *See* in oral part of the lower limb

Ramus: It starts from the body and passes upward, forwards and medially to join with the inferior pubic ramus.

Surfaces

i. **Anterior or external surface:** Directed towards the thigh, continuous with the anterior surface of the inferior pubic ramus.

ii. **Posterior or pelvic surface**

a. Divided into three areas—upper, intermediate and lower by upper and lower bony ridges

b. It is continuous with posterior surface of inferior pubic ramus.

Borders

i. Upper—it forms the margin of the obturator foramen

ii. Lower—it forms the lateral boundary of the urogenital triangle (Fig. 3.3).

Pubis

i. It is the anteroinferior part of the hip bone.

ii. It consists of body, superior and inferior rami.

iii. Anterior one-fifth of the acetabulum is formed by the pubis.

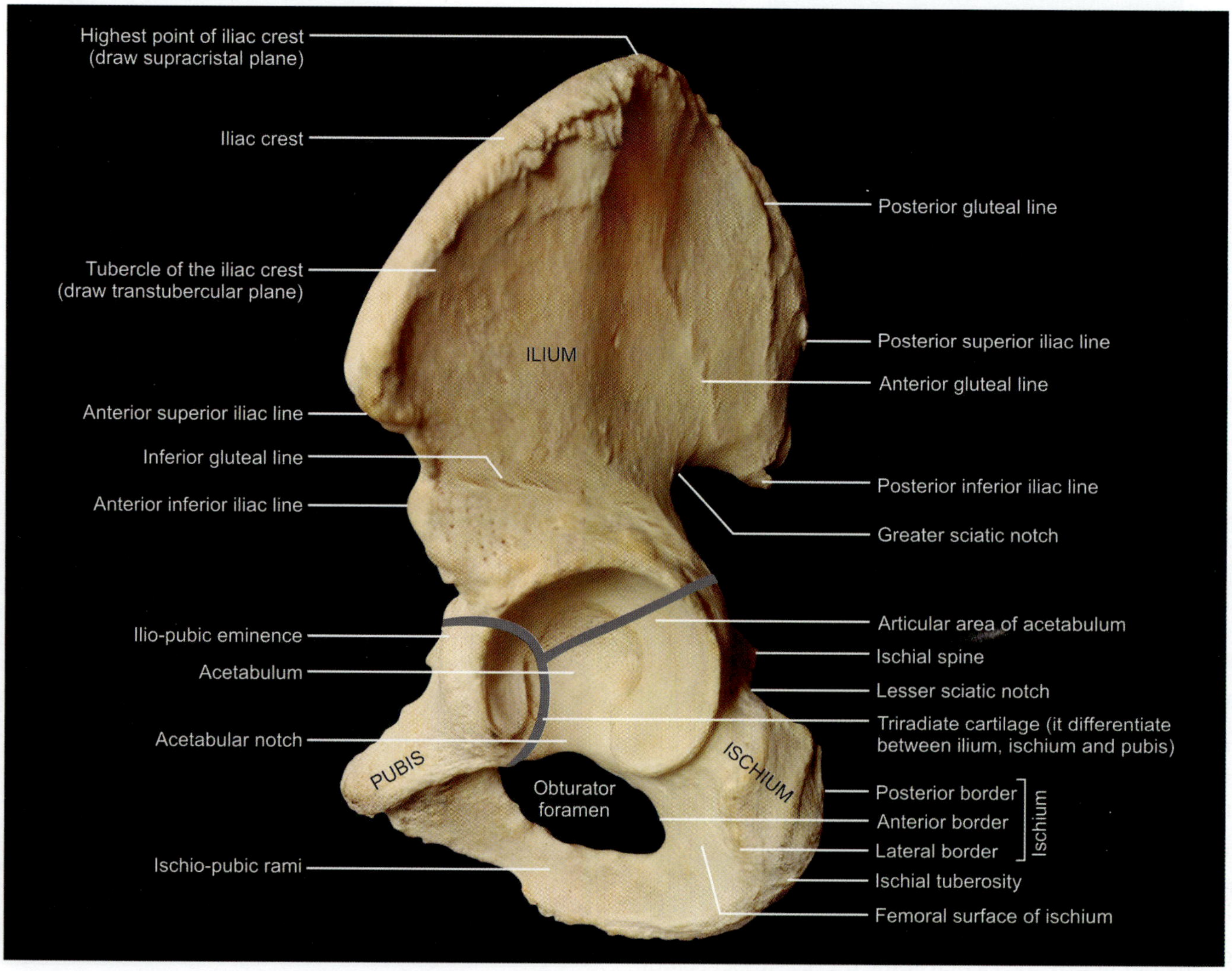

Fig. 3.3: Left hib bone (lateral view)

Body

i. It is flattened anteroposteriorly.
ii. It connects with the superior and inferior rami.
iii. Lies medial to the obturator foramen.

Surfaces

Anterior surface: Directed downward, forwards and laterally.

Posterior surface: Smooth and forms the anterior wall of the true pelvis.

Symphyseal surface: Rough, elongated and articulates with the similar surface of the opposite side to form the symphysis pubis.

Border

Upper border

i. It is thick called pubic crest
ii. On the lateral end of the upper border have a tubercle called pubic tubercle.

Superior ramus: It lies above the obturator foramen.

Borders

Anterosuperior border or obturator crest

a. Begins from the anterior part of the pubic tubercle
b. Then goes laterally and ends at the anterior part of the acetabulum.

Posterosuperior border or pectineal line

a. It is sharp and well-marked
b. Begins from the posterior part of the pubic tubercle
c. Then goes laterally and backwards, continuous with the arcuate line.

Inferior border: It forms the upper boundary of the obturator foramen.

Surfaces

Pectineal surface (with its boundaries)

Anteriorly: Obturator crest.

Posteriorly: Pectineal line.

Laterally: Iliopubic eminence.

Medially: Pubic tubercle.

Obturator surface: It lies between the obturator crest and inferior border, there is a groove called the obturator groove.

Pelvic surface: It lies between the pectineal line and the inferior border, continuous with pelvic surface of the body of the pubis.

Inferior ramus: It lies medial to the obturator foramen continuous with ischial ramus.

Surfaces

Anterior surface: Directed downwards, forwards and laterally.

Posterior surface

i. Continuous with the posterior surface of the ramus of ischium below and posterior surface of the body of the pubis above.
ii. This surface is subdivided into three areas by two oblique ridges
   a. Lateral
   b. Intermediate
   c. Medial.

Obturator foramen

i. It is oval and larger in male.
ii. It is small and triangular in female.

Acetabulum

i. It is a cup-shaped cavity.
ii. Head of the femur articulates.
iii. Its periphery gives attachment to acetabular labrum except below where forms the acetabular notch.
iv. Two ends of acetabular notch gives attachment transverse acetabular ligament and the base of the ligamentum teres femoris.
v. Ilium contributes two-fifths, ischium contributes two-fifths and pubis contributes one-fifth of the acetabulum.

ATTACHMENTS OF HIP BONE

Ilium

Upper end (iliac crest) (Fig. 3.5)

From outside inwards:

i. **Fascia lata:** Including the iliotibial tract (whole length)
ii. **Origin of tensor fasciae latae:** From the anterior superior iliac spine to the tubercle
iii. **Insertion of external obliquus abdominis:** Anterior half of the outer lip
iv. **Origin of latissimus dorsi:** Posterior one-third of the outer lip
v. Between the attachments of external obliquus abdominis and latissimus dorsi the remaining gap of the iliac crest forms the base of the lumbar (Petits) triangle
vi. **Origin of internal obliquus abdominis:** From whole of the intermediate area of the ventral segment
vii. **Origin of transversus abdominis:** From the anterior two-thirds and quadratus lumborum from posterior one-third of the inner lip.

viii. **Anterior and middle layers of thoracolumbar fascia:** Attached medial and lateral to the quadratus lumborum respectively

ix. **Fascia iliaca and iliacus muscle:** Attached below the transversus abdominis and quadratus lumborum

x. **Origin of gluteus maximus and fascia lata:** From the outer sloping area of the dorsal segment

xi. **Origin of erector spinae (sacrospinalis):** From the inner sloping area

xii. **Origin of sartorius and lateral end of inguinal ligament:** From the anterior superior iliac spine.

Anterior border of ilium (Fig. 3.4)

i. **Origin of straight head of the rectus femoris:** In the upper part of the anterior inferior iliac spine

ii. **Stem of the iliofemoral ligament:** In the lower part of the anterior inferior iliac spine.

Posterior border of ilium

i. **Sacrotuberous ligament:** Posterior superior iliac spine with posterior border extends to posterior inferior iliac spine.

ii. **Origin of piriformis:** From the upper border of greater sciatic notch.

iii. **Structures transmit through the greater sciatic foramen** (*see in oral part of lower limb*)

Sacropelvic surface (Fig. 3.4)

i. **Origin of Iliacus:** From the upper two-thirds of the iliac fossa.

ii. **Nutrient foramen:** It presents at the posterior inferior part of the iliac fossa.

iii. **Insertion of psoas minor:** Middle of the arcuate line.

iv. **Iliac tuberosity** gives attachments to following ligaments from anterior to posterior:
   a. Iliolumbar ligament
   b. Dorsal sacroiliac ligament
   c. Interosseous sacroiliac ligament.

v. **Auricular surface:** It articulates with the lateral mass of sacrum.

vi. **Preauricular sulcus:** It gives attachment to the ventral sacroiliac ligament.

vii. **Origin of obturator internus:** From the lower pelvic surface.

Gluteal surface

Origin of (Fig. 3.5)

i. **Gluteus maximus:** Area behind the posterior gluteal line.

ii. **Gluteus medius:** Between the posterior and anterior gluteal lines.

iii. **Gluteus minimus:** Area between the anterior and inferior gluteal lines.

iv. **Reflected head of the rectus femoris:** Between the inferior gluteal line and acetabular margin (Fig. 3.4).

Ischium

Body

Femoral surface (Fig. 3.5)

Origin of:

i. **Obturator externus:** Femoral surface and adjoining obturator foramen.

ii. **Quadratus femoris:** Just in front of the lateral border of the femoral surface.

iii. **Ischiofemoral ligament:** To the upper part of lateral border and adjoining part of the acetabular margin.

Dorsal surface

Origin of

i. **Semimembranosus:** From the lateral part of the upper quadrilateral area.

ii. **Common origin of the long head of the biceps femoris and the semitendinosus:** From the lower medial area.

iii. **Adductor magnus:** From the lateral area of the lower triangular part.

iv. **Sacrotuberous ligament:** Medial margin of the medial area of the lower triangular area.

Pelvic surface (Fig. 3.4)

Origin of

i. **Obturator internus:** Close to the obturator foramen.

ii. **Pudendal (Alcock's) canal:** It lies on the lateral wall of the ischiorectal fossa formed by the splitting of the obturator fascia containing:
   a. Internal pudendal vessels
   b. Pudendal nerves with its divisions the dorsal nerve of penis or clitoris and the perineal nerve.

In the ischial spine (Fig. 3.4)

i. **Sacrospinous ligament:** Tip of the ischial spine

ii. **Origin of levator ani:** In its pelvic surface.

iii. **Origin of gemellus superior:** Lower border of spine

iv. Dorsal surface of the spine crossed by the
   a. Internal pudendal vessels
   b. Nerve to the obturator internus.

Ramus

i. **Anterior surface of the ramus:** Origin of obturator externus laterally and adductor magnus medially.

ii. **Origin of gracilis and adductor brevis:** Extends to this surface from the inferior ramus of the pubis.

33

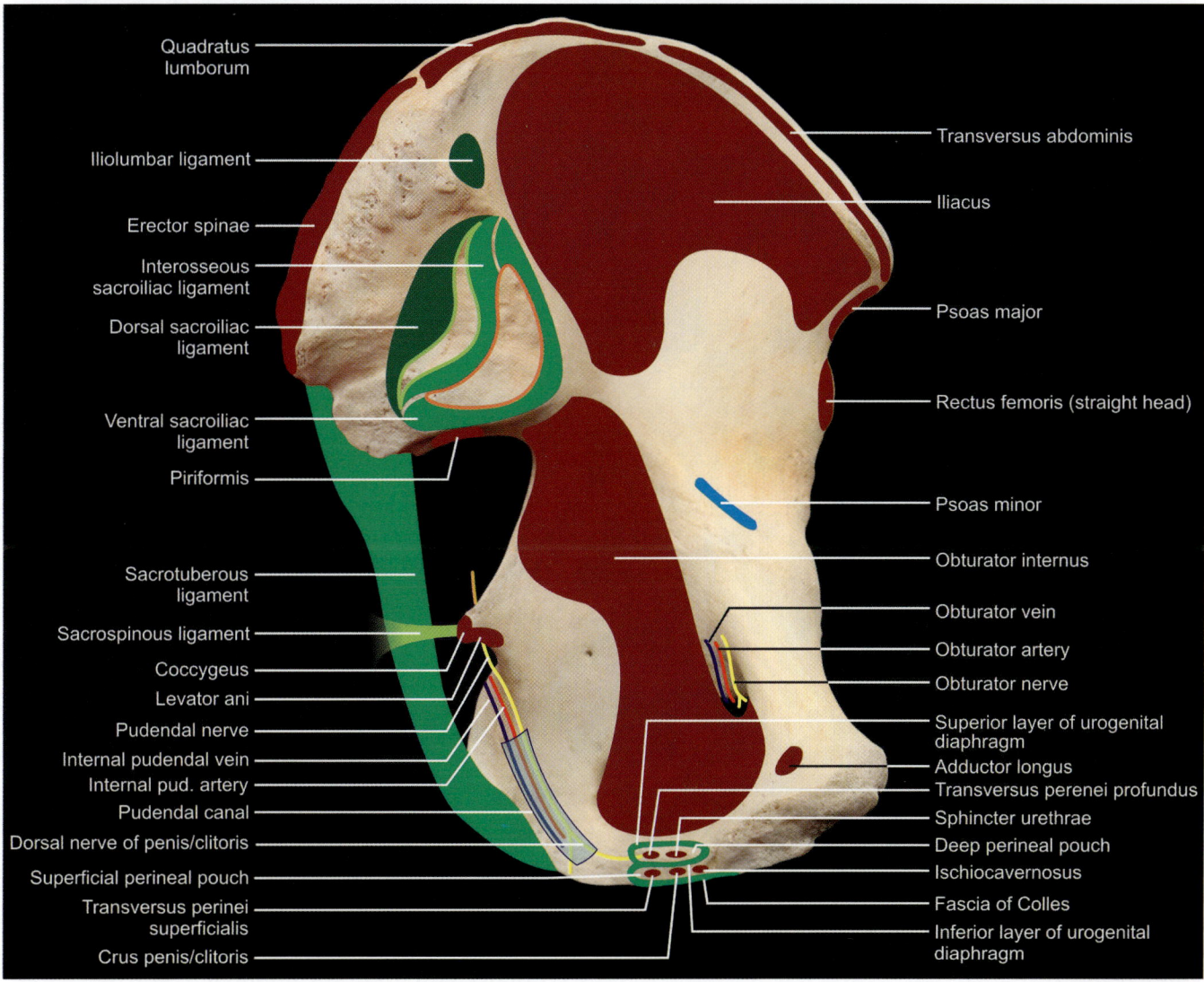

Fig. 3.4: Attachments of left hip bone (medial view)

iii. Posterior or pelvic surface of the ramus:

a. **Upper ridge:** Attachment to the superior fascia of the urogenital diaphragm

b. **Lower ridge:** Attachment to the perineal membrane or inferior fascia of urogenital diaphragm

c. **The upper area:** Origin of obturator internus

d. **The intermediate area:** Origin of
   a. Sphincter urethra in front
   b. Transversus perinei profundus behind.

e. **The lower area:** From before backwards origin of
   – Crus penis or clitoris
   – Ischiocavernosus
   – Transversus perinei superficialis.

f. **Upper border of ramus:** Attachment to obturator membrane

g. **Lower border of ramus:** Attachments fascia of Colles and fascia lata (Fig. 3.4).

PUBIS

Body

Anterior surface (Fig. 3.5)

i. **Origin of adductor longus:** Immediately below the junction of pubic crest and pubic tubercle

ii. **Rest of the surface:** Medial to lateral
   a. Gracilis
   b. Adductor brevis
   c. Obturator externus.

All three muscles extend to the external surface of the ischiopubic rami.

Posterior surface

i. Medial puboprostatic ligament

ii. **Origin of levator ani:** Close to center of the surface

iii. **Origin of obturator internus:** Lateral part of the surface

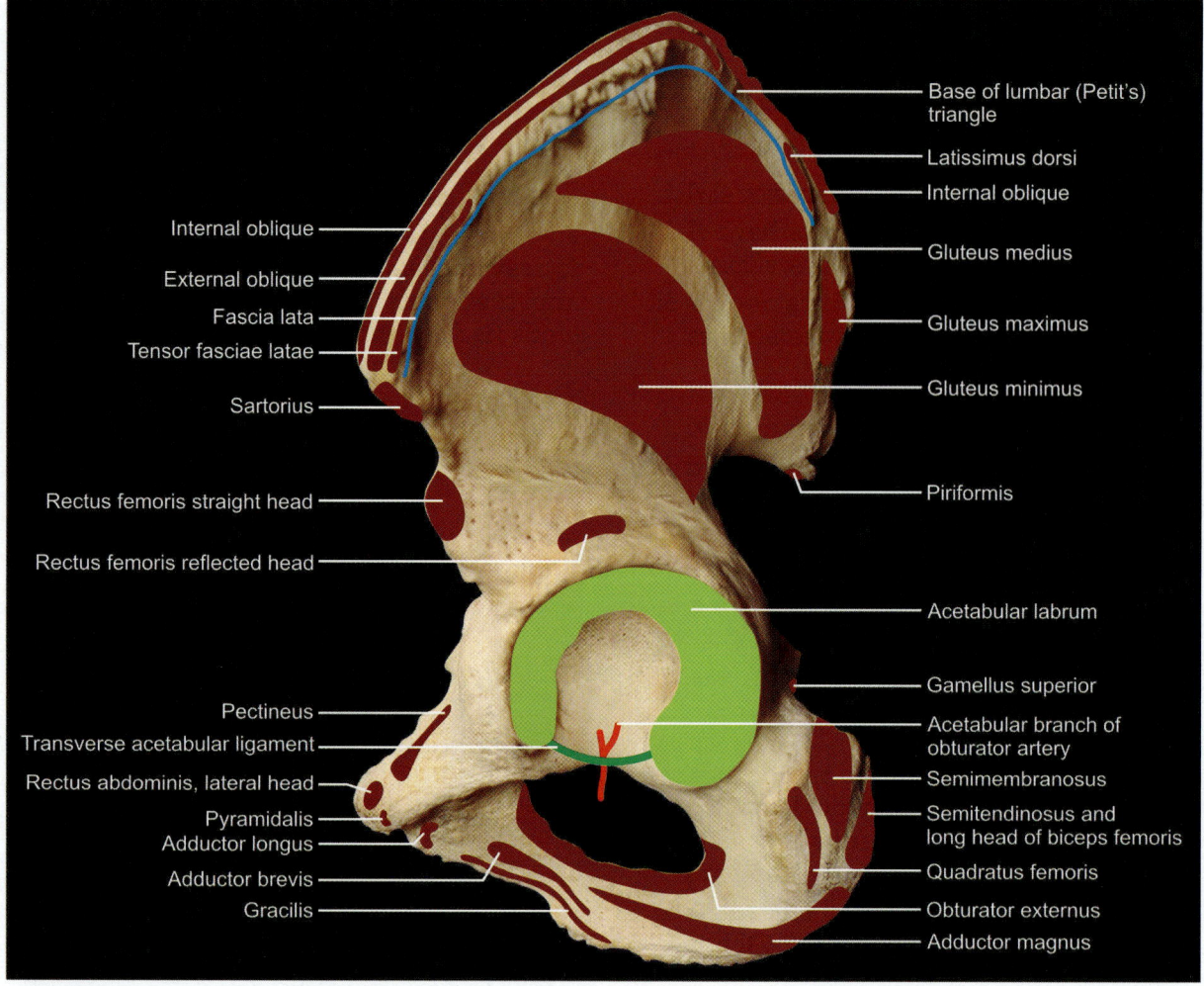

Fig. 3.5: Attachments of left hip bone (lateral view)

Medial surface

i. Covered by hyaline cartilage

ii. Between the two symphyseal surfaces lies the fibrocartilage and forms the symphysis pubis which is a secondary cartilaginous joint.

Pubic crest

i. Fascia lata

ii. Anterior wall of the rectus sheath

ii. **Origin of** lateral head of rectus abdominis and pyramidalis (if present) muscles

iv. Conjoint tendon

v. Fascia transversalis

vi. Linea alba.

Pubic tubercle

i. Medial end of inguinal ligament

ii. Lateral crus of the superficial inguinal ring

iii. Apex of the lacunar ligament

iv. Reflected part of the inguinal ligament

v. Upper loop of the cremaster muscle

vi. Anterior wall of the rectus sheath.

Superior ramus

Pelvic surface

i. Medial part of the pectineal line: From anterior to posterior

  a. Lacunar ligament

  b. Conjoint tendon.

ii. Lateral part of the pectineal line:

  a. Pectineal ligament

  b. Pectineal fascia.

iii. **Obturator crest and iliopubic eminence:** Pubofemoral ligament.

iv. **Inferior border:** Attachment of obturator membrane.

Pectineal surface: Medial part—origin of pectineus muscle.

Inferior ramus

Anterior surface

Medial to lateral: Origin of gracilis, adductor brevis, adductor magnus and obturator externus (Fig. 3.5).

Posterior surface (Fig. 3.4)

   i. **Perineal membrane:** To the ridge between the medial and intermediate areas.
  ii. **Superior layer of urogenital diaphragm:** To the ridge between the intermediate and lateral areas.
 iii. **Crus penis or clitoris:** To the medial area.
  iv. **Origin of sphincter urethrae:** To the intermediate area.
   v. **Origin of obturator internus:** To the lateral area.

Borders

Lateral border: Obturator membrane.
Medial border: Fascia lata and fascia of Colles.

Obturator foramen

   i. It is oval and larger in male.
  ii. It is small and triangular in female.
 iii. Obturator membrane is attached along the margin of the foramen except in the above.
  iv. The obturator groove transmits
       From above downwards
       a. Obturator nerve
       b. Obturator artery
       c. Obturator vein.

Subpubic angle (in articulated pelvis)
In male—70–75°
In female—90–100°

OSSIFICATION

   i. **Three primary centers**
      a. For the ilium about second month of intra-uterine life

      b. For the body of pubis between fourth and fifth months of intrauterine life
      c. For the body of ischium about fourth month of intrauterine life.

  ii. **Secondary centers**
      a. The centre of ossification for illiac crest appears by 14th year in female and 17th years in male and fuses with the body by 17th to 19th years in female and 19th to 20th years in male
      b. The center of ossification for ischial tuberosity appears by 14th to 16th years in female and 16th to 18th years in male and fuses with the body by 20th year in both male and female.
      c. Triradiate cartilage disappears by 14th year in female and 15th to 16th years in male (Fig. 3.3).

CLINICAL ANATOMY

   i. Hip bone fractures and dislocations are uncommon but fractures may occur in high-energy motor vehicle accident, falls during skipping and ice dancing.
  ii. Anterior and posterior compression of the hip bones pubic rami fracture commonly occurs.
 iii. Lateral compression of the pelvis may cause fracture of acetabulum.
  iv. **Nélaton's line:** In dislocation of hip joint the tip of the greater trochanter shifted above the Nélaton's line (line joining between the anterior superior iliac spine and prominent part of the ischial tuberosity).
   v. **Importance of ischial spine:** By digital examination per vagina on its lateral fornix the ischial spine is palpable and at the same level external os of cervix lies. If external os descends into the vagina below the level of ischial spine, indicates prolapse of uterus.

Table 3.1:	Difference between the male and female hip bones
Male	**Female**
i. It is heavier and muscular impressions are more prominent	i. It is lighter and muscular impressions are less prominent
ii. Iliac fossa more concave	ii. Iliac fossa is sallow
iii. Obturator foramen is large and oval	iii. Obturator foramen is small and triangular
iv. Ischiopubic rami are thick and more everted	iv. Ischiopubic rami are thin and not more everted
v. Preauricular sulcus is very less marked	v. Preauricular sulcus is more prominent especially in parous women.
vi. Articulates with upper three sacral vertebrae	vi. Articulates with the upper two sacral vertebrae
vii. Anterior superior iliac spine is interned	vii. Anterior superior iliac spine directed anteriorly
viii. Acetabulum is large	viii. Acetabulum is small
ix. Greater sciatic notch is narrower	ix. Greater sciatic notch is wider
x. Ischial tuberosity is inverted	x. Ischial tuberosity is everted

vi. **Lumbar hernia:** Occasionally hernia occurs through the lumbar (Petits) triangle.

vii. **Pudendal block:** Pudendal nerve crosses the ischial spine. The pudendal nerve can be blocked by two ways, by transvaginal or perineal approach, with patient in lithotomy position.

a. **Transvaginal approach:** First the ischial spine palpated per vaginum. The needle is then guided through the vaginal wall towards the ischial spine and the anesthetic agent is injected in the sacrospinous ligament. This procedure is repeated on the other side.

b. **Perineal approach:** At first the ischial tuberosity is palpated through skin and the needle is introduced along the medial surface of the tuberosity depth of 2.5 cm. The anesthetic agent blocks the pudendal nerve in the pudendal canal. The procedure is repeated on the opposite side.

Indications of pudendal nerve block: During second stage of labor, application of forceps in difficult child birth or other operations on perineum.

viii. **Pubic tubercle is an important landmark:** The inguinal hernia lies above and medial to the pubic tubercle whereas femoral hernia lies below and lateral to the pubic tubercle.

ix. **Low back pain during pregnancy:** This results from strain on ligaments of sacroiliac joints.

FEMUR

▌ INTRODUCTION

The femur or thigh bone is the longest and strongest bone in the body having a body or a shaft and two ends (upper and lower).

ANATOMICAL POSITION

i. Head looks upwards, medially and slightly forwards.
ii. Convex surface should be anteriorly.
iii. Expanded end having two condyles directed downwards.

SIDE DETERMINATION

After holding the bone in anatomical position the head on which side belongs will determine the opposite side of the bone.

GENERAL FEATURES

Parts

i. Upper end
ii. Shaft
iii. Lower end.

Upper End

The upper end consists of head, neck, greater and lesser trochanters (Fig. 3.6).

Head

i. It forms two-thirds of a sphere.
ii. Near the center of head presents a rough depression called fovea capitis femoris or pit.

Neck

i. It is broad and flattened from before backwards.
ii. It connects the head with shaft.
iii. **Inter-trochanteric line:** It is the junction between the neck and the shaft anteriorly.
iv. **Intertrochanteric crest:** It is the junction between the neck and the shaft posteriorly. On its midpoint presents a tubercle called quadrate tubercle.
v. **Angle of inclination:** Long axis of neck makes an angle with the long axis of shaft about 127° in adult. The angle is less in female due to wider pelvis.
vi. **Angle of torsion or the angle of declination:** It is obtained by the meeting of two lines through the long axis of the neck and other through the centers of the two condyles of femur. The mean angle is 14.01 degree.
vii. **Calcar femorale:** It is bony lamellae which strengthen the bone. It extends from the linea aspera to the posterior wall of neck of the femur medially to the greater trochanter laterally.

Greater trochanter (Fig. 3.6)

i. It is a quadrangular elevation.
ii. It projects upwards from the junction of the neck and the shaft.

Surfaces: Anterior, lateral and medial.

Anterior surface

i. It is rough and irregular.
ii. Separates from the lateral surface by an indistinct ridge.

Lateral surface

i. It is quadrilateral.
ii. Presents an oblique ridge from the posterosuperior angle and divides the lateral surface into upper and lower triangular areas.

Medial surface

i. Presents a deep depression at its junction with the neck called trochanteric fossa.

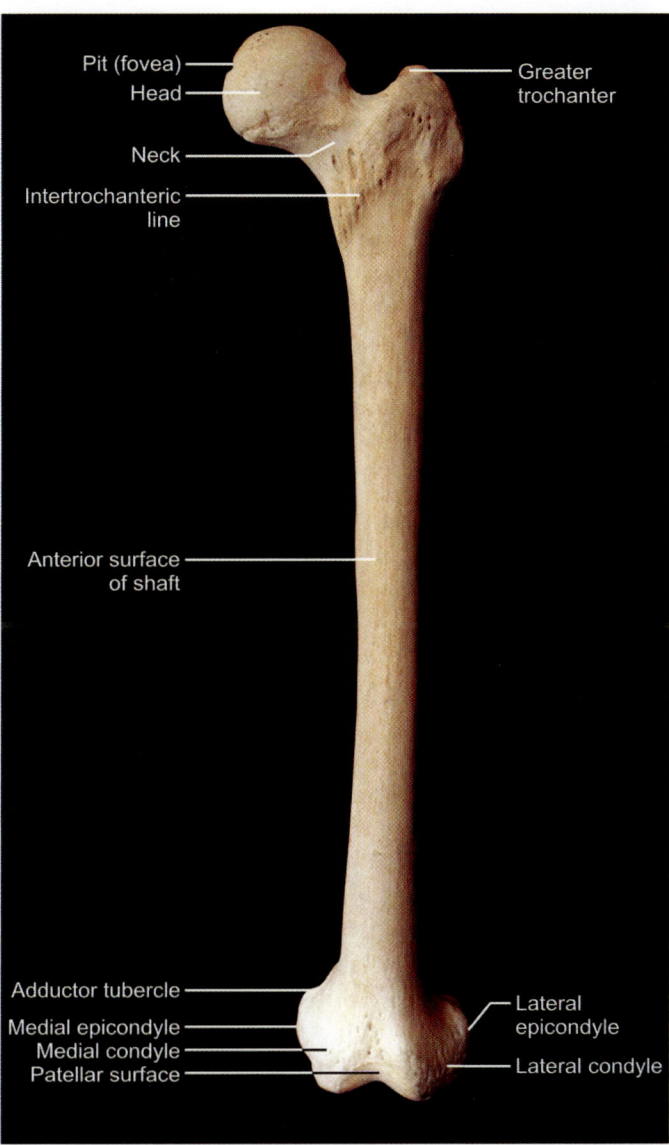

Pit (fovea)
Head
Neck
Intertrochanteric line
Anterior surface of shaft
Adductor tubercle
Medial epicondyle
Medial condyle
Patellar surface
Greater trochanter
Lateral epicondyle
Lateral condyle

Fig. 3.6: Anterior view of the left femur showing general features

ii. Above the trochanteric fossa presents, another depression for muscular attachment.

Borders: Superior and posterior.

Superior border
i. It is prominent.
ii. At its anterior part presents a muscular impression.

Posterior border: It is continuous with the intertrochanteric crest.

Lesser trochanter: It is conical in shape situated on the inferomedial part at the junction between the neck and shaft (Fig. 3.7).

Shaft
i. The shaft is convex in front, which is more in its middle one-third.

ii. It is narrow in the middle but expands both above and below.
iii. **Borders:** Medial, lateral and posterior (middle one-third).
iv. **Surfaces:** Anterior, medial, lateral, upper posterior and lower posterior.

Medial and lateral borders
i. These borders are ill-defined and rounded.
ii. The medial border separates the anterior from the medial surfaces.
iii. The lateral border separates the anterior from the lateral surfaces.

Posterior border (Fig. 3.7)
i. Opposite the middle one-third presents a crest, called linea aspera
ii. Linea aspera consists of lateral and medial lips and an intermediate area
    a. The lateral and medial lips diverge each other both upwards and downwards to forms the upper and lower posterior surfaces
    b. Inferiorly the lateral and medial lips form prominent margins to reach into lateral and medial condyles of the lower end called lateral and medial supracondylar lines respectively
    c. Superiorly the lateral lip reach to the root of the greater trochanter as a rough ridge, called gluteal tuberosity (often it is called third trochanter)
    d. The medial lip superiorly continuous with the spiral line.

Anterior surface: It is convex, lies between the medial and lateral borders.

Medial surface: Lies between the medial border and linea aspera.

Lateral surface: Lies between the lateral border and linea aspera.

Upper posterior surface (Fig. 3.7)
Situation: Lies between the gluteal tuberosity laterally and spiral line medially.

Lower posterior surface (Fig. 3.7)
i. It lies between the lateral supracondylar line laterally and medial supracondylar line medially.
ii. This surface is also called popliteal surface of the femur.
iii. This surface presents two tubercles laterally and medially in its lower part (Fig. 3.7).

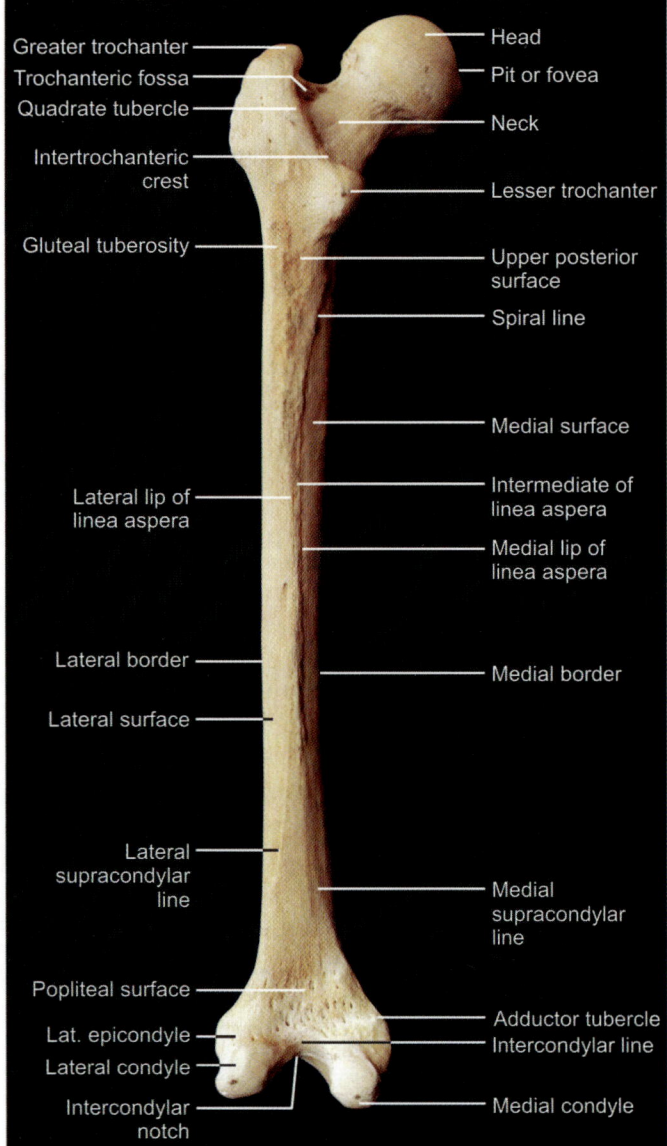

Fig. 3.7: Posterior view of left femur showing general features

Lower End

i. It is broad and expanded (Fig. 3.6).

ii. It consists of lateral and medial condyles.

iii. The two condyles articulate with the patella in front and corresponding condyles of the tibia below and behind.

iv. The outer surfaces of the condyles is rough and convex and the most prominent part of the convexity is called epicondyles (medial and lateral).

v. Just above the medial part of the posterior end of the medial epicondyle presents a small tubercle called adductor tubercle.

vi. The condyles having articular and nonarticular parts.

vii. Anterior articular surface of the two condyles form a saddle-shaped articular area called patellar surface, which articulates with the posterior surface of the patella.

viii. The patellar articular surface of the lateral condyle raised more on the anterior aspect than the medial condyle.

ix. The inferior and posterior articular surfaces of each condyle form the tibial articular surface.

x. The tibial articular surfaces are separated from each other by intercondylar notch.

xi. The medial condyle descends 0.5 cm more than the lateral condyle.

xii. Posteriorly, the intercondylar notch is separated from the popliteal surface by a transverse ridge called intercondylar line.

xiii. Between the lateral epicondyle and articular margin posteriorly presents a groove.

ATTACHMENTS OF FEMUR

Upper End

Head

Articulation: Head articulates with the acetabulum of the hip bone to form the hip joint.

Ligament: Ligament of the head of the femur (ligamentum teres femoris)—to the fovea capitis femoris or pit (which is intracapsular but extrasynovial).

Neck

Capsular ligament (Fig. 3.8)

Attachments

Anteriorly: In front to the intertrochanteric line.

Posteriorly: About 1.3 cm medial and parallel with the intertrochanteric crest,

Superiorly: Close to the junction with the greater trochanter.

Inferiorly: Above the root of the lesser trochanter.

Greater trochanter

Insertion of (Fig. 3.8)

  i. Gluteus minimus: To the anterior surface

  ii. Gluteus medius: To the oblique ridge on the lateral surface

Medial surface

Insertion of

  i. Obturator externus: At the trochanteric fossa.

  ii. Common tendon of obturator internus, gemellus superior and inferior: To another depression above the trochanteric fossa.

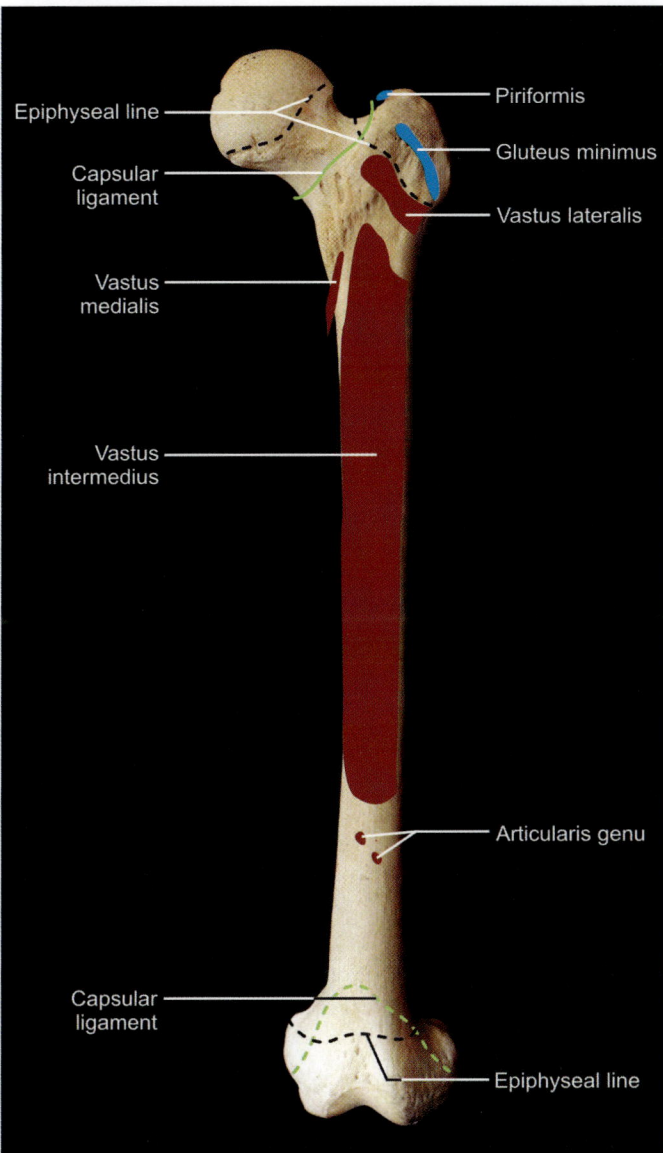

Epiphyseal line

Capsular ligament

Vastus medialis

Vastus intermedius

Piriformis

Gluteus minimus

Vastus lateralis

Articularis genu

Capsular ligament

Epiphyseal line

Fig. 3.8: Anterior view of left femur showing attachments

Superior border

Insertion of: Piriformis.

Lesser trochanter

Insertion of

  i. Psoas major: On its tip.

  ii. Iliacus: To the inferomedial part of its base which also extends to the upper posterior surface.

Intertrochanteric line

Origin of (Fig. 3.8)

  i. Vastus lateralis: From the upper half of the line.

  ii. Vastus medialis: From the lower half of the line.

Ligaments

  i. Capsular ligament: Attached to its inner part in its whole length.

  ii. Lateral and medial bands of iliofemoral ligament: Attached outside the capsular ligament.

Intertrochanteric crest

Insertion of

Quadratus femoris: On the quadrate tubercle (Fig. 3.9).

Shaft

Posterior border (linea aspera): Arrangements of attachment—from medial to lateral (Fig. 3.9)

  i. Medial intermuscular septum: On the medial lip.

  ii. Origin of vastus medialis: More medial to the medial intermuscular septum.

  iii. Posterior intermuscular septum: On the intermediate area.

  iv. Insertion of adductor brevis and longus: Between the medial and posterior intermuscular septa of which brevis in upper part longus is in the lower part.

  v. Insertion adductor magnus: More lateral to the adductor brevis and longus.

  vi. Lateral intermuscular septum: On the lateral lip.

  vii. Origin of vastus lateralis: More lateral to the lateral intermuscular septum.

  viii. Origin of short head of biceps femoris: Between the posterior and lateral intermuscular septa, and also upper two-thirds of the lateral supracondylar line.

From the surfaces

Origin of (Fig. 3.8)

  i. Vastus intermedius: From the upper three-fourths of the anterior and lateral surfaces.

  ii. Articularis genu: From the upper part of the lower one-fourth of the anterior surface.

  iii. Upper posterior surface (Fig. 3.9)

    Insertion of: following muscles from medial to lateral:

    a. Vastus medialis

    b. Iliacus

    c. Pectineus

    d. Adductor brevis

    e. Adductor magnus

    f. Gluteus maximus

  iv. On the popliteal surface (Fig. 3.9)

    Origin of:

    a. **Plantaris**—from the tubercle on the lower lateral part

    b. **Medial head of gastrocnemius**—from the tubercle on the lower medial part

c. **Short head of biceps femoris**—from the lateral supracondylar line in the upper two-thirds.

d. **Plantaris, and lateral head of gastrocnemius**- from lower one-third of the lateral supracondylar line.

c. **Vastus medialis**—from the upper two-thirds of the medial supracondylar line.

Insertion of

Adductor magnus: From whole length of the medial supracondylar line except in the area of adductor hiatus.

v. **Lateral intermuscular septum**—whole length of the lateral supracondylar line.

vi. **Medial intermuscular septum**—whole length of the medial supracondylar line (Fig. 3.9).

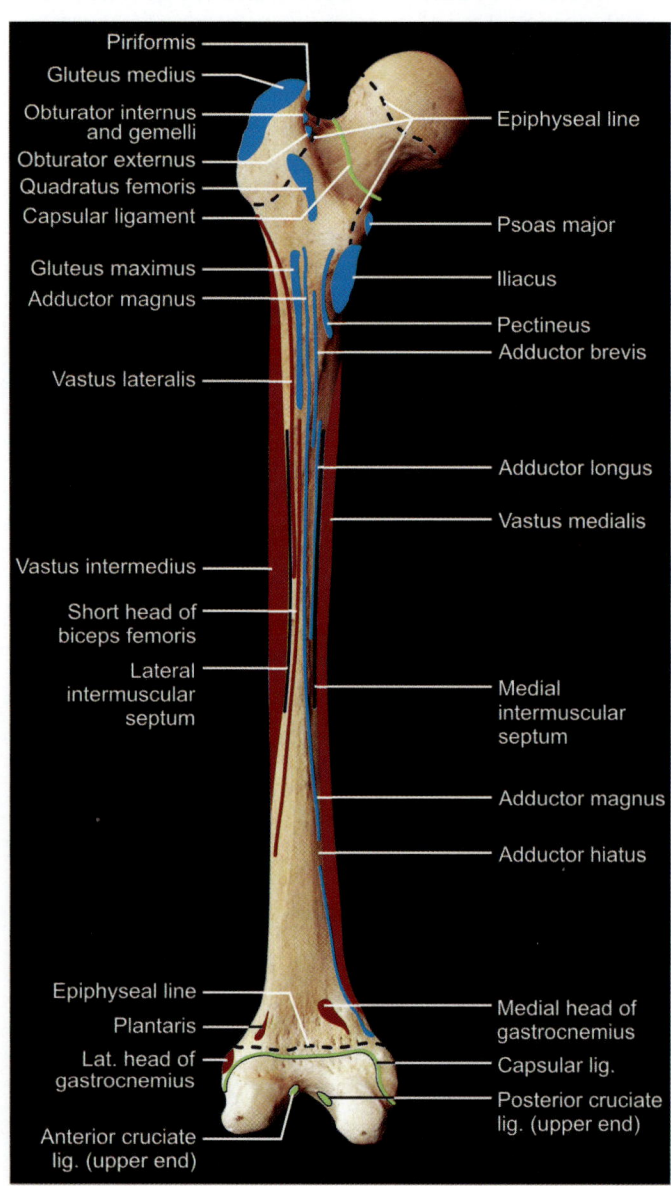

Fig. 3.9: Posterior view of left femur showing attachments

Lower End (Fig. 3.9)

Ligaments

i. **Menisci or semilunar cartilages (medial and lateral)**—between the articular surfaces of the femur and tibia.

ii. **Tibial collateral ligament**—at the medial epicondyle.

iii. **Fibular collateral ligament**—at the lateral epicondyle.

iv. **Oblique popliteal ligament**—at the lateral part of the intercondylar line.

v. **Capsular ligament**—at the intercondylar line.

vi. **Anterior cruciate ligament (upper end)**—to the medial surface of the lateral condyle

vii. **Posterior cruciate ligament (upper end)**—to the lateral surface of the medial condyle.

Muscles

Origin of

i. **Popliteus:** From the anterior part of the groove on the lateral condyle.

ii. **Lateral head of gastrocnemius**—groove on the posterosuperior part of the lateral epicondyle.

Insertion of

Adductor magnus: to the adductor tubercle of the medial condyle.

OSSIFICATION

i. **Primary center:** One primary center appears in middle of the shaft about seventh week of embryonic life.

ii. **Secondary centers**

a. One for the lower end—appears in the nine month of fetal life.

b. For the head sixth month to one year after birth

c. For the greater trochanter—about forth year

d. For the lesser trochanter—about fourteenth year:

– The lesser trochanter unites with the diaphysis during sixteenth year

– The greater trochanter unites with the diaphysis during seventeenth year

– The head unites with the diaphysis during eighteenth year.

The aboves help in age determination.

CLINICAL ANATOMY

i. Fracture of neck of the femur

a. The femoral neck is more susceptible to fracture in insignificant trauma than the shaft of the femur among postmenopausal women due to no estrogen is secreted by the senile ovaries as a result producing osteoporosis and degeneration of calcar femorale.

b. Fractures of neck of femur are of two types:

Intracapsular—it is serious and most complicated due to retinacular arteries are injured leading to delay in healing or nonunion or may leads to avascular necrosis of head of the femur

– In intracapsular fracture, the affected side of the limb is shortened and laterally rotated with toes pointing laterally, shortening is due to pulled by rectus femoris, hamstring and adductor muscles and lateral rotation is due to contraction of gluteus maximus.

Extracapsular—in this fracture, the blood supply is retained hence there is no avascular necrosis of the head.

ii. In children and adolescents the epiphysis of the head of the femur may slip away the neck due to weakness of the epiphyseal plate.

iii. The angle of inclination (neck-shaft angle) normally in adult 125° and children 160°, its abnormality produces two conditions:

a. **Coxa valga:** When neck-shaft angle is increased found in congenital dislocation of hip, results in adduction of the hip joint to be limited

b. **Coxa vara:** When neck-shaft angle is decreased found in fracture in neck of the femur, results in abduction of the hip joint to be limited

iv. When fracture in the shaft makes into fragments it is difficult to keep them together due to pull of the muscles attached to the femur.

v. Fracture between the greater and lesser trochanters called intertrochanteric fracture or through the trochanters called pertrochanteric fracture, these fractures also commonly seen in above 60 years.

vi. **Medicolegal importance:** Secondary center of ossification for lower end has medicolegal importance. Presence of this center in X-ray is a proof of the viability or maturity of the fetus.

PATELLA

▌ INTRODUCTION

i. Patella is the largest sesamoid bone in the body
ii. Situated in front of the knee joint
iii. It develops in the tendon of quadriceps femoris muscle.

ANATOMICAL POSITION

i. Pointed apex looks downwards.
ii. Articular surface looks backwards.

SIDE DETERMINATION

After holding the bone in anatomical position the larger part of the articular surface on which side belongs will determine the side of the bone.

GENERAL FEATURES

i. It is flattened from before backwards
ii. Somewhat triangular in shape
iii. Its pointed apex directed downwards
iv. Broad base directed upwards
v. Anterior surface is subcutaneous, rough and nonarticular with presence of numerous vascular foramina and marked by numbers of longitudinal ridges
vi. Posterior surface divides into:
   a. Large, smooth articular part above.
   b. Narrow, rough, depressed nonarticular part below (close to the apex)
vii. The articular part divided by a vertical ridge into large and deeper lateral and small medial parts (Fig. 3.10).

ATTACHMENTS OF PATELLA

i. **Ligamentum patellae:** To the apex and lower part of the nonarticular area on the posterior surface
ii. **The base receives insertion of:** Following muscles From anterior to posterior—
   a. Rectus femoris
   b. Vastus medialis on the medial one-third and vastus lateralis on the lateral two-thirds in a same plane
   c. Vastus intermedius
iii. **Medial border**
   a. **Insertion of vastus medialis:** On upper two-thirds (Fig. 3.11)
   b. **Medial patellar retinaculum:** On lower one-third

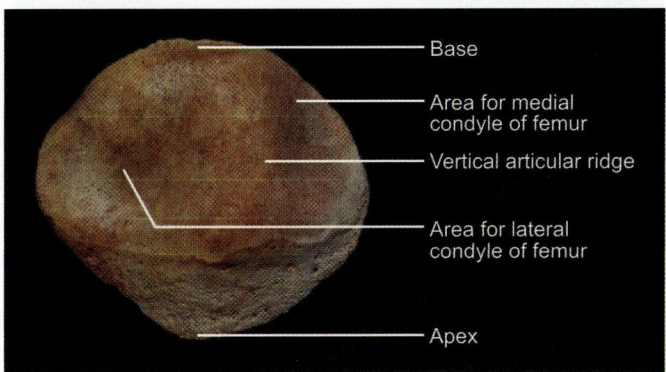

Fig. 3.10: Posterior view of right patella showing general features

Base
Area for medial condyle of femur
Vertical articular ridge
Area for lateral condyle of femur
Apex

iv. **Lateral border** (Fig. 3.11)
   a. **Insertion of vastus lateralis:** On the upper one-third
   b. **Lateral patellar retinaculum:** On the rest part of the lateral border.
v. **Anterior surface:** Present a subcutaneous prepatellar bursa, which separates the anterior surface from the skin.
vi. **Posterior surface**
   a. The larger lateral articular part of the posterior surface articulates with the lateral condyle of the femur
   b. The smaller medial articular part of the posterior surface articulates with the medial condyle of the femur
   c. The vertical ridge on the articular part of the posterior surface fits into the groove on the patellar surface of the femur
   d. The nonarticular part of the posterior surface subdivided into upper and lower parts:
      – The upper part gives attachment to the infrapatellar pad of fat
      – Lower part together with the apex gives attachment to the ligamentum patellae.

OSSIFICATION

i. It ossifies from the several centers, they appear during the third to sixth years, and unite quickly
ii. Ossification completes at puberty.

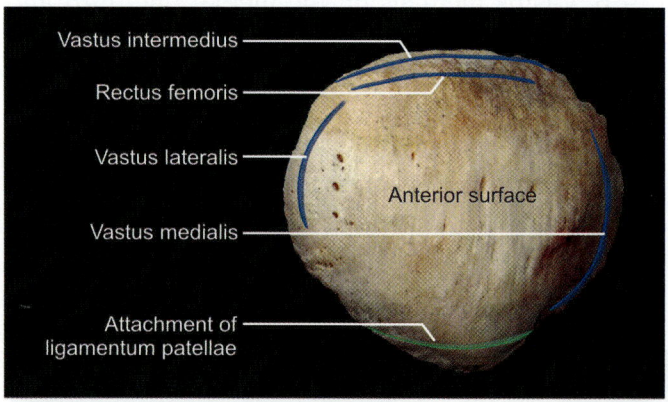

Fig. 3.11: Anterior view of right patella showing attachments

CLINICAL ANATOMY

i. **Patella fracture**
   a. Patella fractured as a result of direct violence commonly in an automobile accident where patella is broken into many small pieces.
   b. Patella may fracture as a result of indirect violence caused by the sudden powerful contraction of the quadriceps femoris in semiflexed or flexed knee.
   c. Patella may also be fractured due to repeated stress, occurs in ballet dancers and long distance runners, etc.
ii. **Congenital dislocation of patella:** Congenital recurrent dislocation of patella commonly occurs laterally due to following factors:
   a. Due to underdevelopment of the lateral condyle of the femur.
   b. Due to lateral angulations between long axis of the thigh and leg.
   c. Also due to poor development of vastus medialis. The dislocation is prevented by following factors:
   d. Large size forward projection of the lateral condyle of the femur
   e. Insertion of vastus medialis on the medial border of the patella extends lower level than the vastus lateralis on the lateral border.
iii. **Multiple patella:** Failure of fusion of several ossification centers results in partition of patella, so that it consists of two or more bony areas. This anomaly occurs bilaterally which helps to distinguish it from a fracture. In patella fracture, the fracture lines are irregular but in congenital multiple patella the edges of bones are regular.

TIBIA

INTRODUCTION

i. Tibia is also known as shin bone because shin means the prominent anterior edge of the tibia or leg.
ii. The tibia is the medial bone of the leg
iii. It is the second longest bone in the body.

ANATOMICAL POSITION

i. Broad upper end looks upwards
ii. Sharp border of the shaft anteriorly
iii. Tibial (medial) malleolus will directed downwards and medially.

SIDE DETERMINATION

After holding the bone in anatomical position the medial malleolus will determine the side of the bone.

GENERAL FEATURES

Parts: It consists of upper end, shaft and lower end.

Upper end (Fig. 3.12)

   i. Transversely broader than anteroposteriorly.

   ii. It consists of:

     a. Lateral and medial condyles

     b. A tubercle

   iii. Intercondylar area.

Lateral condyle

   i. It is smaller than medial condyle.

   ii. It projects more on its posterolateral aspect.

   iii. On the inferior part of the posterolateral aspect presents fibular facet for superior tibiofibular joint.

   iv. Superiorly, it presents a circular articular surface,

   v. Its medial part of the superior articular surface prolonged to the lateral aspect of the lateral intercondylar tubercle.

   vi. Posteriorly, it presents a groove for the tendon of popliteus where capsular ligament is deficient.

Medial condyle

   i. It is larger than lateral condyle.

   ii. Superior articular surface is oval.

   iii. Lateral part of the superior articular surface extends over the medial aspect of the medial intercondylar tubercle.

   iv. Posteriorly, it presents a rough horizontal groove for muscular attachments.

Tuberosity of the tibia: It is a prominent bony eminence at the upper end of the anterior border.

Intercondylar area

   i. It is rough area between the articular surfaces of the medial and lateral condyles.

   ii. In the middle the area is narrow, irregular and elevated, called intercondylar eminence.

   iii. The intercondylar eminence is formed by the lateral and medial intercondylar tubercles (Fig. 3.12).

Shaft

It is prismoidal in shape and triangular on transverse section.

Borders: Anterior, lateral (interosseous) and medial.

Surfaces: Lateral, medial and posterior.

Anterior border (Fig. 3.12)

   i. This border also called shin of the tibia.

   ii. Upper two-third is sharp and prominent and lower part is rounded.

Lateral or interosseous border: Begins from the anteroinferior part of the fibular facet, and ends below

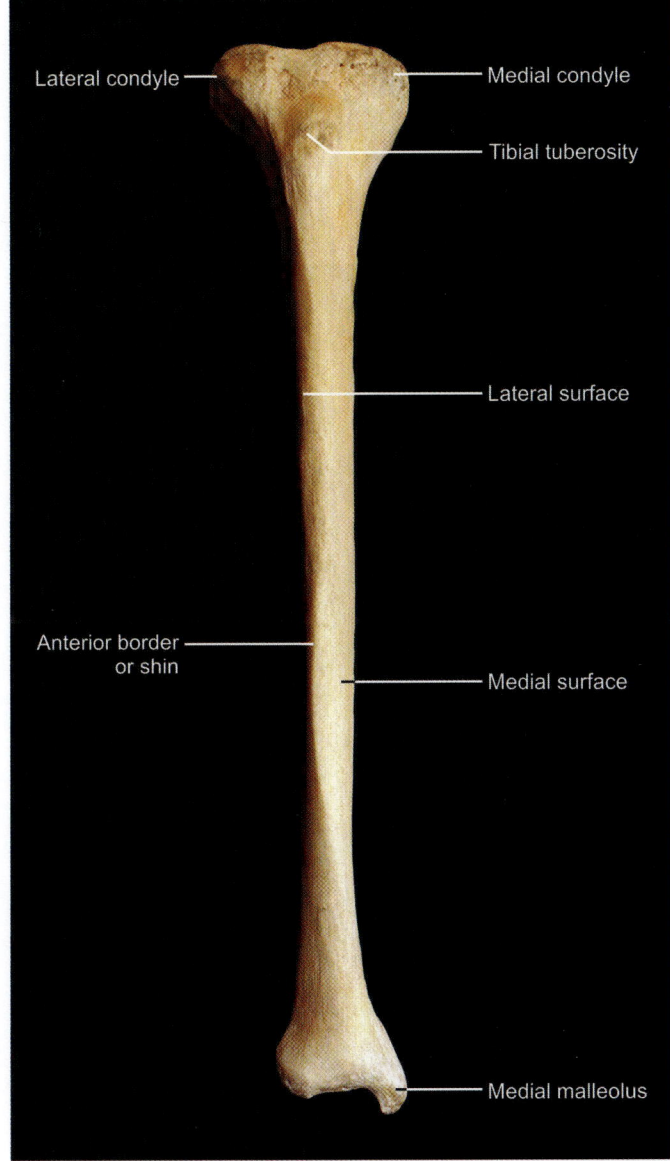

Fig. 3.12: Anterior view of the right tibia showing general features

by dividing to enclose a triangular rough notch at the lateral aspect of the lower end.

Medial border: Begins from the anterior end of the groove on the back of the medial condyle to end in the posterior border of the medial malleolus.

Lateral surface: It lies between the anterior and interosseous borders.

Posterior surface (Fig. 3.13)

   i. It lies between the interosseous and medial borders.

   ii. This surface is divided by the soleal line into upper small triangular and lower larger areas.

   iii. The lower area further subdivided into medial and lateral areas by a vertical ridge.

Relations: The lower one-fourth is related with following:

    i. Tendon of the tibialis posterior

    ii. Tendon of the flexor digitorum longus

Medial surface: It is subcutaneous, lies between the medial and anterior borders (Fig. 3.13).

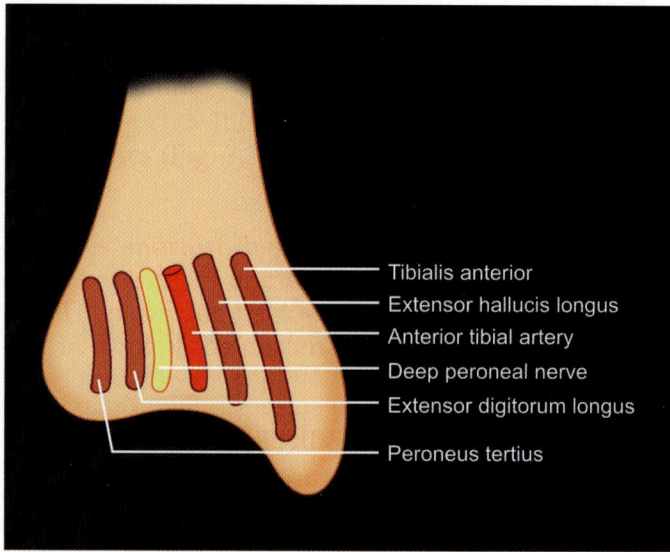

Fig. 3.14: Tendons, artery and nerve related to anterior surface of lower end of right tibia

Relations: From medial to lateral

    i. Tendon of the tibialis anterior

    ii. Tendon of the extensor hallucis longus

    iii. Anterior tibial vessels

    iv. Deep peroneal nerve

    v. Tendon of the extensor digitorum longus

    vi. Tendon of the peroneus tertius

Posterior surface: Separates from the inferior surface by a sharp margin (Fig. 3.15).

Relations: From medial to lateral:

    i. Tendon of the tibialis posterior.

    ii. Flexor digitorum longus.

    iii. Posterior tibial vessels.

    iv. Tibial nerve.

    v. Tendon of the flexor hallucis longus.

Lateral surface: Presents a wide triangular notch called fibular notch of the tibia with sharp anterior and posterior margins.

Medial surface

    i. Convex and subcutaneous.

    ii. It is prolonged downwards to form medial malleolus.

Inferior surface: This surface is smooth and articular and articulates with the superior surface of the body of the talus.

Medial malleolus

    i. It is a short, thick bony projection from the medial aspect of the lower end.

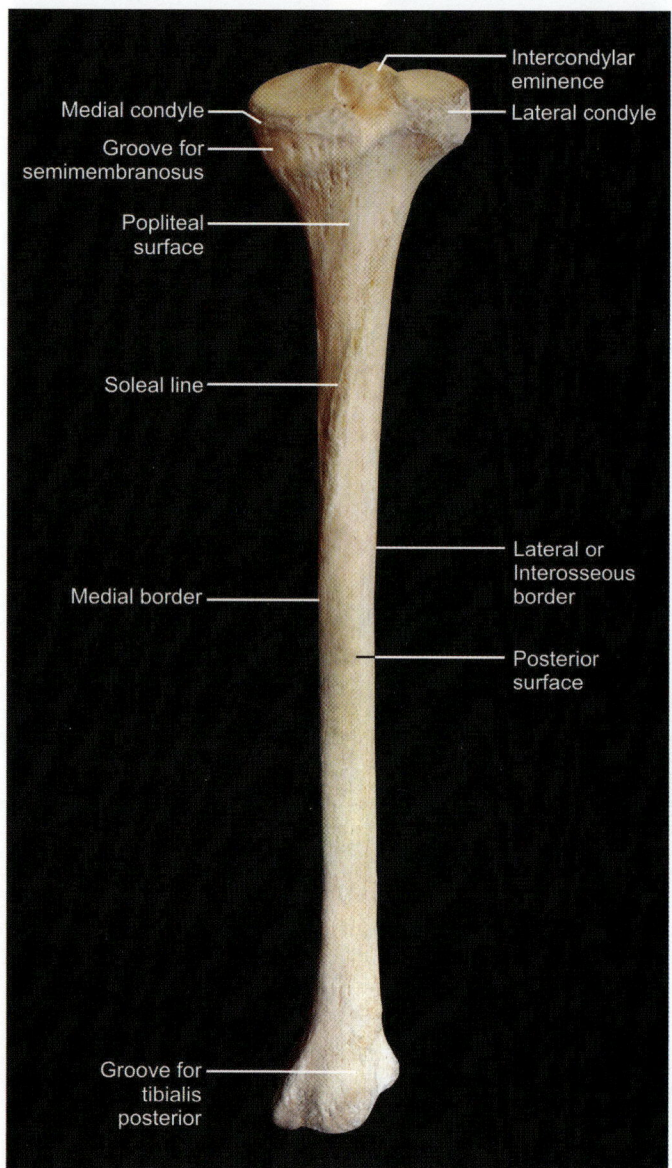

Fig. 3.13: Posterior view of the right tibia showing general features

Lower end

    i. It is broad and expanded.

    ii. Surfaces—anterior, posterior, lateral, medial and inferior.

    iii. Medial malleolus.

Anterior surface: It is convex, separated from the inferior surface by a transverse groove (Fig. 3.14).

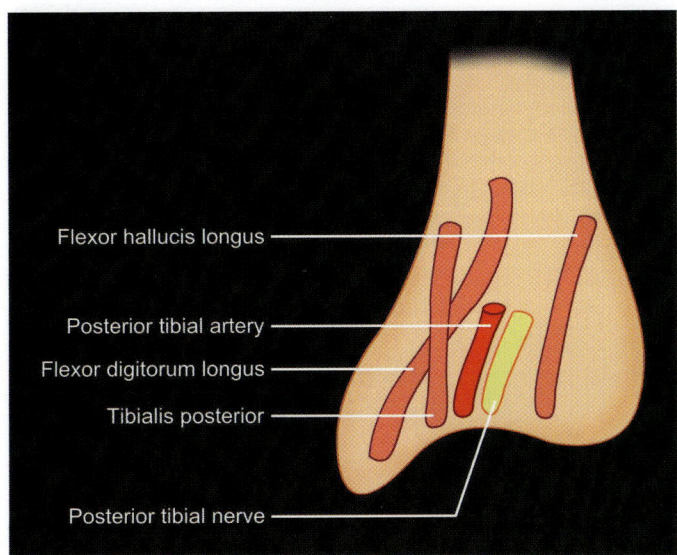

Fig. 3.15: Tendons, artery and nerve related to posterior surface of lower end of right tibia

ii. **Surfaces**—medial, lateral, anterior and posterior.
iii. **Border**—inferior border.

Medial surface: Convex and subcutaneous.

Lateral surface: Presents a comma-shaped articular facet, which articulates with the medial aspect of the body of the talus.

Anterior and posterior surfaces: Marked by shallow grooves.

Inferior border

i. It is pointed in front and behind.
ii. It presents a depressed impression on the middle.

ATTACHMENTS OF TIBIA

Upper End

Lateral condyle (Fig. 3.18)

i. **Origin of** (sometimes): Few fibers of extensor digitorum longus and peroneus longus—to the lateral surface just in front of the fibular facet.
ii. **Insertion of:** Few fibers of biceps femoris—just in front of the fibular facet.
iii. **Lateral meniscus:** It is in contact with the anterior, posterior and lateral margins of the superior articular surface.
iv. **Capsular ligament of the superior tibiofibular joint:** Margins of the fibular facet.
v. **Deep infrapatellar bursa:** It presents on anterior convex surfaces of both the condyles.
vi. **Iliotibial tract and deep fascia of leg:** To the anterior surface of the lateral condyle.

Medial condyle

i. **Insertion of semimembranosus:** To the groove and its lower lip (Fig. 3.18).
ii. **Medial meniscus:** It is in contact with the anterior, posterior and medial margins of the superior articular surface.
iii. Capsular ligament of the knee joint and short posterior fibers of the tibial collateral ligament: at the upper margin of the groove.
iv. **Medial patellar retinaculum:** On the anterior and medial surfaces of the medial condyle.

Tuberosity of the tibia

i. **Ligamentum patellae:** To the upper smooth part (Fig. 3.16 and 3.18).
ii. **Subcutaneous infrapatellar bursa:** It is in contact with the lower part.

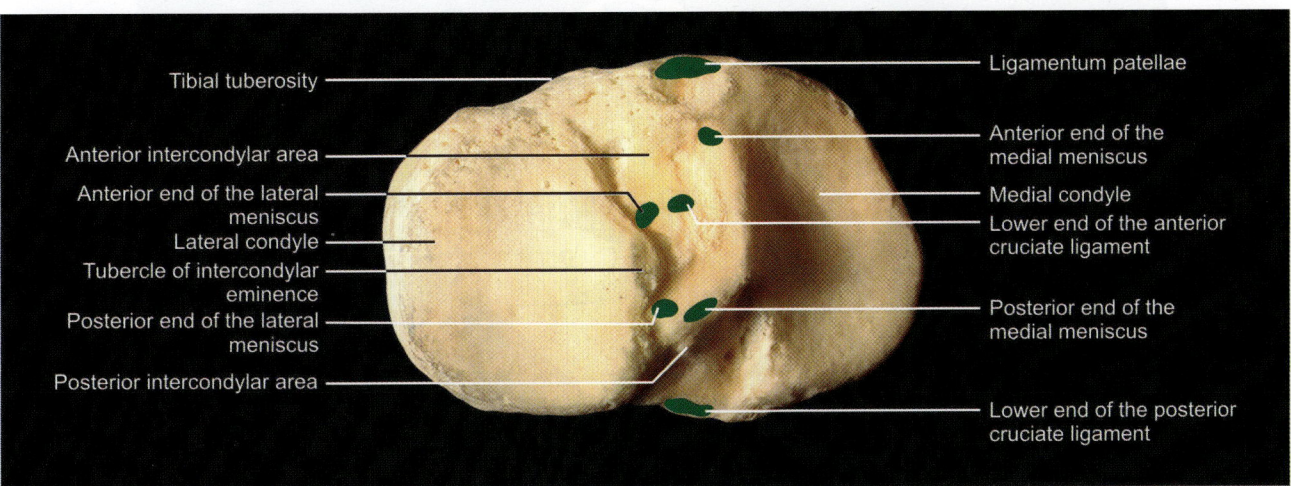

Fig. 3.16: Proximal articular surface of the left tibia, showing the attachments of intercondylar area

Intercondylar area: From anterior to posterior (Figs 3.16 and 3.17)

   i. In front of the intercondylar eminence:

      a. Anterior end of the medial meniscus

      b. Lower end of the anterior cruciate ligament

      c. Anterior end of the lateral meniscus

   ii. Behind the intercondylar eminence:

      a. Posterior end of the lateral meniscus

      b. Posterior end of the medial meniscus

      c. Lower end of the posterior cruciate ligament.

Shaft

   i. Fascia cruris or deep fascia of leg.

   ii. Superior extensor retinaculum immediately above the medial malleolus.

Lateral or interosseous border: Interosseous membrane.

Medial border: From above downward:

   i. Tibial (medial) collateral ligament of the knee joint and **insertion of** few fibers of the semimembranosus.

   ii. Fascia covering the popliteus (above the soleal line).

   iii. **Origin of:** Soleus muscle with its fascia (Fig. 3.19).

   iv. Fascia cruris or deep fascia of leg (below the soleal line).

Lateral surface

Origin of

Tibialis anterior: From the upper two-thirds (Fig. 3.19).

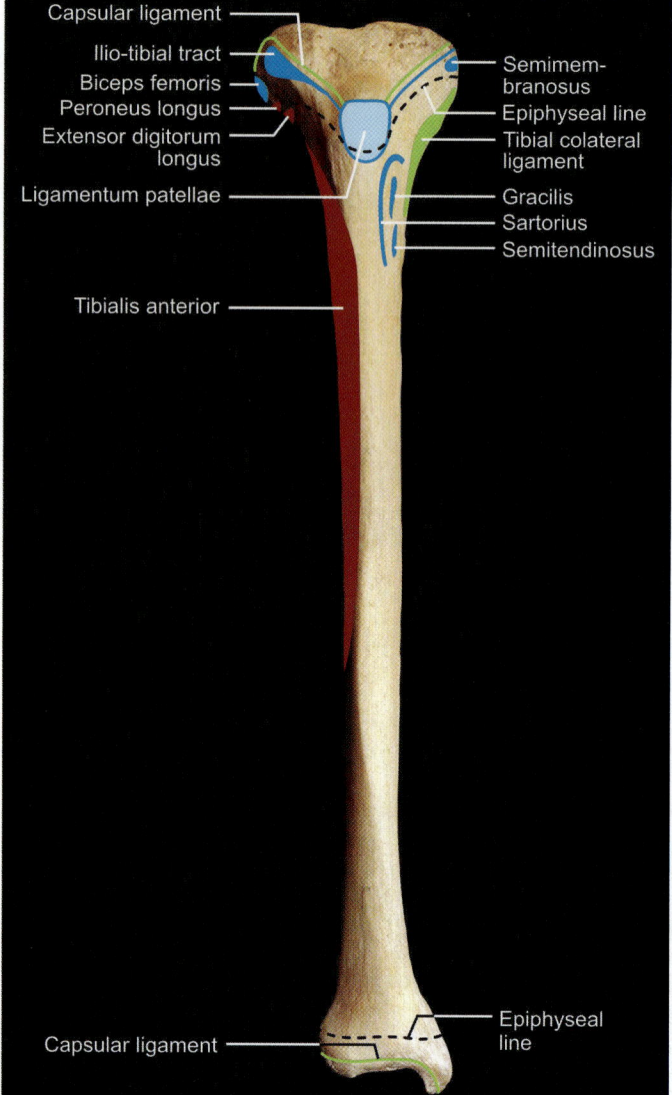

Fig. 3.18: Anterior view of the right tibia showing attachments

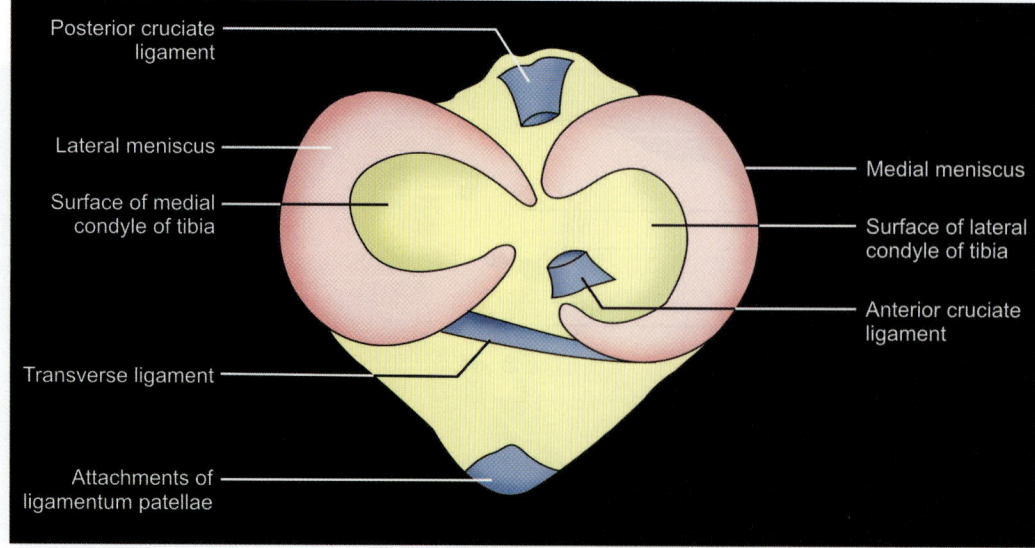

Fig. 3.17: Menisci of the knee joint

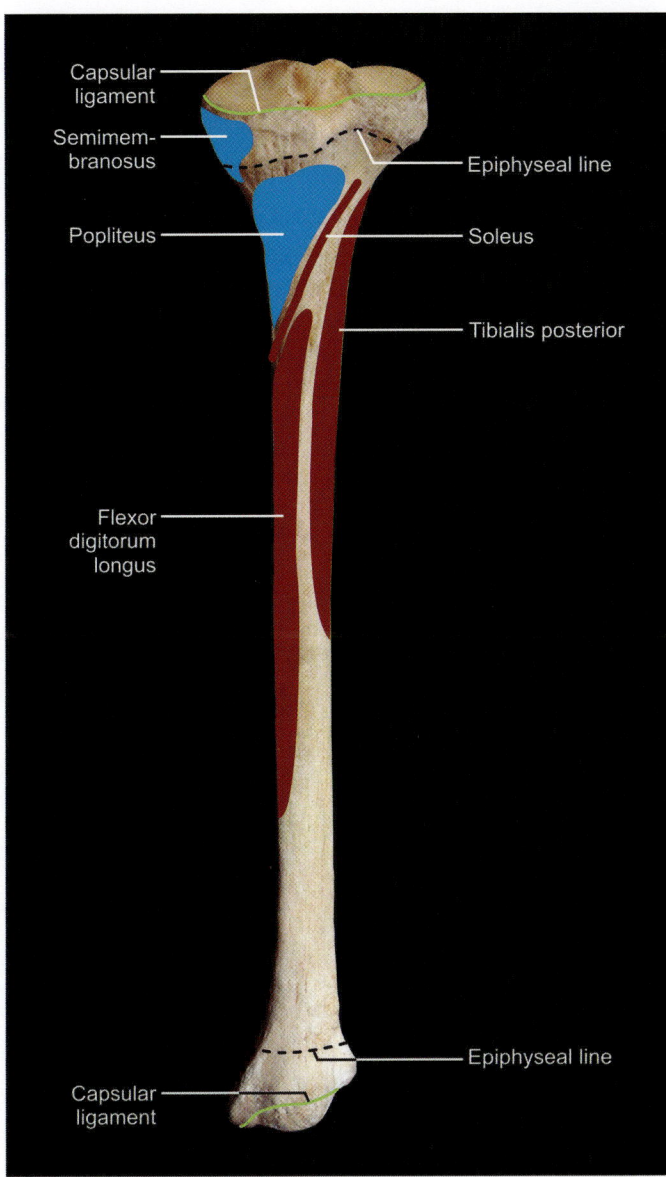

Fig. 3.19: Posterior view of the right tibia showing attachments

Posterior surface

Insertion of

i. **Popliteus:** On the part above the soleal line.

Origin of

ii. **Soleus:** From the soleal line.

The soleal line also attached following fasciae:

a. Fascia covering the soleus

b. Fascia covering the popliteus

c. Deep fascia of the leg.

iii. **Tibialis posterior:** From the lateral area of the lower part in its upper three-fourths.

iv. **Flexor digitorum longus:** From the medial area of the lower part.

Medial surface

i. Deep fascia of the leg.

ii. **Insertion of:** Semimembranosus and tibial collateral ligament—area in front of the upper part of the medial border.

iii. **Insertion of:** In front of the semimembranosus from before backwards following muscles (Fig. 3.18):

a. Sartorius

b. Gracilis

c. Semitendinosus.

Lower end

Anterior Surface: Capsular ligament of the ankle: to the transverse groove.

Posterior Surface

i. **Capsular ligament of the ankle:** At the sharp margin separates the posterior from the inferior surfaces (Fig. 3.19).

ii. **Flexor retinaculum of the leg:** At the sharp margin of the vertical groove.

Lateral surface

i. **Articulation:** Lower end of the fibula articulates with the fibular notch of the tibia.

ii. **Anterior and posterior tibiofibular ligaments:** At the sharp anterior and posterior margins of the fibular notch of the tibia.

Medial malleolus

Inferior border

Ligaments

i. **Deep part of the deltoid ligament:** At the depressed impression.

ii. **Superficial part of the deltoid ligament:** More superficially.

iii. **Capsular ligament of the ankle:** To the anterior, posterior and inferior margins.

OSSIFICATION

i. **Primary center:** One primary center appears in the shaft (near the middle) at about seventh week of intrauterine life.

ii. **Secondary centers:** Secondary center for the upper end—appears at birth or shortly after birth.

iii. Secondary center for the lower end—appears between the one and two years.

iv. The lower epiphysis fused with the shaft—about fifteen to sixteen years.

v. The upper epiphysis fused with the shaft about seventeen and eighteen years, helps in age determination

CLINICAL ANATOMY

i. **Fracture of the tibia**

   a. Fracture of the shaft of the tibia is often open because whole length of the medial surface is only covered by the skin and fasciae.

   b. Commonest site of tibial fracture: It is commonly occur at the junction of the upper two-thirds and lower one-third of the shaft as this part is narrowest.

   c. Fracture of the lower one-third of the shaft is prone to delayed or nonunion as the blood supply to this part is poor.

ii. **Osteomyelitis:** Upper end of the tibia is one of the commonest site of acute osteomyelitis.

iii. **Bone graft:** Sometimes a piece of bone is grafted from the medial surface of the shaft as this surface is subcutaneous.

iv. **Rickets with bowleg (genu varum):** In rickets there is calcium deficiency, its effects particularly shows in tibia and maximum effect is seen at its narrowest part, at the junction of the upper two-thirds and lower one-third of the shaft producing outward bending of the tibia and the condition is known as bowleg (genu varum).

v. **Pott's fracture (fracture dislocation of ankle) and trimalleolar fracture:** These occur when the foot is caught in the rabbit hole and the foot is everted forcibly. Depending on the severity of injury, following are the order of fractures:

   i. Fracture of lateral malleolus.

   ii. Fracture of medial malleolus.

   iii. Fracture of the posterior margin of the lower end of the tibia (third malleolus).

When fractures involving the medial and lateral malleoli the condion is called Pott's fracture, and when fractures all the above mentioned three sites, called trimalleolar fracture.

FIBULA

INTRODUCTION

i. The fibula is a long, slender and lateral bone of the leg.

ii. Fibula does not transmit body weight.

ANATOMICAL POSITION

i. Head looks upwards.

ii. The malleolar fossa lies below and behind the triangular articular facet on the medial aspect of the lower end.

iii. Fibular (lateral) malleolus directed downwards and laterally.

SIDE DETERMINATION

Fibular (lateral) malleolus will determine the side of the bone.

GENERAL FEATURES

Parts: It consists of upper and lower ends and the intervening portion is called shaft or body.

Upper End: Its upper end constitutes the head and neck.

Head

   i. It is expanded in all sides.

   ii. Superiorly presents an oval or circular facet.

   iii. From the posterolateral aspect of the head presents a bony process projects upwards called styloid process (Fig. 3.20).

Neck: It is the constricted portion of the junction between the head with the shaft (Fig. 3.20).

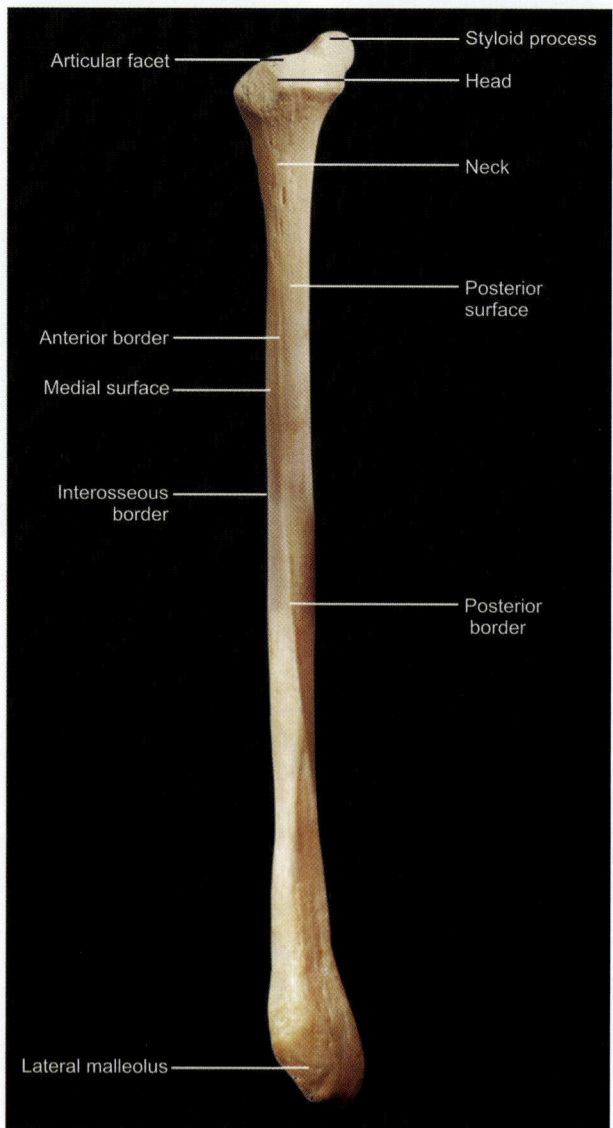

Fig. 3.20: Anterior view of the left fibula showing general features

Shaft

i. **Borders:** Anterior (extensor), interosseous and posterior.
ii. **Surface:** Anterior, posterior and lateral.

Anterior border

Begins from the lower part of the anterior aspect of the head and ends below, where it divides into two limbs to form a triangular area at the lateral aspect of the lower end.

Interosseous border

i. It is medial and parallel to the anterior border.
ii. Opposite the lower one-fourth this border divides to form a rough triangular area lies just above the medial surface of the lower end.

Posterior border

i. It is thick, rounded and less prominent.
ii. It begins from the lower part of the posterior aspect of the head and ends at the medial margin of the groove on the back of the lateral malleolus.

Anterior/medial/extensor surface

i. Between the anterior and interosseous borders.
ii. It is narrower above than below.
iii. Its upper one-third is represented by a ridge.

Posterior/flexor surface

i. Between the interosseous and posterior borders.
ii. A vertical medial crest subdivides the surface into two areas.
iii. Medial crest present only on the middle one-third.

Lateral/peroneal surface: It is subcutaneous, lies between the anterior and posterior borders (Fig. 3.21).

Lower End

i. The lower end of the fibula projects downwards below the level of the lower end of the tibia known as lateral malleolus.
ii. **Surfaces:** Lateral, medial and posterior.
iii. **Borders:** Anterior, posterior and inferior.

Lateral surface: It is smooth, nonarticular, convex and subcutaneous.

Medial surface

i. Presents a triangular articular surface in front.
ii. Below and behind the triangular articular facet a deep nonarticular fossa called malleolar fossa (Fig. 3.21).

Posterior surface: It presents a vertical groove.

Anterior border: It is rounded.

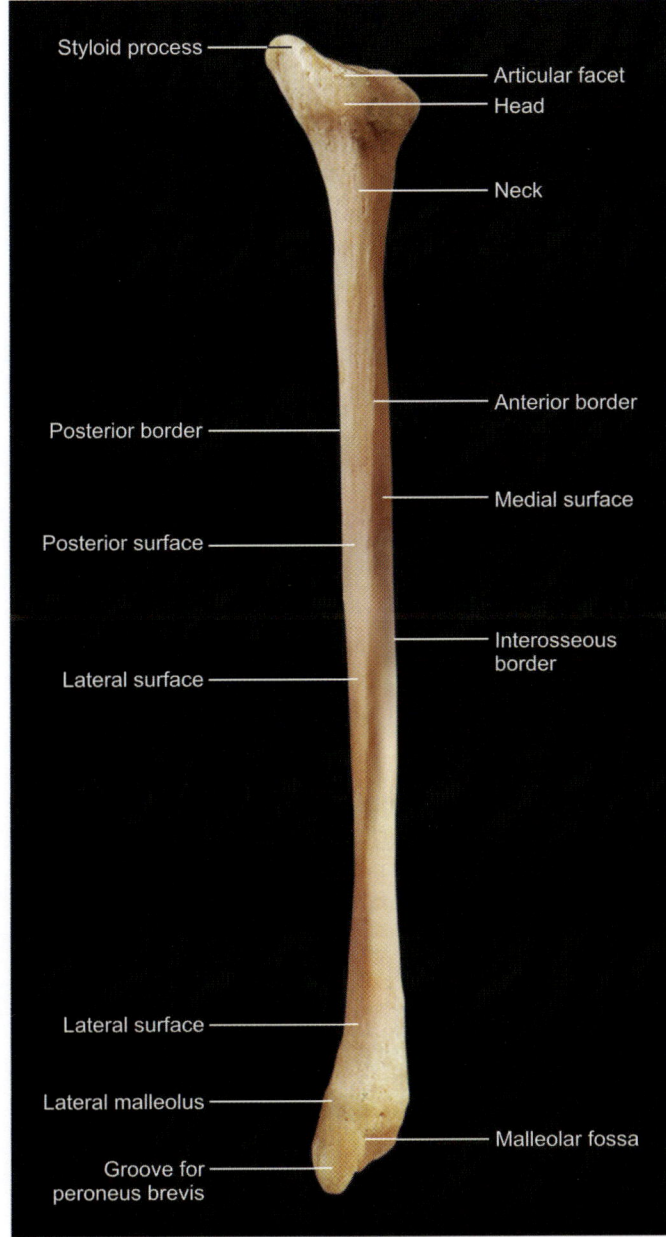

Fig. 3.21: Posterior view of the left fibula showing general features

i. **Posterior border:** It is less distinct and forms medial margin of the posterior surface.
ii. **Inferior border:** It continuous with the anterior margin and presents a notch in its middle part.

ATTACHMENTS OF FIBULA

Head

Origin of

i. **Extensor digitorum longus:** From anteriorly.
ii. **Soleus:** From posteriorly.
iii. **Peroneus longus:** From laterally.

Insertion of

Biceps femoris (anterior fibers): To laterally.

Ligaments

   i. **Fibular collateral ligament:** Laterally.
   ii. **Capsular ligament of superior tibiofibular joint:** Margins of the articular facet.

Neck

Relations

   i. **Laterally:** Common peroneal nerve,
   ii. **Medially:** Anterior tibial vessels.

Shaft

Anterior border

   i. **Intermuscular septum:** Between the extensor and peroneal muscles in upper three-fourths.
   ii. **Superior extensor retinaculum:** At the anterior limb of the lower triangular area.
   iii. **Superior peroneal retinaculum:** At the posterior limb of the lower triangular area.

Interosseous border

   i. **Anterior and posterior tibiofibular ligaments:** To the anterior and posterior limbs of the rough triangular area respectively.
   ii. **Interosseous tibiofibular ligament:** To the rough triangular area.
   iii. **Interosseous membrane:** From below the head to the apex of the rough triangular area.

Posterior border: Posterior intermuscular septum.

Anterior/medial/extensor surface

Origin of (Fig. 3.22)

   i. **Extensor digitorum longus:** From upper three-fourths.
   ii. **Extensor hallucis longus:** From middle two-fourths medial to the extensor digitorum longus.
   iii. **Peroneus tertius:** From the lower one-fourth.

Posterior/flexor surface

Origin of (Fig. 3.23)

   i. **Tibialis posterior:** From anterior to the medial crest.
   ii. **Soleus:** From behind the medial crest in its upper one-fourth.
   iii. **Flexor hallucis longus:** From behind the medial crest in its rest three-fourths.

Others

Deep intermuscular septum: To the medial crest.

Relations: Peroneal vessels related with medial crest.

Lateral/peroneal surface

Origin of

   i. **Peroneus longus:** From upper two-thirds.
   ii. **Peroneus brevis:** From the middle one-third.

Relations: Lower one-third related with the tendons of:

   i. Peroneus longus
   ii. Peroneus brevis

Lower End

Medial surface

Articulation: Triangular articular facet articulates with the lateral surface of the body of the talus.

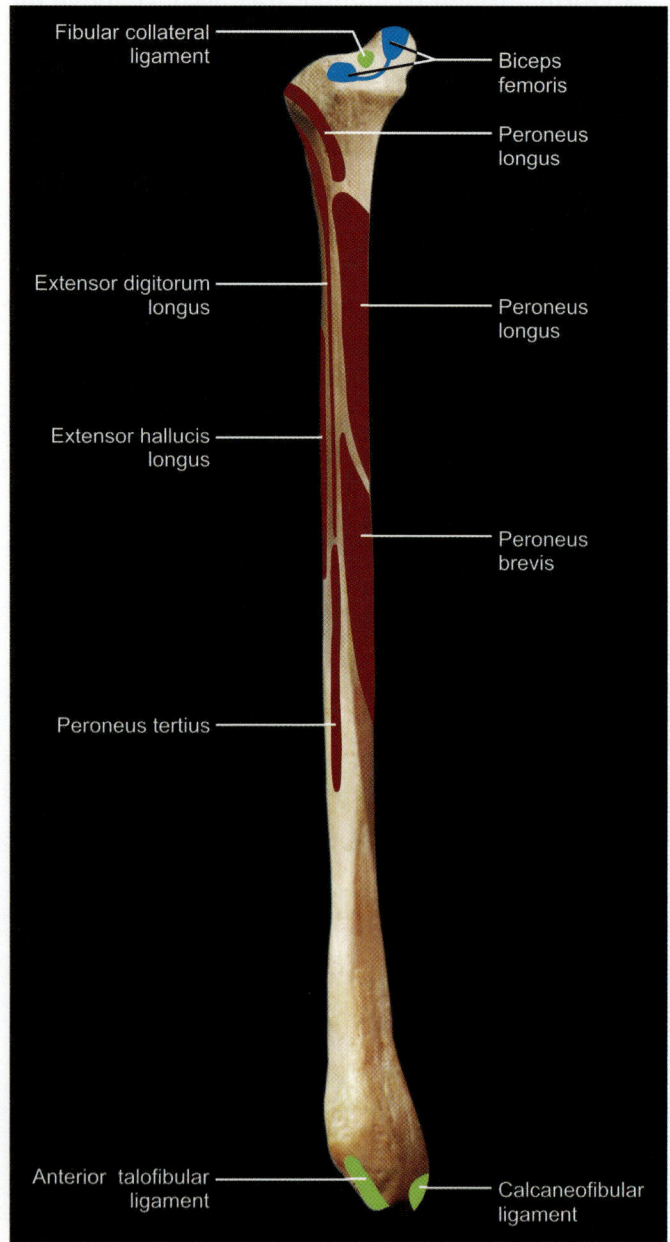

Fig. 3.22: Anterior view of the left fibula showing attachments

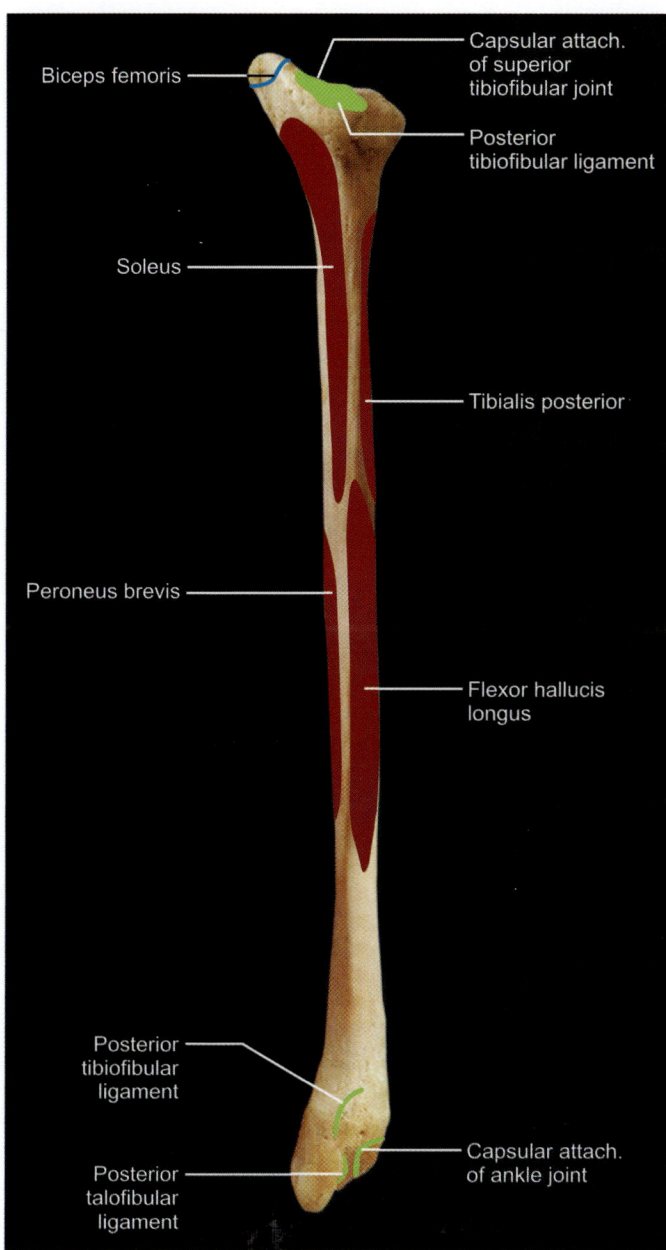

Fig. 3.23: Posterior view of the left fibula showing attachments

Labels on figure:
- Biceps femoris
- Capsular attach. of superior tibiofibular joint
- Posterior tibiofibular ligament
- Soleus
- Tibialis posterior
- Peroneus brevis
- Flexor hallucis longus
- Posterior tibiofibular ligament
- Posterior talofibular ligament
- Capsular attach. of ankle joint

Ligaments (Fig. 3.23)

  i. Posterior tibiofibular ligament: In the upper part of the malleolar fossa.

  ii. Posterior talofibular ligament: In the lower part of the malleolar fossa.

Posterior surface: Superior peroneal retinaculum.

Anterior border: Anterior talofibular ligament.

Posterior border: Posterior talofibular ligament.

Inferior border: Calcaneofibular ligament in the notch of the inferior border.

OSSIFICATION

  i. **Primary center:** One primary center for the shaft appears eighth week of the intrauterine life.

  ii. **Secondary centers:** For the lower end appears between one to two years.

  iii. Secondary center for the upper end appears between three to four years.

  iv. The lower epiphysis unites with the shaft between fifteen to seventeen years (in fibula law of union of epiphysis is violated because the epiphysis, which begins to ossify, first unites with the diaphysis last).

  v. The upper epiphysis unites with the shaft between seventeen and nineteen years.

  The aboves help in age determination.

CLINICAL ANATOMY

  i. **Bone grafting:** Fibula is a common bone for grafting, because it does not transmit body weight. Therefore, fibula is an ideal bone for bone grafting. The bone graft is taken from the site of nutrient foramen so that the graft will have its own artery in the new location.

  ii. If part of the fibula is removed a person can walk, run, and jump normally.

  iii. **Injury of the common peroneal nerve:** At the lateral aspect neck of the fibula, the common peroneal nerve winds round the fibular neck superficially. So fracture or injury of the neck of the fibula may injure the common peroneal nerve.

SKELETON OF THE FOOT

It consists of tarsal, metatarsal, and phalanges. The tarsal bones are seven in number:

  a. Calcaneus

  b. Talus

  c. Navicular

  d. Three cuneiform (medial, intermediate and lateral)

  e. Cuboid

    i. Among the tarsal bones, three cuneiform bones are wedge-shaped and form an important part of the transverse arch of the foot.

    ii. The talus forms the key bone (arch of foot) among the tarsus.

    iii. Superiorly, talus articulates with the bones of the leg and anteriorly with the navicular bone.

    iv. Navicular bone articulates in front with the cuneiform bone.

    v. Calcaneus articulates in front with cuboid bone.

    vi. The cuneiform bones and the cuboid articulated in front with metatarsal bones.

vii. All these bones are so arranged that two arches are formed:
   a. Longitudinal
   b. Transverse

viii. Talus is placed at the summit of the arch and transmits body weight.

ix. Tarsal bones are arranged in three rows but arrangement is not regular.

x. Here calcaneus and talus form the bones of proximal row and the cuneiform bones form the distal row.

xi. The navicular bone is interposed between the talus and cuneiform bones, cuboid is placed laterally in front of calcaneus (Fig. 3.24).

INTRODUCTION

i. These are short bones, seven in number.

ii. The bones are the talus, calcaneus, navicular, the medial, intermediate and lateral cuneiform and the cuboid

iii. All these bones are arranged in three rows.
   a. Proximal row—talus and calcaneus
   b. Middle row—navicular
   c. Distal row—cuneiform (medial, intermediate and lateral) and cuboid.

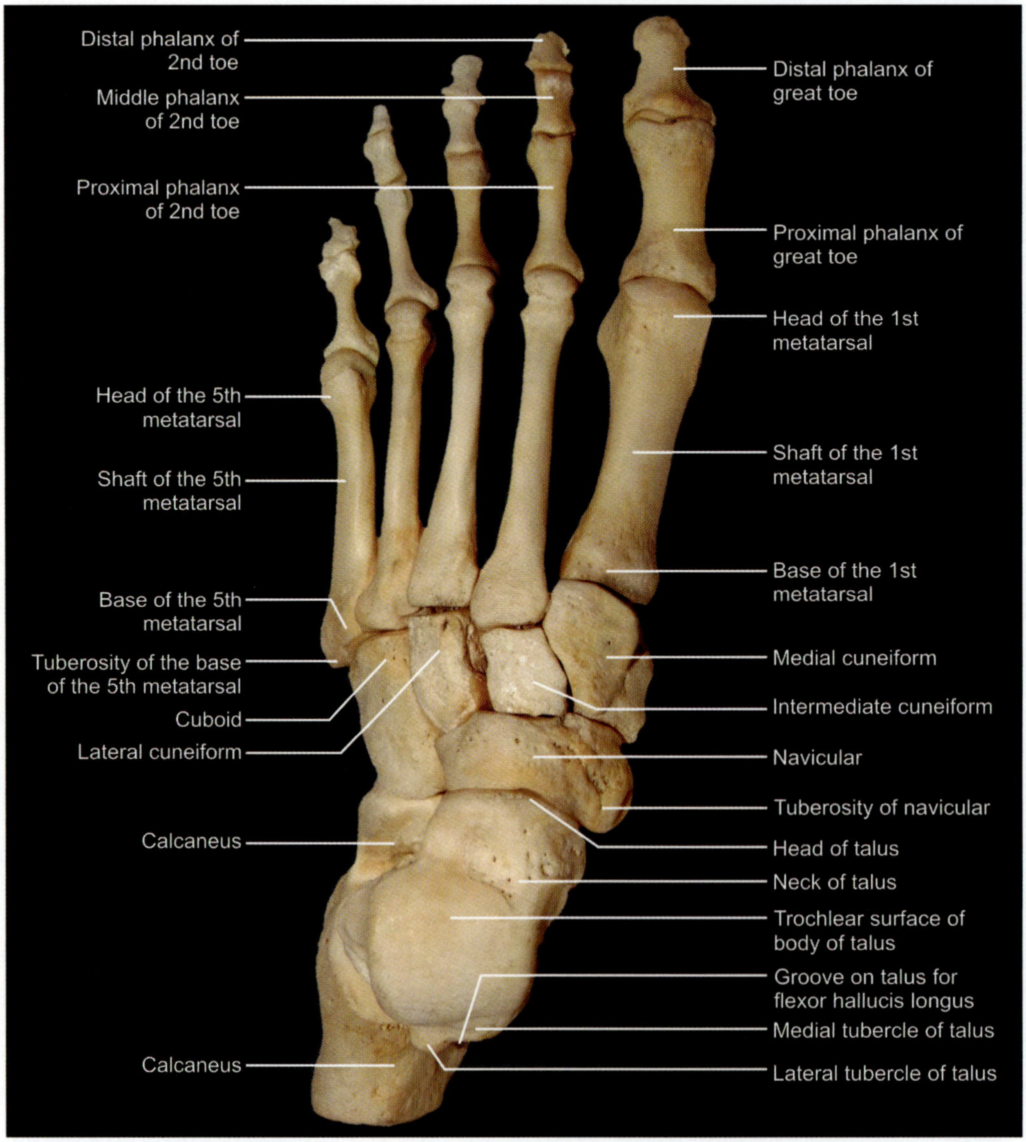

Fig. 3.24: Skeleton of the left foot (dorsal view)

TALUS

INTRODUCTION

i. It is the principal bone connecting between the foot and the bones of the leg
ii. It takes an important role in formation of the talocrural/ankle joint
iii. It has no muscular attachments

ANATOMICAL POSITION

i. Its rounded head looks forwards, downwards and slightly medially
ii. Superior convex surface of the body looks upwards
iii. The triangular facet on the lateral surface of the body
iv. Comma-shaped facet on the medial surface

SIDE DETERMINATION

After holding the bone in anatomical position the triangular facet on the lateral surface of the body, will determine the side of the bone.

GENERAL FEATURES WITH ATTACHMENTS

Head

i. It is the anterior rounded part of the bone
ii. Its anterior or distal surface has an oval, convex articular surface which articulates with the proximal or posterior surface of the navicular bone.
iii. Its plantar or inferior surface is marked by three articular impressions:
    a. The most posterior one is largest, and oval articulates with the similar facet on the upper surface of sustentaculum tali of calcaneus.
    b. Infront and lateral to the posterior impression there is another facet which articulates with the similar facet on the superior surface of the calcaneus.
    c. Medial to the calcaneal facets a rounded impression, contact with the spring ligament or the plantar calcaneonavicular ligament.

Neck

It is the short, constricted part, connects the head with the body.

Surfaces

i. **Upper surface:** It is rough for ligamentous attachments.
ii. **Inferior or plantar surface:** Presence of a groove, the "sulcus tali".

Attachments

Dorsal aspect of the neck: From before backwards—
    a. The capsular ligament of the talocalcaneonavicular joint
    b. The dorsal talonavicular ligament
    c. The capsular ligament of the ankle joint
Plantar aspect of neck: Interosseous talocalcaneal ligament.
Lateral aspect of the neck: Anterior talofibular ligament.
Body: It is broad, expanded and cuboidal in shape.

Surfaces

Dorsal surface or superior surface (Fig. 3.25)
i. It is also called trochlear articular surface
ii. It is convex from before backwards and concave from side to side

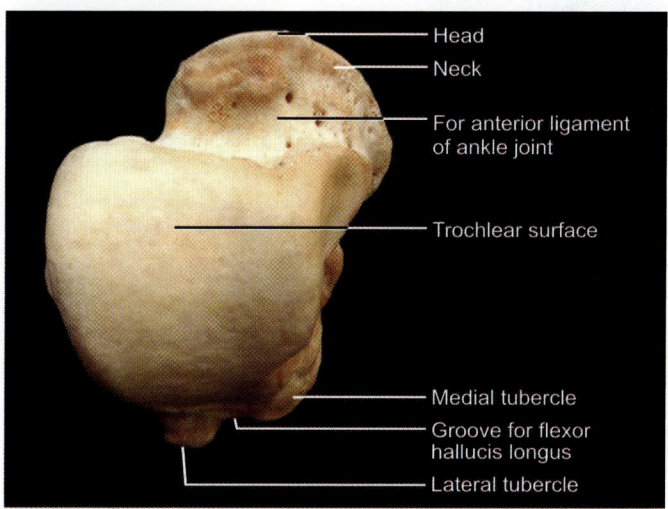

Fig. 3.25: Left talus showing dorsal aspect

Articulation: Articulates with the lower end of the tibia, forming talocrural joint or ankle joint .

Plantar or inferior surface: It is an oval, concave articular surface (Fig. 3.26).

Articulation: It articulates with the intermediate part of the dorsal surface of calcaneus, forming subtalar joint.

Lateral surface (Fig. 3.27)

Articulation: It is fully articulates with the lateral malleolus.

Medial surface (Fig. 3.28)

It has articular and nonarticular parts:
    a. Upper part comma-shaped articular surface— articulates with the medial malleolus.
    b. Lower part—rough, depressed and non-articular.

Attachment: It gives attachment to deep part of the deltoid ligament.

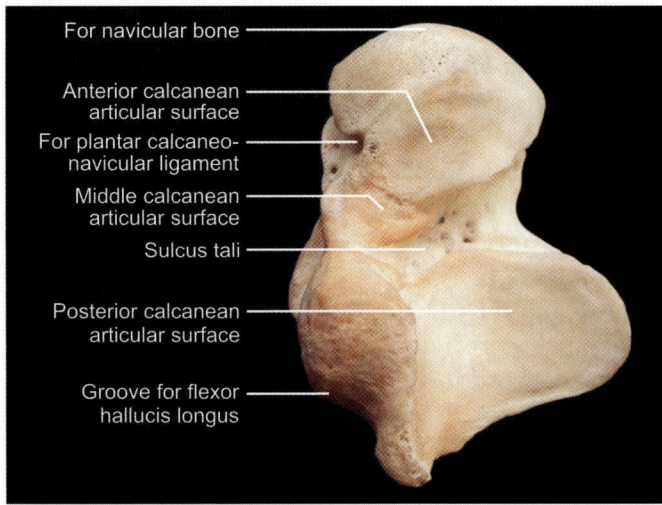

Fig. 3.26: Left talus showing plantar aspect

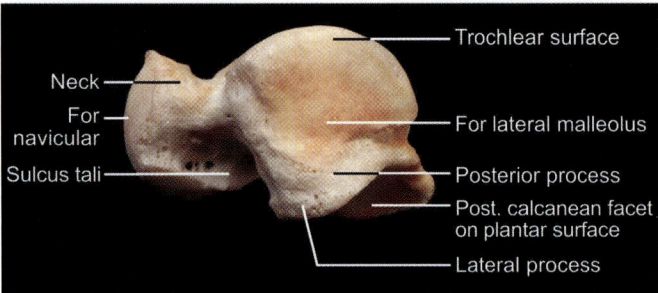

Fig. 3.27: Left talus showing lateral aspect

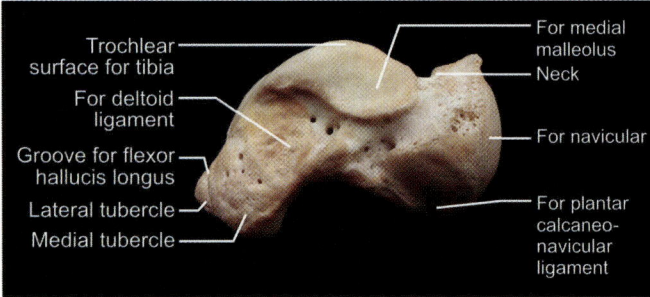

Fig. 3.28: Left talus showing medial aspect

Posterior surface: It is rough marked by a shallow groove, bounded by medial and lateral tubercles.

Lodges: This groove lodges the tendon of flexor hallucis longus.

Medial tubercle: Lies on the medial side of the groove of posterior surface.

Medial tubercle

i. **Dorsal aspect:** Superficial fibers of the deltoid ligament
ii. **Lower margin:** Medial talocalcaneal ligament

Lateral tubercle or process—lies on the lateral side.
Attachments: For lateral talocalcaneal ligament.

Posterior process/tubercle

Attachment: It gives attachment to the posterior talocalcaneal ligament.

Movements of talus: Above the talus, the movements are dorsiflexion and plantar flexion at the ankle joint.

Below, it takes part in the movement of eversion and inversion of foot.

OSSIFICATION

i. This appears during six to eight months in intrauterine life
ii. Then it fuses quickly.

CLINICAL ANATOMY

i. **Fracture of neck of the talus:** It occurs during sever dorsiflexion of ankle.
ii. **Dislocation of talus:** Dislocation of talus is rare but if it occurs it is usually posteriorly.
iii. **Os trigonum:** Sometimes during ossification the lateral tubercle of the talus fails to unite with the body of the talus, in radiological view it may confused with fracture of talus. But os trigonum is differentiated with fracture that it is bilateral.

CALCANEUS/CALCANEUM

INTRODUCTION

i. It is the largest and strongest of all the tarsal bones
ii. It transmits the weight of body to the ground
iii. It provides the leverage for the action of calf muscles attached to the posterior surface
v. Anterosuperiorly, there is a shelf like projection, called sustentaculum tali

ANATOMICAL POSITION

i. Anterior surface bears a triangular facet looks forwards and upwards
ii. The posterior surface is large and rough
iii. Laterally, the superior surface bears a facet in its intermediate area looks upwards

SIDE DETERMINATION

After holding the bone in anatomical position the sustentaculum tali will determine the opposite side of the bone.

GENERAL FEATURES WITH ATTACHMENTS

Surfaces

Anterior surface: It is small, bears an oblique facet.

Articulation: To the cuboid bone forming calcaneo-cuboid joint.

Attachment: Its margin gives attachment to the capsular ligament of calcaneocuboid joint.

Posterior surface: It is divided into upper, middle and lower areas (Fig. 3.29).

Attachments

i. **The rough impression on the middle area:** Insertion of the tendocalcaneus
ii. **The medial margin of the middle area:** Insertion of plantaris muscle
iii. **The upper area:** Covered by bursa
iv. **The lower area:** Attachment to some fibrofatty tissue.

Medial surface

i. It is overhang above by the sustentaculum tali.
ii. **Sustentaculum tali:** It is a shelf-like bony projection passes medial-wards and forwards form anteromedial part and overhang the anterior part of the medial surface (Fig. 3.30).

Attachments

i. **Two facets on the upper surface:** To articulate with the head of the talus.
ii. **Lower surface is grooved for:** The tendon of the flexor hallucis longus
The medial surface of the sustentaculum tali provides attachments to:

a. Anteriorly, the spring ligament
b. Some fibers of deltoid ligament
c. Medial talocalcaneal ligament posteriorly
d. A slip of insertion of the tibialis posterior

Plantar or inferior surface: It is rough, and irregular, bounded posteriorly by the calcaneal tuberosity which is divisible into lateral and medial processes (tubercles) and anteriorly, by the anterior tubercle.

Attachments

i. **The medial tubercle:** Origin of abductor hallucis
ii. **At the medial margin:** Flexor retinaculum
iii. **At the anterior margin:** Origin of flexor digitorum brevis
iv. **Behind:** Plantar aponeurosis
v. **The anteromedial aspect of the lateral process:** Origin of abductor digiti minimi
vi. **The anterior tubercle:** Attachment to short plantar ligament
vii. **Between anterior and posterior process/tubercle:** Attachment to long plantar ligament
viii. **The area in front of the lateral process:** Origin of lateral head of the flexor digitorum accessorius (Fig. 3.31).

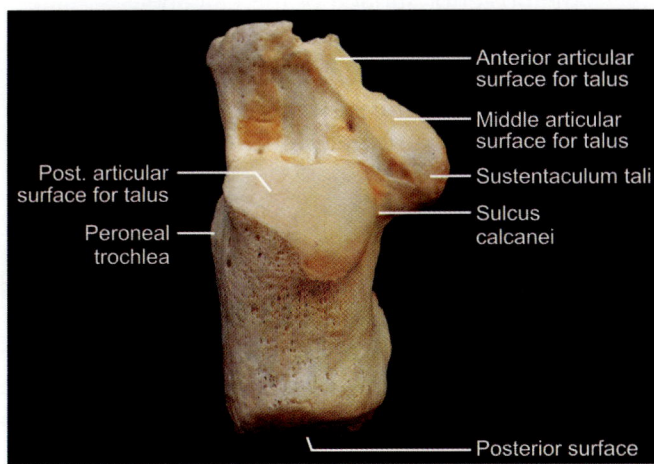

Fig. 3.29: Left calcaneus showing dorsal aspect

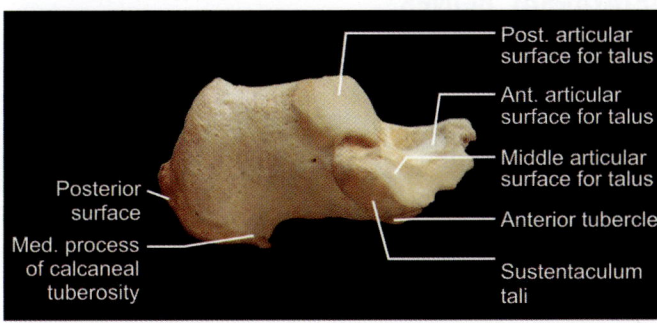

Fig. 3.30: Left calcaneus showing medial aspect

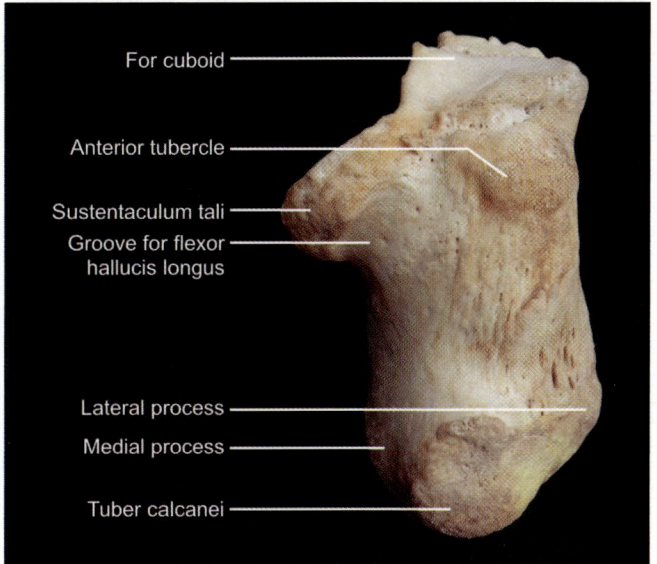

Fig. 3.31: Left calcaneus showing plantar aspect

Lateral surface

   i. It is flat, marked by two tubercles, called peroneal trochlea (tubercle) anterior and posterior.

   ii. It can be palpable at about 2 cm below the tip of the lateral malleolus.

Attachments

   i. The anterior tubercle or peroneal trochlea: The inferior peroneal retinaculum

   ii. The posterior tubercle: Calcaneofibular ligament.

Dorsal or superior surface: It is also divided into anterior, posterior and intermediate areas.

Posterior area: It is rough, convex and nonarticular.

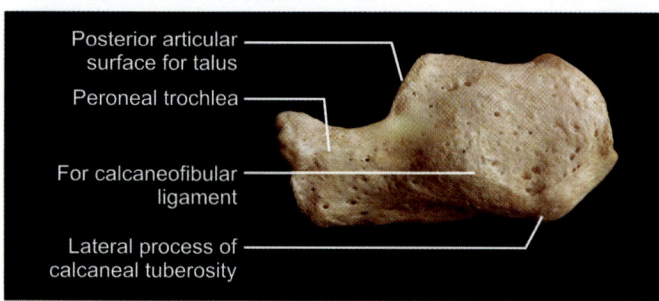

Posterior articular surface for talus

Peroneal trochlea

For calcaneofibular ligament

Lateral process of calcaneal tuberosity

Fig. 3.32: Left calcaneus showing lateral aspect

Attachments

   i. It is covered by fibrofatty tissue,

   ii. It gives attachment to the dorsal talocalcaneal ligament.

Intermediate area: It occupied by an oval facet, posterior facet for the talus.

Anterior area: It bears a groove, the sulcus calcanei.

Attachments: The anterior part of the dorsal surface, attachment to:

   i. Interosseus talocalcaneal ligament, in front of the groove: Attachment to the:

     a. Anterior talocalcaneal ligament

     b. Inferior extensor retinaculum

     c. Stem of the bifurcated ligament

     d. Dorsal calcaneocuboid ligament

     e. Some fibers of the extensor digitorum brevis (origin) on its dorsal portion.

OSSIFICATION

   i. This appears during five to six months in intrauterine life.

   ii. Then it fuses quickly.

CLINICAL ANATOMY

   i. Fracture of the calcaneus: It occur when fall from a ladder on the heal or landing on the heel from high place

   ii. Calcaneal tendinitis: It is caused by the microscopic tears of collagen fibers in the tendocalcaneus results pain during walking especially when wearing rigid soled shoes.

   iii. Ruptured tendocalcaneus

     a. The rupture occurs in the narrowest part about 5 cm above its insertion

     b. It causes sudden pain in calf with a audible snap

     c. Cause of rupture is due to sudden dorsiflexion of a plantar foot, frequently occurs among tennis players

     d. *Features:* A gap is palpable on the tendon in incompletely ruptured tendon, and a lump appears in the calf due to shortening of the calf muscles,

     e. In a complete rupture case, patient can not easily plantar flex the foot but dorsiflexed the foot.

   iv. Calcaneal bursitis

     a. It is also called retroAchilles bursitis situated between the tendocalcaneus and upper part of the posterior surface of the calcaneus

     b. It is commonly seen among the long distance runner, basketball players, etc.

   v. Inflammation of the superficial calcaneal bursa: It is caused by the repeated microtrauma produced by the back of a shoe.

METATARSAL BONES

INTRODUCTION

The metatarsal bones are five in number and they are named by number from medial to lateral,. Each metatarsal bone is a miniature long bone.

COMMON CHARACTERISTICS OF THE METATARSAL BONES

   i. Body is prismatic in shape and gradually narrows from base to head.

   ii. Body is convex dorsally and concave ventrally.

   iii. Base is (directed backwards) much larger than the head

   iv. Head presents a tubercle and a depression on either side for the attachments of collateral ligaments of the metatarsophalangeal joints.

PHALANGES

The phalanges of the each side are fourteen, two for the great toe and three for each of the other toes.

Phalanges of the foot: The phalanges of the toes are divided into three groups namely:

   i. Phalanges of proximal row

  ii. Phalanges of middle row

 iii. Phalanges of distal row.

Characteristic Features of the Phalanges

Proximal Row

   i. The body is cylindrical, it is convex dorsally but concave on its plantar aspects.

  ii. The base presents a single concave facet for articulation with the head of the corresponding metatarsal bone.

 iii. The head presents a pulley-shaped facet articulates with proximal surface of middle row of phalanx.

Middle Row

They are of same shape as those of proximal row, the difference being that they are:

   i. Smaller in size.

  ii. The base presents two facets.

Distal Row

   i. They are much smaller.

  ii. Base is broad with two facets.

 iii. Distal end is nonarticular.

 iv. Presents a rough tuberosity on its plantar aspect.

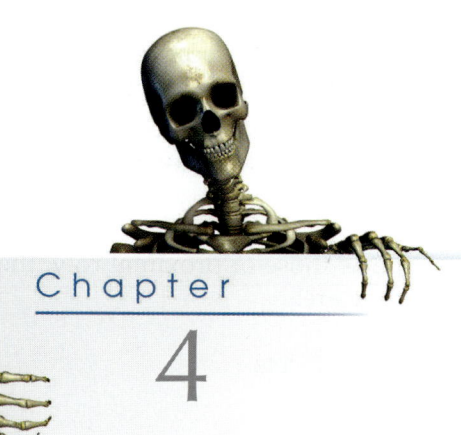

Ribs and Sternum

RIBS

INTRODUCTION

Ribs are elongated, arch, flat bones and form the major part of the thoracic cage.

NUMBER

Twelve pairs (they are numbered from above downwards).

CLASSIFICATION OF RIBS

i. **True ribs (vertebrosternal):** The first seven pairs. They articulate anteriorly with the sternum and posteriorly with the upper seven thoracic vertebrae.

ii. **False ribs:** The last (lower) five pairs. False ribs are further subdivided into:

  a. **Vertebrochondral:** The eighth, ninth and tenth pairs, they articulate anteriorly with the costal cartilages of the above and posteriorly with the vertebral column.

  b. **Vertebral (floating ribs):** The eleventh and the twelfth pairs, they articulate posteriorly with the vertebral column but anteriorly they are free.

iii. **Longest rib:** Seventh rib.

iv. **Maximum oblique rib:** Ninth rib.

v. **The maximum diameter of the thorax:** At the level of eighth rib.

vi. **Typical ribs:** Third to ninth ribs are typical ribs.

vii. **Atypical ribs:** First, second, tenth, eleventh and twelfth ribs.

TYPICAL RIBS

Each typical rib consists of:

  i. Anterior or sternal end

  ii. Posterior or vertebral end

  iii. Body or shaft.

ANTERIOR END

  i. It is lower than the vertebral end.

  ii. Presents a cup shaped depression, which articulates with its own costal cartilage.

POSTERIOR END

It consists of: Head, neck and tubercle (Fig. 4.1).

Head

Features (Fig. 4.1)

  i. It has upper and lower facets separated by a crest

  ii. Lower facet articulates with the numerically corresponding thoracic vertebra.

  iii. The upper facet articulates with vertebra above.

  iv. Crest corresponds with the intervertebral disk.

Attachments

  i. **Capsular ligament of the costovertebral joint:** Along the peripheral margins of the head.

  ii. **Radiate ligament:** To the anterior margin of the head (also adjoining anterior surface of the neck).

  iii. **Intra-articular ligament:** To the crest of the head.

Relations

The anterior surface of the head of the lower ribs related to the sympathetic trunk.

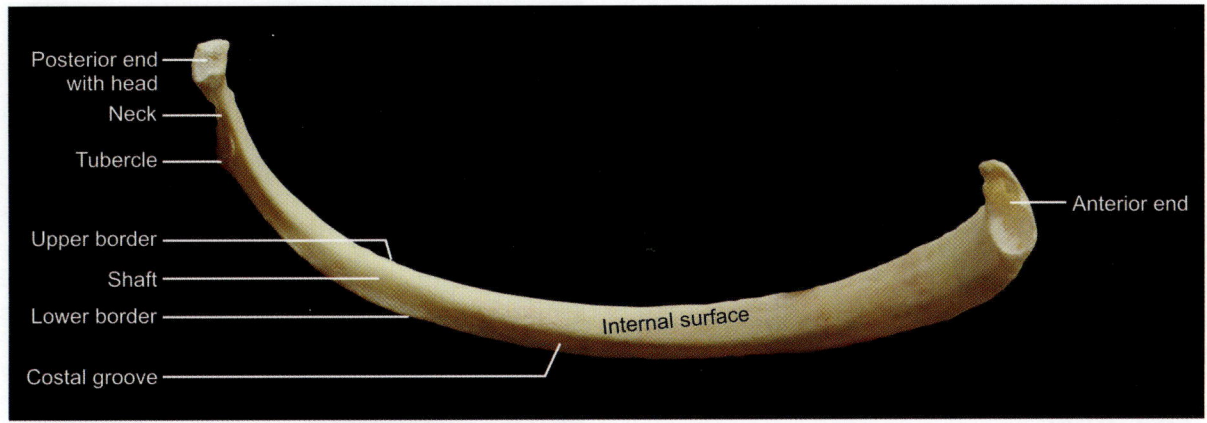

Fig. 4.1: General features of Typical rib (right side)

Neck

Features

i. It is flattened from before backwards.

ii. It is just succeeds the head.

iii. Its length about 2.5 cm.

iv. It lies opposite the corresponding transverse process of the thoracic vertebra.

v. *Surfaces:* Anterior and posterior.

vi. *Borders:* Superior and inferior.

vii. The upper border of the neck is called crest

viii. Tubercle of the rib situated on the lateral part of the posterior surface (demarcation between neck and shaft).

ix. The tubercle of the neck presents medial articular part and lateral nonarticular part.

x. The medial articular part having facet articulates with the transverse process of the numerically corresponding vertebra.

Attachments

i. **Superior costotransverse ligament:** To the crest of the neck.

ii. **Inferior costotransverse ligament:** To the posterior surface.

iii. **Internal intercostal membrane:** To the inferior border and ridge on the anterior surface.

iv. **Lateral costotransverse ligament:** To the non-articular part of the tubercle.

v. **Costal pleura:** To the anterior surface.

SHAFT OR BODY

i. It is flat.

ii. **Surfaces:**

a. Outer or external: It is convex

b. Inner or internal: It is concave

iii. **Borders**

a. Upper

b. Lower.

iv. It is bent and twisted.

v. At the bent and twisting on the outer surface presents an angle, marked by an oblique ridge which is about 5 cm from the tubercle, known as angle of the rib.

vi. Close to the anterior end of the outer surface marked by a faint ridge known as anterior angle.

vii Presents the costal groove close to the lower border of the inner surface.

viii. Costal groove become deficient beyond the junction between the anterior and middle third of the rib.

ix. Lower border is sharp.

x. Upper border divided into outer and inner lips.

Attachments

i. **Origin of**

a. **External obliquus abdominis:** Anterior to the anterior angle of the lower eight ribs.

b. **Serratus anterior:** Posterior to the anterior angle of the third to eight ribs.

c. **Latissimus dorsi:** Posterior to the anterior angle of the ninth and tenth ribs.

d. **Intercostalis intimus:** To the upper margin of the costal groove.

e. **Intercostalis internus:** To the floor of the costal groove.

f. **Intercostalis externus:** To the lower border of the costal groove.

ii. **Insertion of**

a. **Levator costarum:** To the area between the tubercle and the angle.

    b. Intercostalis internus and intercostalis intimus: To the inner lip of the upper border.

    c. Intercostalis externus: To the outer lip of the upper border.

  iii. **Thoracolumbar fascia and iliocostocervicalis:** To the ridge at the anterior angle of the shaft.

  iv. **Structure lodges in the costal groove:** From above downwards
    a. Intercostal vein
    b. Intercostal artery
    c. Intercostal nerve

▌ ATYPICAL RIBS

FIRST RIB

Anatomical Position

i. Anterior expanded end looks forwards and downwards.

ii. The head looks downwards, forwards and medially.

iii. The convex border outwardly.

iv. The superior surface having two grooves, directed upwards.

Side Determination

After holding the bone in anatomical position the outer convex border will determine the side to which side the bone belongs.

Special Features

i. It is the most curved and strongest of all ribs.

ii. Consist of outer and inner borders.

iii. Outer border is convex and inner border is concave.

iv. It has superior and inferior surfaces.

v. It is shortest of all the true ribs.

vi. Head is small and only one facet.

vii. Neck is rounded directed upwards, backwards and laterally.

viii. Its angle coincides with the tubercle.

ix. The rib is bent at the point of angle.

x. Superior surface of the body is rough irregular with two grooves (Fig. 4.2).

xi. Inferior surface is smooth and no costal groove (Fig. 4.3).

xii. Presents of a tubercle, on the inner border called scalene tubercle.

Features with Descriptions

i. **Facet on the head, its margin:** Attachment to capsular ligament of the first costovertebral joint.

ii. **Anterior margin of the head:** Attachment to radiate ligament.

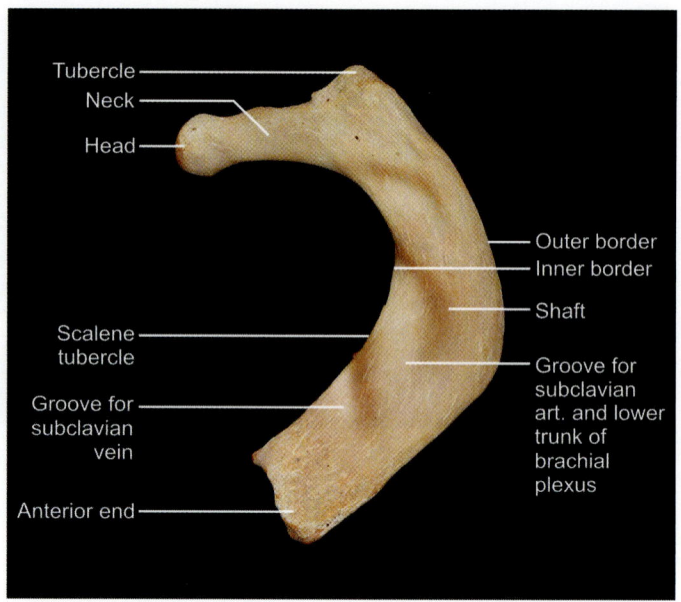

Fig. 4.2: Superior surface of left first rib (general features)

iii. **Posterior margin of the neck:** Attachment to inferior costotransverse ligament.

iv. **Superior margin of the neck:** Attached to superior costotransverse ligament.

v. **Lateral part of the tubercle:** Lateral costotransverse ligament.

vi. **Relations of the anterior aspect of the neck:** Crossed longitudinally from lateral to medial by:
  a. First thoracic nerve.
  b. First posterior intercostal vein.
  c. Superior intercostal artery.
  d. Sympathetic trunk with the first thoracic ganglion.
  e. Sometimes stellate ganglion: It is formed by the first thoracic sympathetic ganglion with the inferior cervical sympathetic ganglion.
  f. Apex of the lung.
  g. Cervical pleura
  h. Suprapleural membrane (Fig. 4.4)

vii. **The anterior groove on the superior surface lodges:** The subclavian vein (Fig. 4.6).

viii. **The posterior groove on the superior surface lodges:** Subclavian artery with lower trunk of the brachial plexus (Fig. 4.6).

ix. **Rough area anterior to anterior groove:**
Laterally origin of: Subclavius muscle.
Medially attachment of: Costoclavicular ligament (Figs 4.4)

x. **Insertion of scalenus anterior:** Scalene tubercle with ridge on the superior surface (Fig. 4.4).

xi. **Insertion of scalenus medius:** Rough area posterior to the posterior groove.

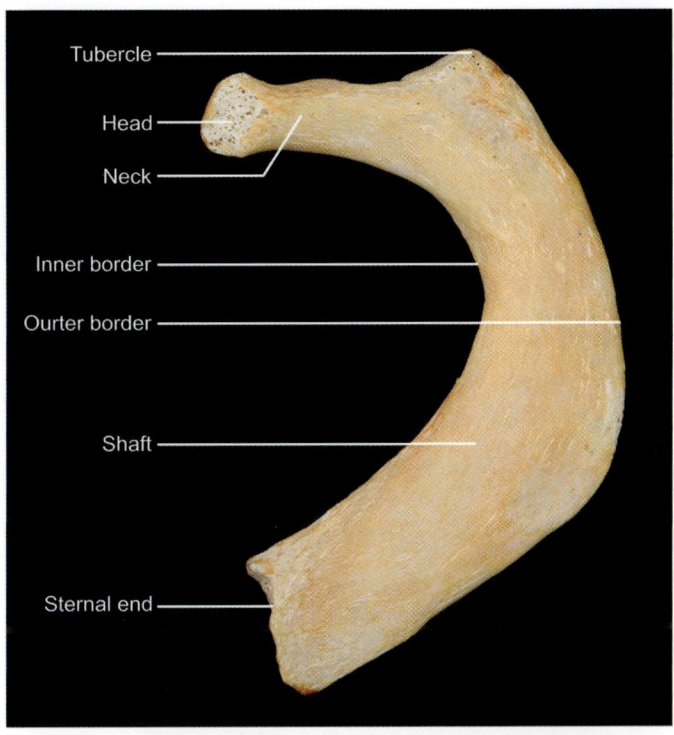

Fig. 4.3: Inferior surface of left first rib (general features)

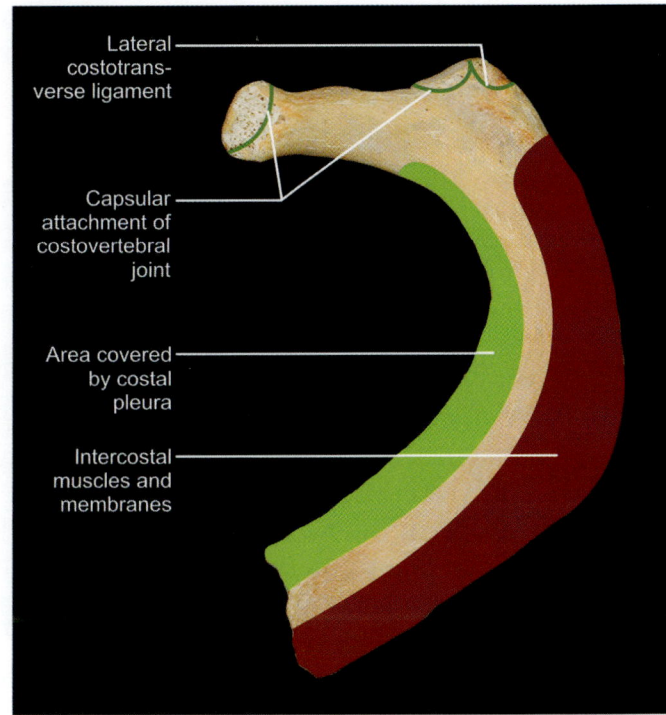

Fig. 4.5: Inferior surface of left first rib (attachments)

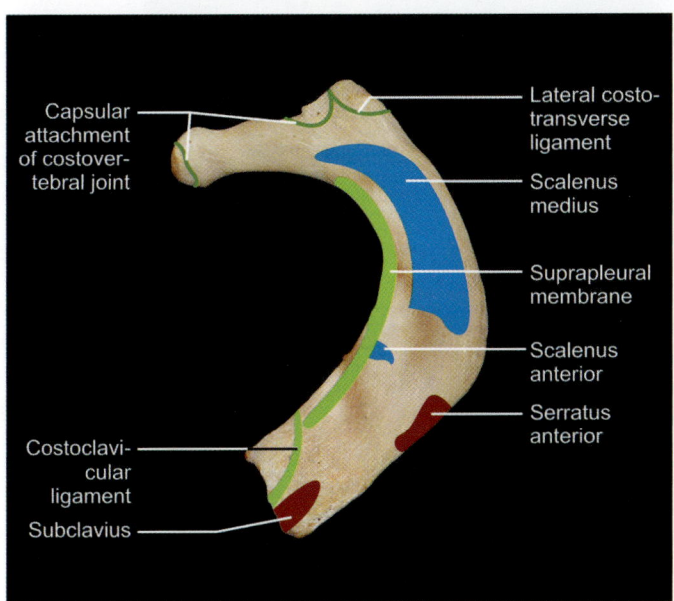

Fig. 4.4: Superior surface of left first rib (attachments)

xii. **Origin of serratus anterior (first digitation):** On the outer border opposite the posterior groove.

xiii. **Whole inner border attachment of:** Suprapleural membrane (Sibson's fascia).

xiv. **Origin of intercostalis externus (outer) and intercostalis internus (inner):** Inferior surface close to outer border.

xv. **Inferior surface:** It is covered by the costal pleura (Fig. 4.5).

SECOND RIB

Features

i. Its curvature is similar to that of first rib

ii. Length is twice the length of first rib

iii. Angle lies close to the tubercle

iv. External surface of the body looks more superiorly than externally

v. The internal surface looks more inferiorly than internally (Fig. 4.7)

vi. There is no twisting

vii. Costal groove is short found only in the posterior part of the internal surface

viii. Head is small with two indistinct facets

ix. When placed on a flat surface the entire rib touches it.

x. On the middle of the external surface presents a muscular impression (Fig. 4.8).

TENTH RIB

Features

i. It presents a single auricular facet on the head.

ii. The other features are similar to a typical rib (Fig. 4.9).

ELEVENTH RIB

Features

i. It presents a single facet on the head.

ii. There is no neck and no tubercle.

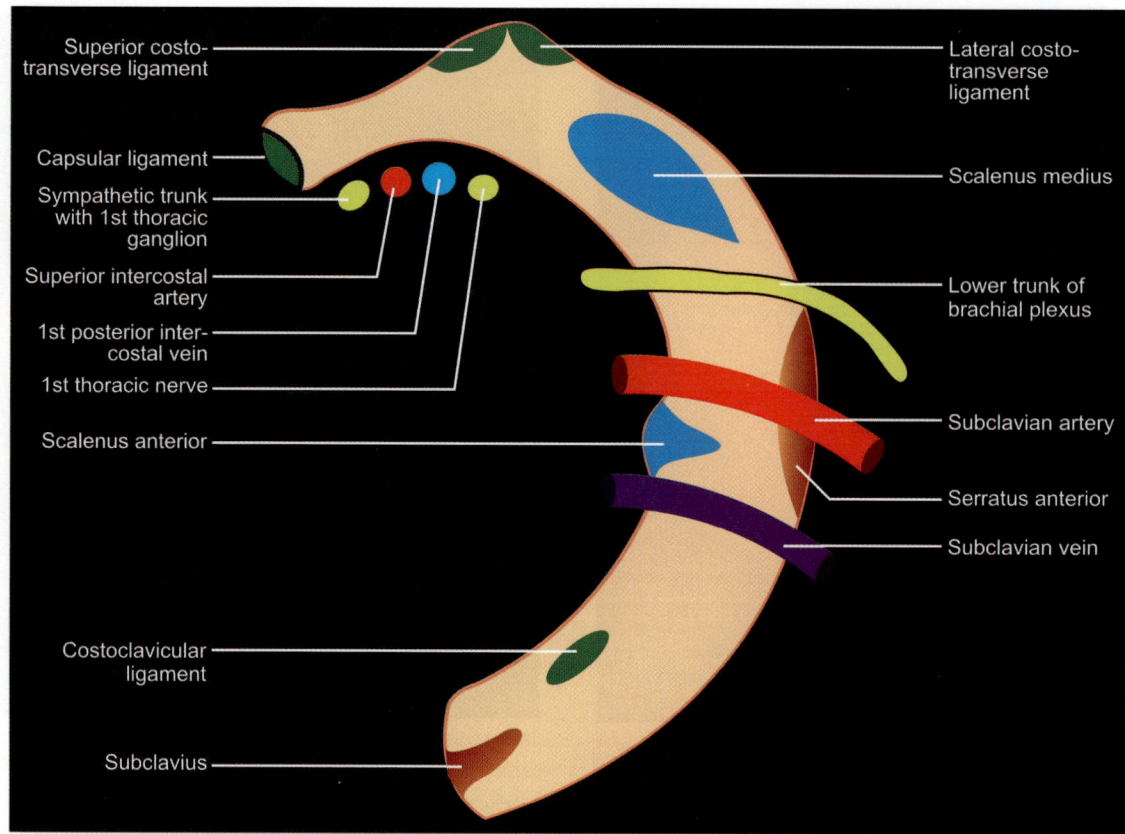

Fig. 4.6: Superior surface of left first rib, showing attachments and relations

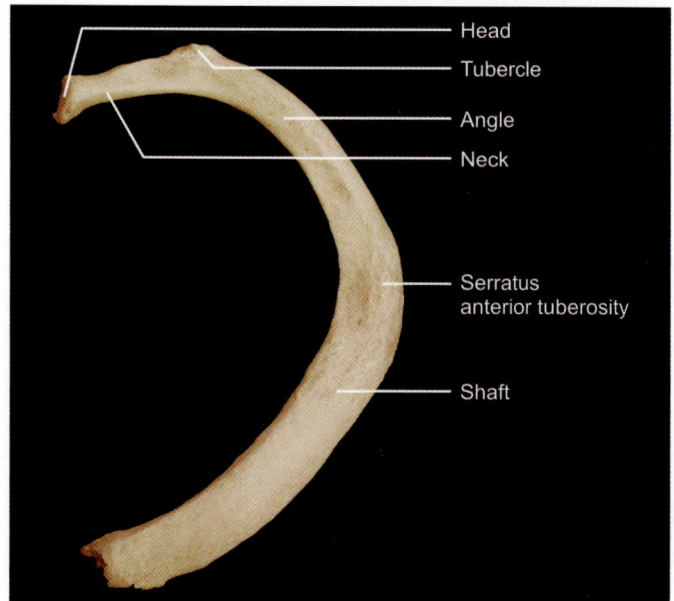

Fig. 4.7: External surface of left second rib (general features)

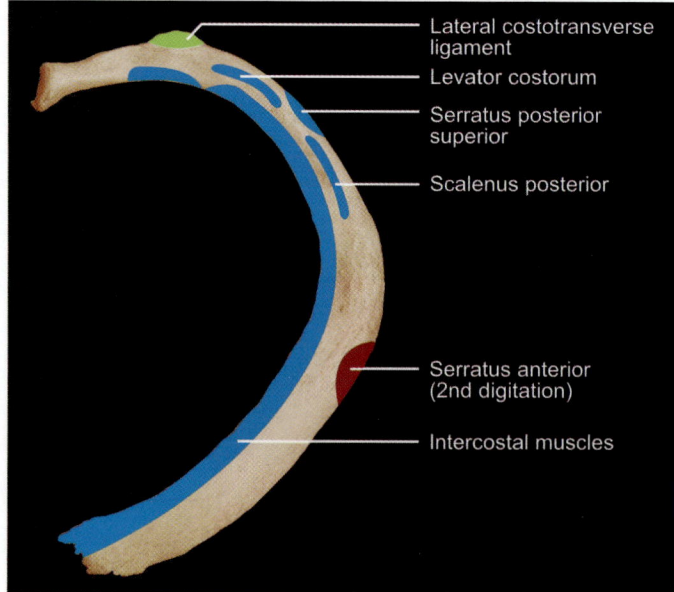

Fig. 4.8: External surface of left second rib (attachments)

iii. Angle is faintly marked on the outer surface.
iv. Faintly marked costal groove on the internal surface.
v. Anterior end is pointed (Fig. 4.10).

TWELFTH RIB

Features

i. Presents a single facet on its head.
ii. Anterior end is pointed.

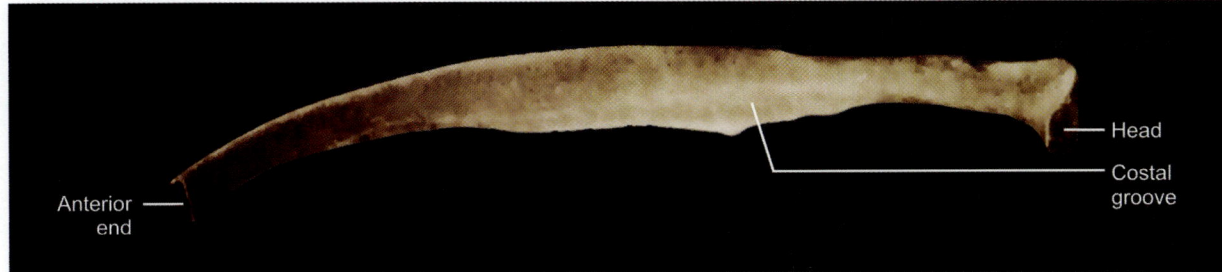

Fig. 4.9: Tenth rib

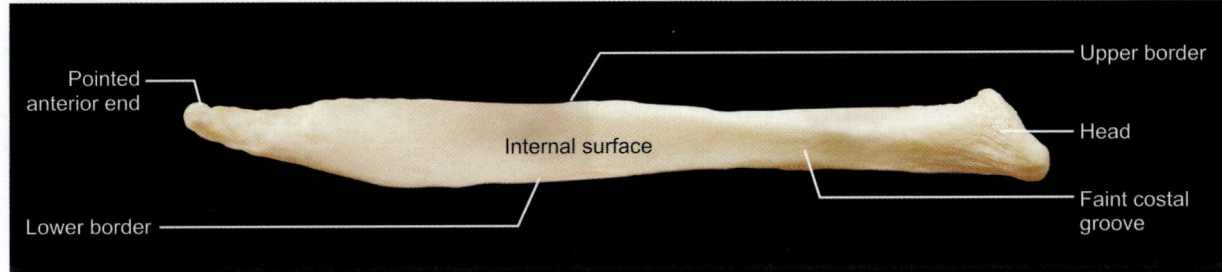

Fig. 4.10: Eleventh rib

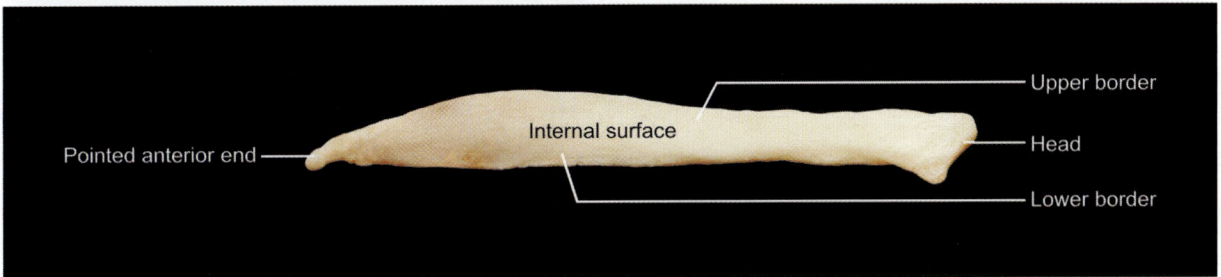

Fig. 4.11: Twelfth rib

iii. It has no neck, no tubercle

iv. It has no angle, no costal groove (Fig. 4.11).

CLINICAL ANATOMY

i. Fracture of ribs
a. Fracture of the middle ribs are most common.
b. The weakest part of the rib just anterior to its angle.
c. The broken end of the fracture rib may injured the lung or spleen.
d. The fracture of the lower ribs may tear the diaphragm results in diaphragmatic hernia.
e. The fracture of the ribs are more painful because of broken parts move with respiration, laughing, coughing and sneezing.

ii. Cervical ribs
a. Cervical ribs are commonly asymptomatic.
b. Clinically cervical ribs very significant as they compress the lower trunk of brachial plexus and cause pain and numbness in the shoulder and upper limb.
c. Cervical ribs may compress the subclavian artery and cause ischemic muscle pain in the upper limb.

iii. **Costovertebral angle:** It presents between the lower border of the 12th rib and the body T12 vertebra. It is occupied by costodiaphragmatic pleural recess.

iv. **Renal angle:** It is formed by the lower border of the 12th rib and the lateral border of erector spine. The renal angle becomes tender on palpation in diseases of kidney.

v. **Notching of the ribs:** This is in X-ray of the ribs where the lower borders of the ribs are eroded produced by tortuosity and dilatations of the posterior intercostal arteries as a result of coractation of aorta or blockage of subclavian or axillary arteries.

vi. **Aspiration of pleural fluid or needle biopsy of liver:** To perform these, the needle is pricked through the lower part of the intercostal space to avoid injury to the neurovascular bundle, which are lodges in the costal groove.

STERNUM

INTRODUCTION

The sternum is an elongated flat bone and is a median bone on the anterior chest wall.

CHARACTERISTICS

i. It is obliquely placed on the anterior chest wall.
ii. Its anterior surface looks upwards and forwards.
iii. It is concave posteriorly.
iv. It is broad, thicker and expanded above and narrow and thinner below.

SEX DIFFERENCES

In males: Body of sternum is more than twice the length of manubrium.

In females: Body of sternum is shorter and less than twice the length of manubrium.

PARTS

i. Manubrium (Fig. 4.12)
ii. Body
iii. Xiphoid process.

Manubrium Sterni

i. It is the upper triangular segment of the sternum.
ii. It is broader and thicker above than below.
iii. Surfaces—anterior and posterior.
iv. Borders—superior, inferior and two lateral borders.

General Features
Anterior surface

i. It is smooth and convex from side to side.
ii. Gently concave from above downwards.

Posterior surface: It is concave.

Superior border

i. It presents a notch on the median plane, called jugular notch (suprasternal notch).
ii. It presents another notches on either side of the jugular notch, called clavicular notch (Fig. 4.12).

Inferior border

i. It is narrow.
ii. It consists of a small oval facet which articulates with the upper end of the body to form a cartilaginous manubriosternal joint.

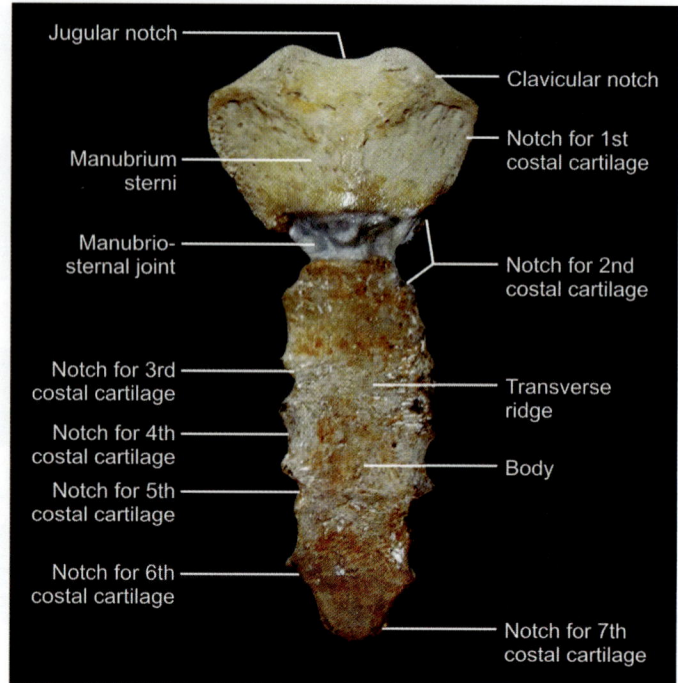

Fig. 4.12: Anterior view of sternum, showing general features

iii. **The sternal angle** (Louis angle): It is formed by the junction of the manubrium sterni and body of the sternum.
    a. It lies opposite the level of the lower border of the fourth thoracic vertebra.
    b. It makes a bony prominence on the anterior chest wall.
    c. It articulates on either side with the second costal cartilages (important for counting the ribs).
    d. Sternal angle in males, it is 163.4° and in females it is 165°.

Lateral borders

i. It presents a cup-shaped depression at its upper part for articulation with the first costal cartilage.
ii. In the lower part close to the sternal angle, presents a small articular facet, which with a similar facet on the upper end of the body of the sternum articulates with the second costal cartilage.

Attachments

To the jugular notch: From before backwards:

i. Anterior investing layer of the deep cervical fascia.
ii. Interclavicular ligament.
iii. Posterior investing layer of the deep cervical fascia. Between the anterior and posterior investing layers of the deep cervical fascia the space is called suprasternal space or space of Burn.

Anterior surface (Fig. 4.13)

i. **Origin of pectoralis major**—on either side of manubrium.

ii. **Origin of sternal head of the sternocleido-mastoid**—close to its upper end on either side of the median plane.

Posterior surface (Fig. 4.14)

i. **Origin of sternohyoid**—from just below the clavicular notch.

ii. **Origin of sternothyroid**—from opposite the level of first costal facet.

To the clavicular notch

i. It articulates with the sternal end of the clavicle to form the sternoclavicular joint.

ii. An articular disk lies in between them.

iii. Capsular ligament—margins of the clavicular notch.

iv. Anterior and posterior sternoclavicular ligaments—to the anterior and posterior margins of the clavicular notch respectively.

Body of the Sternum

i. It is longer and narrower than the manubrium.

ii. On its anterior surface is marked by transverse ridges due to body of sternum having four segmental developments in early embryonic life.

iii. Surfaces—anterior and posterior.

iv. Border—two lateral borders.

v. Ends—upper and lower.

General Features

Anterior surface: It is flat with three transverse ridges.

Posterior surface: It is slightly concave and marked by less distinct transverse ridges.

Lateral borders

i. Marked by four cup-shaped articular depressions for articulation with the third, fourth, fifth and sixth costal cartilages (Fig. 4.12).

ii. The upper part of the lateral border close to the sternal angle presents a small articular facet, which with a similar facet on the lower part of the lateral border of the manubrium articulates with the second costal cartilage.

iii. Seventh costal cartilage articulates with the xiphisternal joint.

iv. Sternopericardial (superior and inferior bands) ligament—to the posterior surface.

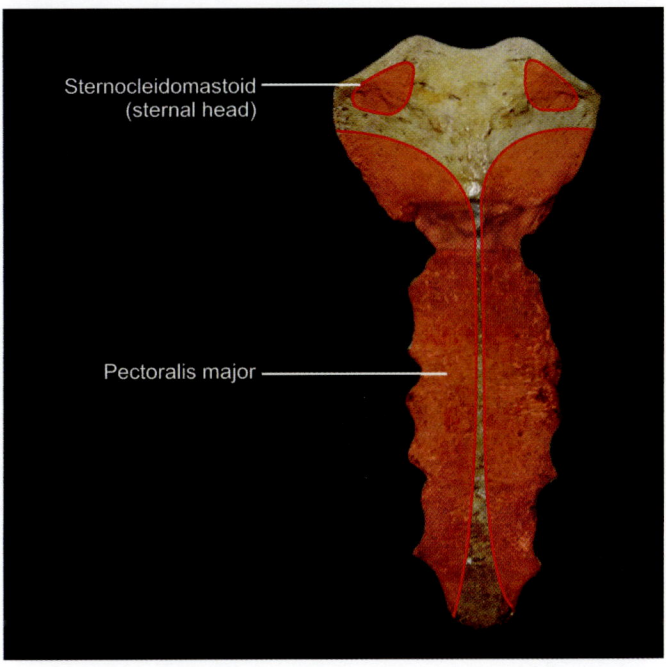

Fig. 4.13: Anterior view of sternum, showing attachments

v. External intercostal membrane—between the costal notches.

Lower end: Articulates with the xiphoid process, which lies opposite the ninth thoracic vertebra.

Upper end: The upper end articulates with the manubrium to form the sternal angle.

Attachments

i. **Origin of pectoralis major**—on either side of the anterior surface (Fig. 4.13).

ii. **Capsular ligament of the sternocostal joints**—on the margins of the costal notches.

iii. **Radiate sternocostal ligament**—anterior and posterior surfaces opposite the costal notches.

iv. **Origin of sternocostalis or transversus thoracis**—on either side of the inferior part of the posterior surface (Fig. 4.14).

Xiphoid Process

General Features

i. It is the smallest and most variable part of the sternum.

ii. It is about half the thickness of the body of the sternum.

iii. It is usually triangular with a pointed caudal end.

iv. It may be curved anteriorly.

v. It may be bifurcated below.

vi. It may be deveated to one or the other side.

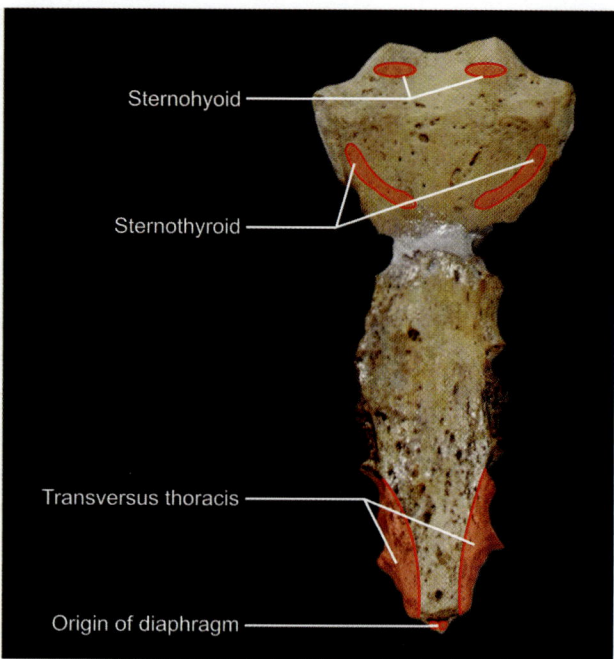

Fig. 4.14: Posterior view of sternum, showing attachments

Attachments

i. Its upper end unites with body to form the xiphisternal joint.
ii. Seventh costal cartilage articulates with the xiphisternal joint.
iii. Lower end or its tip attached to the linea alba.
iv. Lateral borders insertion to the aponeurosis of the internal oblique and transversus abdominis.
v. Anterior surface, insertion of: Medial fibers of the rectus abdominis and aponeurosis of external oblique muscle.
vi. Posterior surface, origin of: The diaphragm and some fibers of the sternocostalis muscle.

OSSIFICATION

Primary centers

i. For the manubrium—appears from one to three months of intrauterine life.

ii. One center for each of the first and second sternebrae—appears fifth month of intrauterine life.
iii. For the third and fourth sternebrae two in number—appears in the fifth and sixth months respectively in intrauterine life.

Secondary centers

i. The four pieces body of sternum fuse with one another from below upwards between 14 and 25 years.
ii. Xiphoid process starts to ossify in the third year, which fused with the body about fortieth year.
iii. The manubrium sterni fused with the body about sixtieth years or in extreme old age.
The aboves help in age determination.

CLINICAL ANATOMY

i. Sternal puncture: It is useful to aspirate the red bone marrow for hematological examination.

ii. Ectopic cordis: In this condition heart is partly or completely exposed on the surface of the thorax. It occurs due to faulty development of the sternum where two halves of the sternum remains widely separated.

iii. Pigeon chest with rickety rosary: In some people, the sternum projects anteriorly and the chest become flattened on each side. This malformation is called the pigeon chest which is seen in rickets. This condition may be associated with the proliferative changes at the costochondral junctions this feature is known as rickety rosary.

iv. Funnel chest: In this deformity the lower end of the sternum is depressed and the xiphoid process projects forward.

v. Midsternotomy: It is an operation to divide the sternum along the median plane to access the heart and great vessels for surgery.

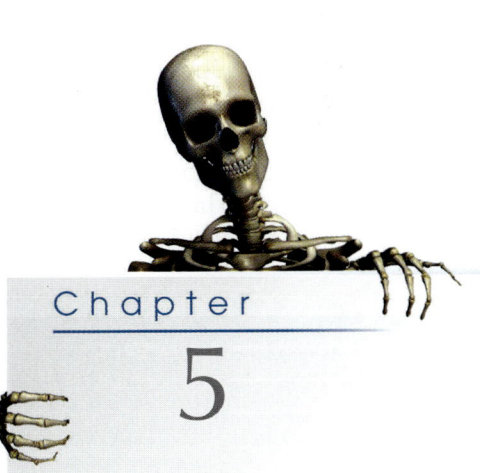

Vertebrae

CLASSIFICATION OF VERTEBRAE

  i. Regional
    a. Cervical: 7
    b. Thoracic: 12
    c. Lumbar: 5
    d. Sacral: 5
    e. Coccygeal: 4
 ii. According to movement
    a. True or movable—upper: 24
    b. False or fixed: 9.

CERVICAL VERTEBRAE

Typical cervical vertebrae: These are third, fourth, fifth and sixth.

Atypical cervical vertebrae: These are first, second and seventh.

CHARACTERISTICS OF TYPICAL CERVICAL VERTEBRAE

Body (Fig. 5.1)

  i. Smallest of all the vertebrae.
 ii. Transverse diameter is greater than the antero-posterior diameter.
iii. On each side of the body of the superior surface presents raised lips.
 iv. On each side of the body of the inferior surface is bevelled.
  v. Anterior and posterior surfaces are flat.
 vi. Lower part of the anterior surface projects inferiorly.

Vertebral foramen: It is large and triangular in shape.

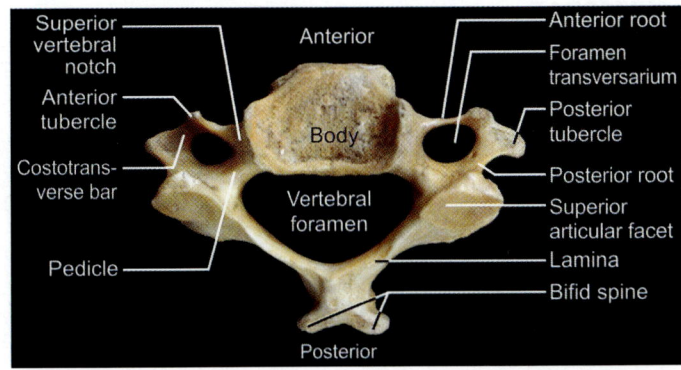

Fig. 5.1: Typical cervical vertebra

Pedicles

  i. Directed backwards and laterally.
 ii. It is attached to the body midway between upper and lower surfaces.
iii. Superior and inferior vertebral notches are equally depth.

Lamina

  i. It is longer, narrower and thinner than the other regions.
 ii. It is directed backward and medially from the pedicle.

Spinous process: It is short and bifided and divided into two tubercles of unequal size.

Articular processes

  i. They projects laterally from the junction of the pedicle and lamina
 ii. The superior articular facet is flat and looks backwards and upwards
iii. The inferior articular facet is looks forwards and downwards.

Transverse process

i. It is directed laterally and slightly forwards

ii. Each transverse process presents an opening, called foramen transversarium transmits following structures (except seventh)
   a. Vertebral artery
   b. Vertebral vein
   c. A branch from the inferior cervical sympathetic ganglion

iii. Foramen transversarium presents anterior and posterior roots

iv. The anterior and posterior roots are joined together by the costotransverse bar

v. The anterior and posterior roots are ends laterally into tubercles called anterior and posterior tubercles respectively.

CHARACTERISTICS OF ATYPICAL CERVICAL VERTEBRAE

FIRST CERVICAL VERTEBRA

Identifications (Fig. 5.2)

i. It is also called Atlas because it supports the globe of the head.

ii. It is ring like.

iii. It has no body no spine.

iv. It has two lateral masses.

v. Lateral masses are connected anteriorly by the anterior arch and posteriorly by the posterior arch.

vi. Anterior arch presents a tubercle opposite the median plane on its anterior surface, called anterior tubercle.

vii. Posterior surface of the anterior arch presents a facet for articulation with the dens of the axis.

viii. Immediately behind the lateral mass on the upper surface of the posterior arch presents a shallow groove.

ix. Posterior aspect of the posterior arch presents posterior tubercle.

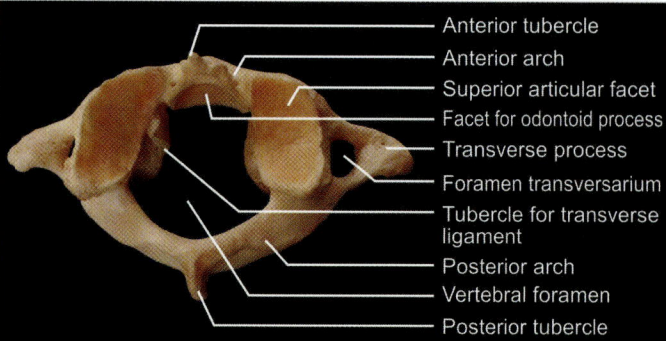

Fig. 5.2: First cervical vertebra (Atlas) superior view

x. Presents kidney-shaped deeply concave articular facet on the superior part of the lateral mass to form the atlanto-occipital joint.

xi. Presents another circular facet on the inferior part of the lateral mass, for articulation with the superior facet of the second cervical vertebra (Fig. 5.3).

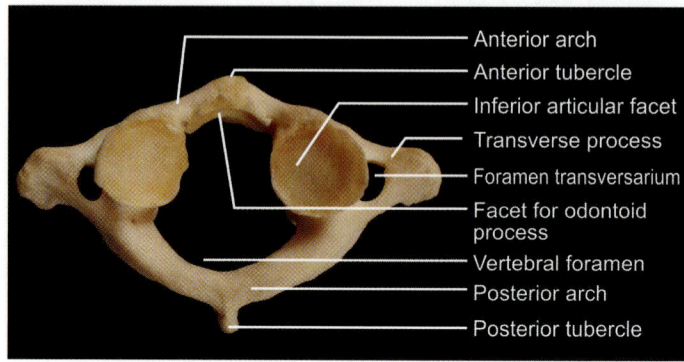

Fig. 5.3: First cervical vertebra (Atlas) inferior view

Relations (Fig. 5.4)

i. **Foramen transversarium:** The vertebral artery passes upwards.

ii. **Over the posterior arch:** The vertebral artery passes medially through the groove, accompanied by the vertebral vein and the sympathetic plexus of nerves

iii. **Deep to the vertebral artery:** The first cervical nerve crosses and immediately divides into anterior and posterior primary rami.

iv. **Through the vertebral canal:** Passes spinal cord with its coverings (meninges), and spinal accessory nerve, the anterior and posterior spinal arteries.

Attachments

i. **In front of lateral mass and root of transverse process: Origin of** the rectus capitis anterior

ii. **Anterior aspect of upper surface of transverse process: Origin of** the rectus capitis lateralis

iii. **Posterior tubercle: Origin of** the rectus capitis posterior minor

iv. **Posterior aspect of upper surface of transverse process: Origin of** the obliquus capitis superior

v. **Inferior aspect of transverse process: Insertion of** the obliquus capitis inferior and splenius cervicis

vi. **The lateral margin of transverse process: Origin of** the levator scapulae

vii. **Anterior tubercle: Insertion of** the longus colli.

viii. **The margins of the facets:** Aattachment of the capsule of the atlanto-occipital and atlantoaxial joints.

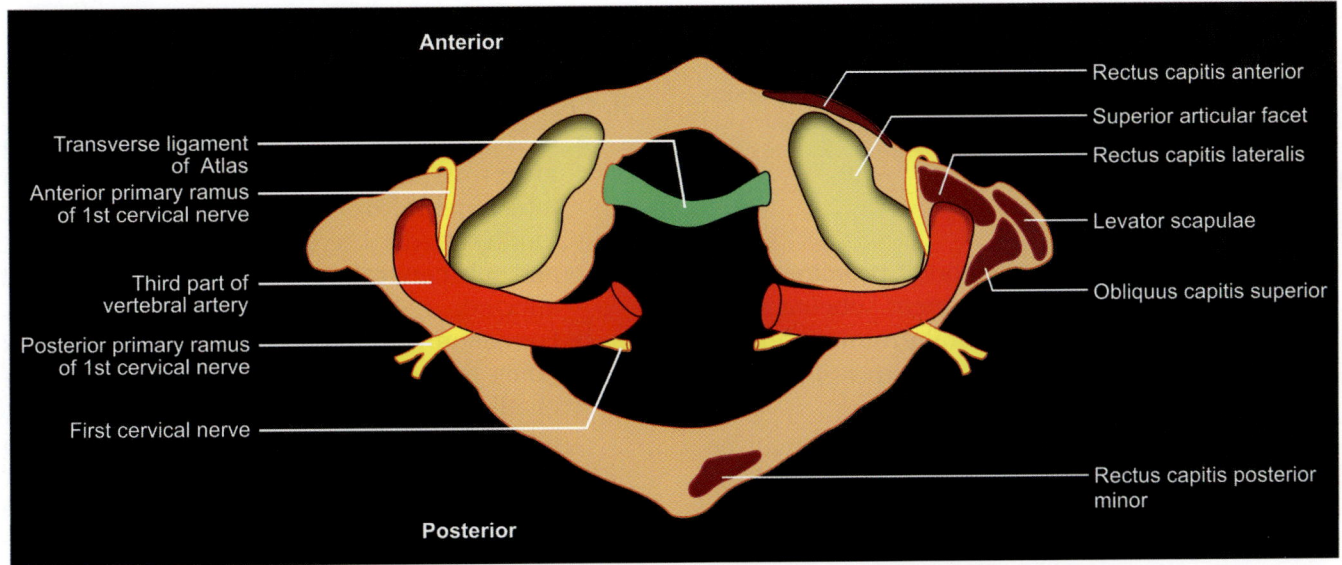

Fig. 5.4: Atlas or first cervical vertebra superior view showing relations and attachments

ix. **Upper margins of the arches of atlas**: Attachments of anterior and posterior atlanto-occipital membranes.

x. **Medial side of lateral masses**: Attachment of transverse ligament.

xi. **Tip of the posterior tubercle**: Attachment to the ligamentum nuchae.

xii. **Lower border of posterior arch:** Attachment to the highest part of ligamentum flavum.

SECOND CERVICAL VERTEBRA

Identifications (Fig. 5.5)

i. It is also called axis.

ii. It presents a tooth-like process, called dens or odontoid process, which projects upwards from the body.

iii. On each side of the dens presents a large oval facet on the upper surface of the body, which articulates, with the inferior facet of the lateral mass of the Atlas.

iv. Lamina is very thick and strong.

v. Spinous process is thick.

vi. Pedicles are too short.

vii. Transverse process short and ends into a tubercle.

viii. Superior vertebral notches are absent.

ix. Inferior vertebral notches are too deep.

Attachments

i. **Posterior edge of spine: Origin of** the rectus capitis posterior major.

ii. **Sides of spine: Origin of** the obliquus capitis inferior.

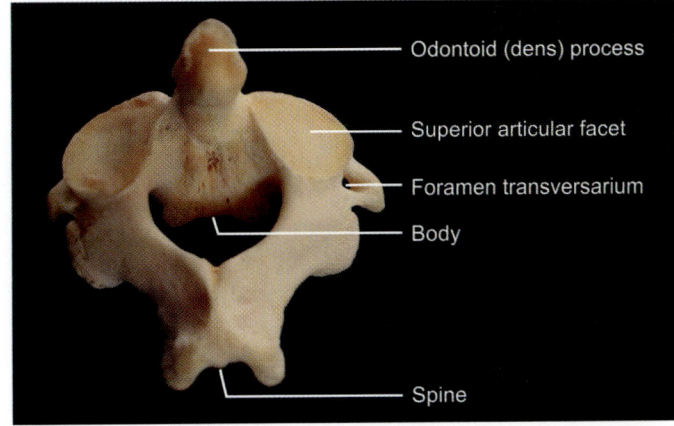

Fig. 5.5: Second cervical vertebra (axis) superior view

iii. **Anterior aspect of transverse process: Origin of** the scalenus medius.

iv. **Lateral aspect of transverse process: Origin of** the levator scapulae.

v. **Lower aspect of spine and the lamina: Insertion of** the semispinalis cervicis.

vi. **Posterior aspect of transverse process: Insertion of** the splenius cervicis.

vii. **Anterior aspect of the body: Attachment of** the vertical part of the longus colli.

viii. **Spine: Attachments of** spinalis cervicis, and the interspinalis muscles.

ix. **Apex of dens or odontoid process: Attachment of** apical ligament.

x. **Depression of dens: Attachments of** the right and left alar ligaments.

xii. **Posterior surface of body: Attachment of** the lower end of membrana tectoria.

Relations

Through the foramen transversarium: It passes vertebral artery, vertebral vein, and sympathetic plexus of nerves.

SEVENTH CERVICAL VERTEBRA

Identification (Fig. 5.6)

i. Spinous process is long, horizontal, prominent and not bifided (it forms a prominent subcutaneous bony landmark called vertebral prominence).

ii. Posterior root of the transverse process is much shorter.

iii. Foramina transversarium is small and may be double transmits only accessory vertebral vein.

iv. Distance between the two transverse processes is much longer than any other cervical vertebrae.

Attachments

i. **Anterior part/aspect of body:** Attachments of the longus colli muscle and anterior longitudinal ligament.

ii. **Posterior aspect of body:** Attachments of posterior longitudinal ligament.

iii. **Posterior tubercle on the transverse process:** attachments of scalenus minimus and the apex of the suprapleural membrane or Sibson's fascia.

iv. **Lower border of the transverse process:** Origin of first pair of levator costarum (Fig. 5.6).

CLINICAL ANATOMY

i. Dislocation of the cervical vertebrae
  a. Cervical vertebrae can be dislocated by a little force of injuries than is required to fracture
  b. Due to large vertebral canal in the cervical region, slight dislocation may damage the spinal cord

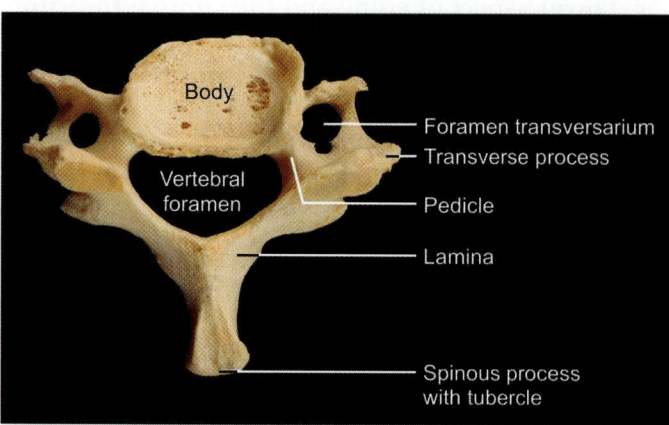

Fig. 5.6: Seventh cervical vertebra

Body

Foramen transversarium
Transverse process
Vertebral foramen
Pedicle
Lamina
Spinous process with tubercle

  c. Dislocated cervical veretebra may self reduced (return to place).

ii. Cervical spondylosis
  a. It is the most common clinical condition affecting the neck. Degeneration of the intervertebral discs, often during the third or fourth decade. The disc space between the 5th and 6th cervical vertebrae is most frequently affected.
  b. Formation of osteophytes to joints of Luschka (joints between the lateral margins of the bodies of adjacent vertebrae) which project backwards into the intervertebral foramen as a result, the cervical nerve roots are compressed by osteophytes leading to pain along their distribution.

iii. Dizziness in cervical spondylosis: Cervical spondylosis causes distortion of the vertebral artery leading to vertebrobasilar insufficiency which clinically presents as dizziness.

iv. Prolapse of intervertebral disc in the cervical region: It usually involves the disc between C5 and C6 or C6 and C7. The nucleus pulposus generally herniates in the posterolateral direction and compresses a nerve root. The herniated disc between C5 and C6 compresses C6 nerve root, hence patient feels pain in the thumb, whereas herniated disc between C6 and C7 compresses C7 nerve root and consequently there is pain, tingling and numbness on the posterior aspect of arm, forearm, middle and index fingers.

v. Fracture of axis
  a. The dens of axis may be fractured by the road traffic accidents or a fall from the hight.
  b. The fractured dens may compress the spinal cord or injure the vital centers of the medulla oblongata, ultimately leads to death.

vi. Hangman's fracture
  a. The fracture occurs through the pedicles of the axis.
  b. Sudden over extension of the neck as produced by the knot of a Hangman's rope beneath the chin, is the reason for common name.

vii. Death by hanging: The dens of axis dislocates backwards after tearing the transverse ligament and strikes the lower part of medulla and upper part of spinal cord. This is due to atlantoaxial dislocation without fracture of dens.

viii. Cervical rib: The costal element of C7 vertebra is sometimes detached from the transverse element and grows separately to form as cervical rib which may compress the lower trunk of the brachial plexus and result in Klumpke's paralysis.

THORACIC VERTEBRAE

Typical thoracic vertebrae: These are second to eighth and they have common features.

Atypical thoracic vertebrae: These are first, ninth, tenth, eleventh and twelfth.

CHARACTERISTICS OF TYPICAL THORACIC VERTEBRAE

i. **Body** (Fig. 5.7)

a. Shape—heart-shaped (broader antero-posteriorly than from side to side).

b. On either side of the body presents two articular facets, one above and other below.

c. The superior and inferior facets are half facets but superior one is larger.

d. Superior facet is situated on the upper margin close to the pedicle.

e. Inferior facet is situated on the lower margin close to the inferior vertebral notch.

ii. **Pedicles**

a. It is projected backwards.

b. Vertebral foramen smaller and circular.

iii. **Laminae:** They are thick and overlap one another.

iv. **Spinous process**

a. It is directed downwards and backwards.

b. The spine ends in single tubercle.

v. **Superior and inferior articular process:** Their articular surfaces are flat.

vi. **Transverse process**

a. It is stout and club-shaped.

b. Directed laterally and slightly backwards.

c. Presents an articular facet near its end and articulates with the tubercle of the numerically corresponding rib.

CHARACTERISTICS OF ATYPICAL THORACIC VERTEBRAE

FIRST THORACIC VERTEBRA (Fig. 5.8)

i. **Body**

a. It looks like cervical vertebra which is broader transversely than anteroposteriorly.

b. The posterolateral margins of the upper surface of the body are raised like cervical vertebrae.

c. Costal facet—on the side of the body a circular costal facet above and a half facet below.

ii. **Superior vertebral notches**—they are considerable depth.

iii. **Spinous process**—is long and directed horizontaly.

iv. **Vertebral foramen**—it is large and triangular.

v. Absence of foramen transversarium differentiates from the cervical vertebrae.

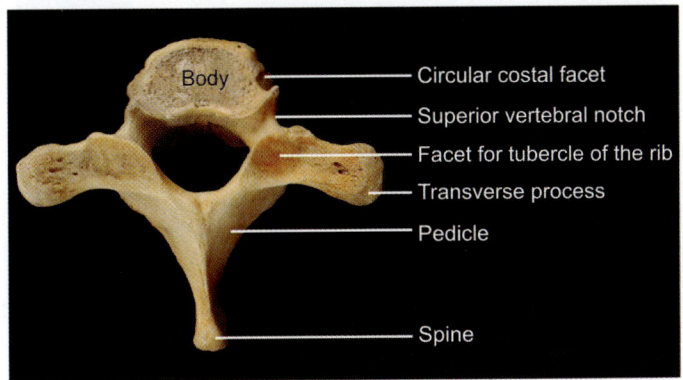

Fig. 5.8: First thoracic vertebra

TENTH THORACIC VERTEBRA

i. **Body:** Presents a single full costal facet close to the upper border at the junction between the pedicle and the body.

ii. Absence of lower costal facet on the body.

iii. Transverse processes present costal facets (Fig. 5.9).

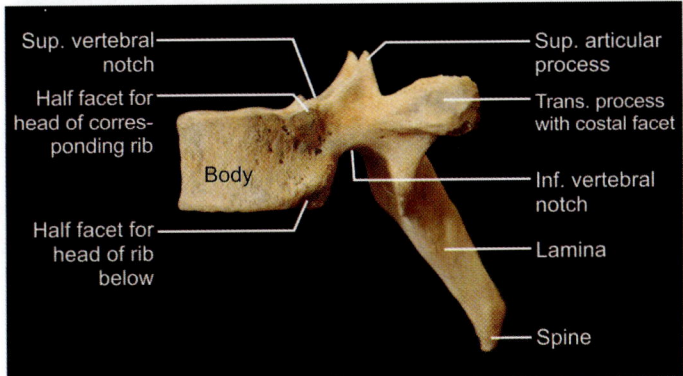

Fig. 5.7: Typical thoracic vertebra

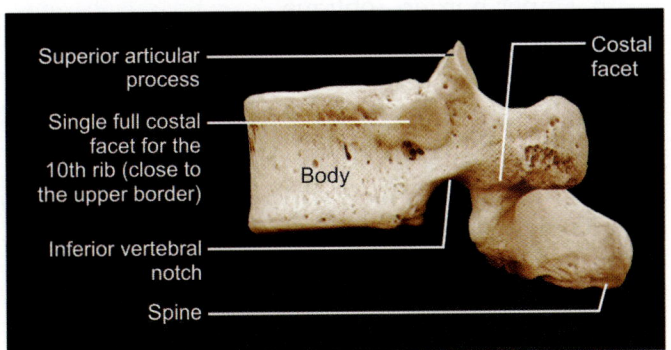

Fig. 5.9: Tenth thoracic vertebra

ELEVENTH THORACIC VERTEBRA

i. Body presents a single full costal facet which is partly on the body and partly on the pedicle.

ii. Transverse processes have no costal facets

iii. Inferior articular facets directed downwards and forwards.

iv. Spinous process:
   a. Shape—triangular.
   b. Upper border—oblique.

v. Lower border—horizontal (Fig. 5.10).

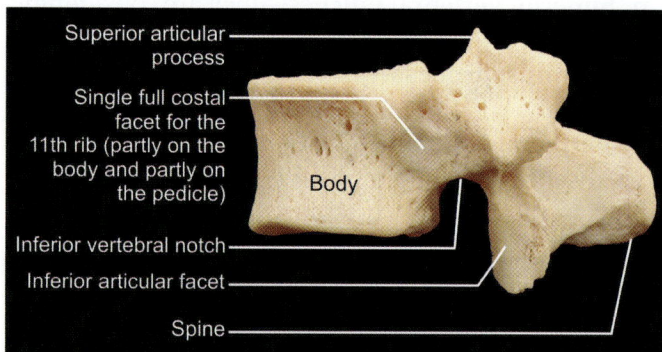

Fig. 5.10: Eleventh thoracic vertebra

TWELFTH THORACIC VERTEBRA

i. **Body:** Broader from side-to-side than antero-posteriorly.

ii. **Costal facet:** There is a single full costal facet on the body which is much below from its upper border, presents mainly on the pedicle and partly on the body.

iii. **Inferior articular facets:** It is convex and twisted laterally.

iv. **Transverse processes**
   a. No costal facets.
   b. It broken into superior, lateral and inferior tubercles.

v. **Spinous process**
   a. Shape—triangular.
   b. Upper border—oblique.
   c. Lower borders—horizontal (Fig. 5.11).

CLINICAL ANATOMY

Tuberculosis of spine (Pott's disease) with cold abscess:

a. It is the tuberculosis of the vertebral column commonly affecting the body of thoracic vertebrae or in a disc space.

b. The pus produced by such disease is called cold abscess, because it does not express the local signs of heat and redness of acute infection.

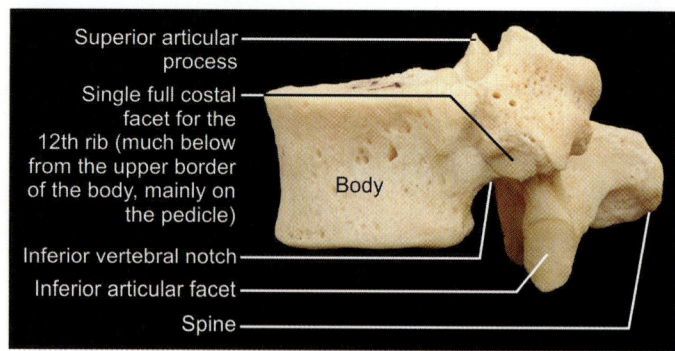

Fig. 5.11: Twelfth thoracic vertebra

LUMBAR VERTEBRAE

Characteristics of the Typical Lumbar Vertebrae (Figs 5.12 and 5.13)

i. **Body**
   a. It is large
   b. Transverse diameter is larger than the anteroposterior diameter
   c. No costal facets on the body.

ii. **Transverse processes**
   a. It is slender elongated and flattened antero-posteriorly
   b. On the posteroinferior aspect presents a tubercle

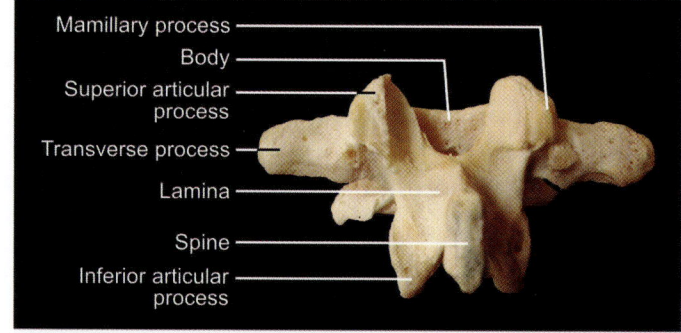

Fig. 5.12: Typical lumbar vertebra (posterior view)

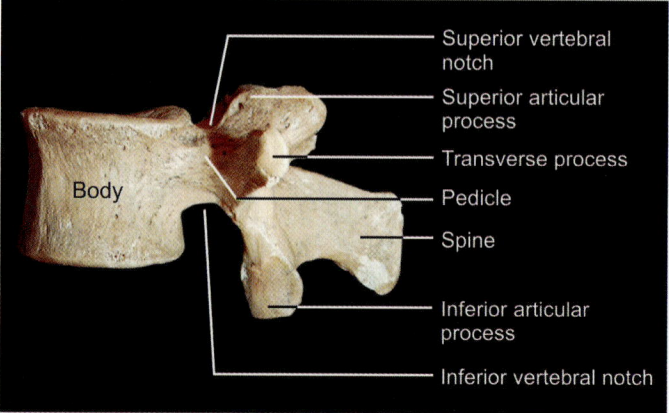

Fig. 5.13: Typical lumbar vertebra (lateral view)

c. Transverse process of the third lumbar vertebra is largest

iii. **Vertebral foramen:** Triangular in shape.

iv. **Superior articular processes:** Concave and directed backwards and medially.

v. **Mamillary processes:** Presents of tubercles called mamillary process placed behind the superior articular processes.

vi. **Inferior articular processes:** They are convex and twisted laterally and close to each other.

vii. **Spinous process:**
   a. Shape—quadrangular
   b. It projects horizontally backwards.

ATTACHMENTS

i. **Anterior and posterior longitudinal ligaments:** They are attached to the upper and lower borders of the front and behind the body respectively.

ii. **Origin of the right and left crus of the diaphragm**
   - **Right crus:** On the right side of anterior longitudinal ligament on bodies of the first, second and third lumbar vertebrae.
   - **Left crus:** On the left side of anterior longitudinal ligament on bodies of the first and second lumbar vertebrae.

iii. **Origin of the psoas major muscle:** Posterior to the origin of the crus of the diaphragm from the all lumbar vertebrae (extends upwards the twelfth thoracic vertebra) and also from the medial areas of the anterior aspects of the transverse processes of all the lumbar vertebrae.

iv. **Posterior layer of the thoracolumbar fascia, supraspinous and interspinous ligaments:** To the posterior border of the spine of the lumbar vertebrae.

v. **Attachments of erector spinae, multifidus, spinalis thoracis and interspinalis muscles:** To the posterior border of the spine of the lumbar vertebrae.

vi. **Anterior layer of the thoracolumbar fascia:** To the anterior aspects of the transverse processes of all the lumbar vertebrae.

vii. **Insertion of the quadratus lumborum:** From lateral areas of the anterior aspects of transverse processes of all the lumbar vertebrae.

viii. **Middle layer of the thoracolumbar fascia:** From the tips of the transverse processes of all the lumbar vertebrae.

ix. **Medial and lateral arcuate ligaments:** From tip of transverse process of the first lumbar vertebra.

x. **Iliolumbar ligament:** From tip of transverse process of the fifth lumbar vertebra.

xi. **Origin of longissimus thoracis:** From the posterior surfaces of the transverse processes.

xii. **Attachment of the intertransverse muscle:** From the upper and lower borders of the transverse processes.

xiii. **Multifidus and medial intertransverse muscles:** From the mamillary process.

FIFTH LUMBAR VERTEBRA

It is atypical lumbar vertebra (Fig. 5.14).

i. **Body**
   a. It is very large
   b. Deeper in front than behind.

ii. **Transverse processes**
   a. Shape-conical.
   b. Stout and bulky.
   c. Mainly arises from the pedicle and encroaches on the body

iii. **Articular processes:** Distance between the superior articular processes and also inferior articular processes are almost equal.

iv. **Spinous process:** It is less substantial and its upper border close to its dorsal end is rounded and down-turned.

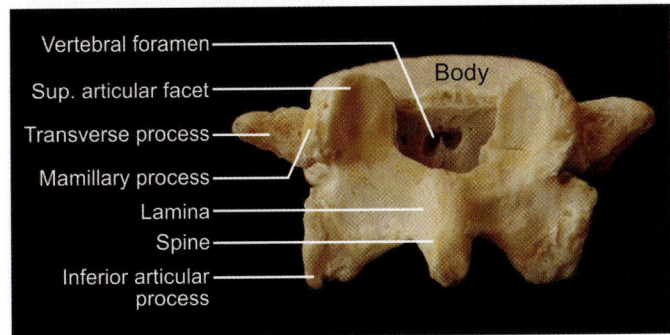

Fig. 5.14: Fifth lumbar vertebra

CLINICAL ANATOMY

i. **Lumbar puncture**
   a. This is the easiest and commonly used method of aspiration of CSF
   b. This is done by passing a needle in between the third and fourth lumbar spines, for the biochemical analysis of CSF for diagnostic purpose
   c. The normal rate of CSF flow is about one drop per second, but when the CSF pressure is increased the CSF escapes in continuous stream

Complication of lumbar puncture

a. **Postlumbar puncture headache:** This starts after the procedure and lasts for 24 to 48 eight hours.

b. **Brain herniation:** Here the lumbar puncture is contraindicated.

ii. Herniation of the nucleus pulposus (Fig. 5.15)

a. It is a condition of herniation or protrusion of the nucleus pulposus (a gelatinous central mass of the intervetebral disc). It is often called slipped disc or ruptured disc

b. About 95% of the lumbar disc herniation occurs between the L4 and L5 or L5 and S1 levels

c. If nucleus pulposus herniate posteriorly into the vertebral canal causes compression of the spinal cord or nerve roots of the spinal cord.

iii. Loss of height in old age:
In old age persons due to dehydration and degeneration of intervertebral discs, their disc spaces become decrease which is responsible for slight loss of height and narrowing of the intervertebral foramina producing compression of the spinal nerve roots. Osteoporotic patients also showing loss of height due to kyphosis and compression of vertebrae.

iv. Lumbago

a. It is an acute mid and low back pain extending downwards along the posterolateral aspect of the thigh and leg

b. It is often results from posterolateral herniation of a lumbar intervertebral disc between the L5 and S1 level that affects the S1 component of the sciatic nerve

c. Ultimately it may leads to sciatica.

v. Sciatica

a. It is pain in the lower part of the back and hip extending back of the thigh into the leg

b. Cause—it is caused by a herniated lumbar intervertebral disc that compresses the L5 or S1 nerve root

c. In the lumbar region intervertebral foramina decrease in size and the lumbar nerves increase in size

d. At the same time, if osteoarthritis (deposition of new bone) occurs further narrows the intervertebral foramina as a result shooting pain is extending the lower limbs.

e. By the flexion or extension of the thigh stretches the sciatic nerve which may exacerbate the pain.

f. Herniated intervertebral disc compressed the nerve roots numbered one below to the disc, such as when L4 and L5 disc herniate the L5 nerve is compressed.

vi. Compression of the lumbar spinal roots

a. The thickest spinal nerve roots are the L5 but their foramina is narrowest

b. This anatomical factor is the main cause of that the nerve roots will be compressed when nucleus pulposus herniation occurs.

vii. Abnormal curvatures of the vertebral column:
To inspect whether any abnormal curvature in the vertebral column person stand in the anatomical position, physician will follow from the person's side.

The abnormal curvature may be due to following causes:

a. Developmental anomalies

b. From pathological process like osteoporosis

c. Atrophy of the skeletal tissues

Following are the abnormal curvature in the vertebral column:

– Kyphosis

– Lordosis

– Scoliosis

– Kyphoscoliosis

Kyphosis or humpback or hunchback

Feature: The abnormal increase in thoracic curvature backward.

Cause: Erosion of the anterior part of one or more vertebrae due to osteoporosis.

Dowayer's hump: It is type of kyphosis in older women caused by wedge fractures of the thoracic vertebrae due to osteoporosis.

Lordosis or hollow back or swayback

Features: In this condition the abnormal increase of lumbar curvature forward.

Causes

a. It occurs due to an anterior rotation of the pelvis in which the upper part of the sacrum tilts anteroinferiorly

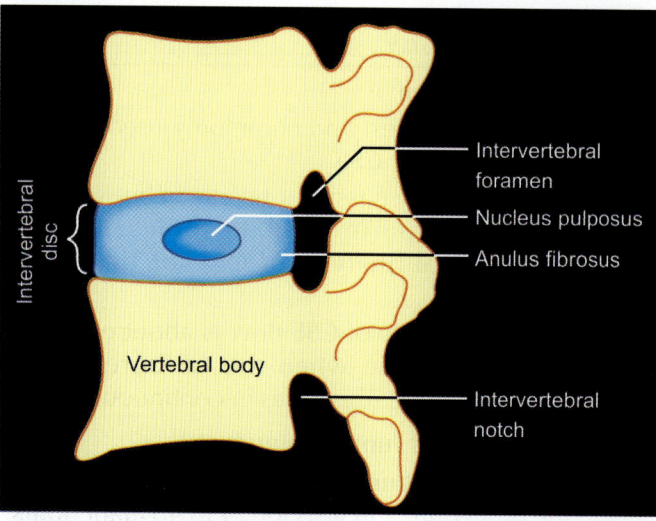

Fig. 5.15: Intervertebral joint

b. This abnormal curvature is often associated with weakness of the trunk musculature.

c. During pregnancy, women develop a temporary lordosis and may cause low back pain which may disappears soon after childbirth

d. Obesity in both sexes can produced lordosis with low back pain which may be corrected by loss of weight

Scoliosis or crooked or curved back

Features: It is an abnormal lateral curvature of the vertebral column.

Causes

a. It is the most common deformity among the pubertal girls

b. Asymmetrical weakness of the intrinsic muscles of back (myopathic scoliosis)

Kyphoscoliosis (sometimes present): It is a combined conditions of kyphosis and scoliosis in which abnormal anteroposterior diameter causes severe restriction of the thorax and lung expansion.

viii. **Abnormal fusion of vertebrae**

a. **Hemisacralization and sacralization of L5 vertebra:** It is a condition where L5 vertebra is partly or completely incorporated into the sacrum.

b. **Lumbarization of S1 vertebra:** In some people the S1 vertebra is more or less separated from the sacrum and is partly or completely fused with L5 vertebra

c. When L5 is sacralized, the L5/S1 level is strong and the L4/L5 level degenerate often producing pain.

ix. **Anomalies of the vertebrae**

a. **Spina bifida occulta**

– In this anomaly, the laminae of L5 and/or S1 fail to develop normally

– In this defect have no back problems

– This defect is concealed by skin, but its position is often indentified by a tuft of hair

b. **Spina bifida cystica**

– It is a severe type of spina bifida caused by improper closer of the neural tube during embryonic life

– The spina bifida cystica associated with meningocele (herniation of the meninges) and/or meningomyelocele (herniation of the spinal cord).

x. If pain of the back is felt on bending forward, the involvement is in the intervertebral disc and pain is felt on backward bending of the vertebral column the involvement is in the intervertebral joint.

SACRUM

INTRODUCTION

i. Sacrum is a large triangular bone formed by the fusion of the five sacral vertebrae. It forms the posterior boundary of the bony pelvic cavity.

ii. It articulates between the two hip bones.

ANATOMICAL POSITION

i. Smooth pelvic surface looks downward and forward and the rough dorsal surface looks upward and backward.

ii. The upper surface of the body of the first sacral vertebra slopes.

iii. The sacral promontory looks forwards as if, lifting something from ground.

GENERAL FEATURES

Base

i. It is directed upwards and forwards with articular and non-articular parts.

ii. Upper surface of the body of first sacral vertebra is articular.

iii. Anterior margin of first sacral vertebra is called sacral promontory.

iv. The non-articular part of the base projects lateralwards on either side of articular part known as ala sacralis.

v. Ala is subdivided into smooth medial part and rough lateral part.

vi. The vertebral foramen is large and triangular which leads into sacral canal.

Apex

i. The apex of the sacrum is formed by the inferior surface of the body of the fifth sacral vertebra.

ii. It bears an oval facet for articulation with the coccyx.

Pelvic Surface (Fig. 5.16)

i. It is concave from above downwards.

ii. Pelvic surface of sacrum presents four pairs of pelvic (anterior) sacral foramina.

iii. The first foramina are the largest and the fourth is the smallest.

iv. Presents four transverse ridges which ends laterally up to sacral foramina (Fig. 5.16).

Dorsal Surface (Fig. 5.17)

Features

i. **Sacral crest:** Opposite the median plane presents a raised crest, on which lies four small tubercles,

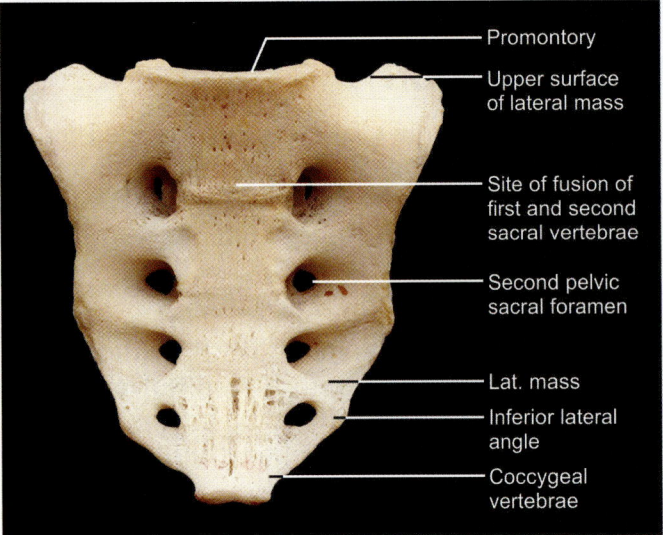

Fig. 5.16: Pelvic surface of sacrum, showing general features

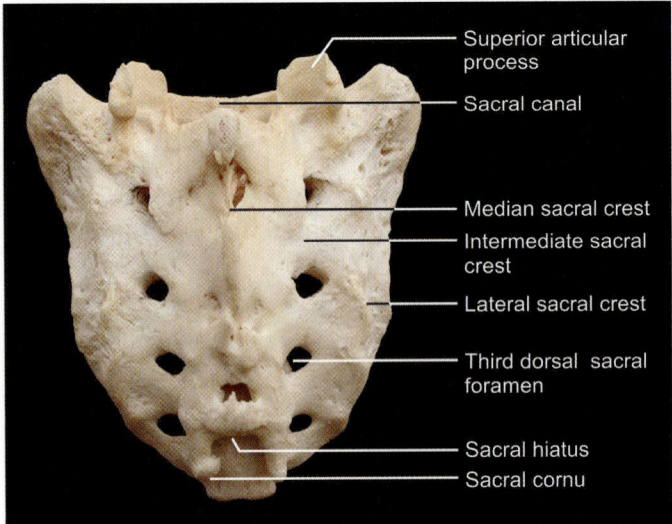

Fig. 5.17: Dorsal surface of sacrum, showing general features

which represents the spinous processes of upper four fused sacral vertebrae.

ii. **Sacral hiatus or hiatus sacralis:** Below the fourth tubercle there is an inverted U-shaped or V-shaped gap called sacral hiatus or hiatus sacralis.

iii. On the lateral part of the dorsal surface presents four posterior sacral foramina.

Intermediate sacral crest

i. Just medial to dorsal sacral foramina there are four artricular tubercles.

ii. They collectively form intermediate sacral crest.

Transverse elevations: Lateral to dorsal sacral foramina prominent lateral sacral crest formed by fused transverse processes of the sacral vertebrae.

Sacral cornu: At the sides of the sacral hiatus two small tubercles looks downwards and forwards called sacral cornu

Sacral canal

i. It is formed by sacral vertebral foramina,

ii. Inferiorly, the canal opens at the sacral hiatus (Fig. 5.17)

Lateral surface (Fig. 5.18)

i. It is formed by the fused transverse processes and the costal elements of the sacral vertebrae .

ii. It is wide above and narrow below.

iii. The upper wider part bears auricular surface (ear shaped) for articulation with the ilium forming sacroiliac joint (Fig. 5.18).

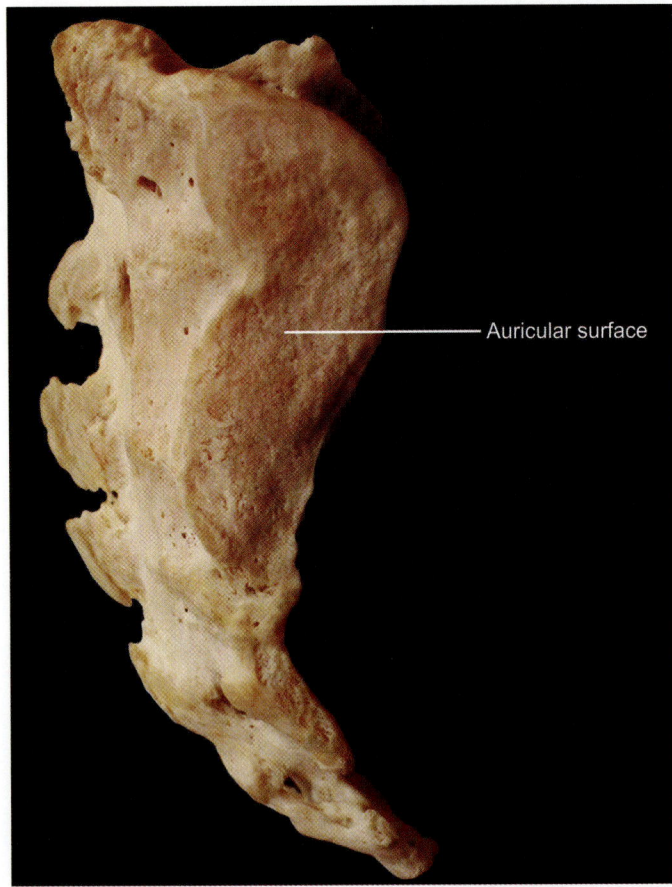

Fig. 5.18: Lateral surface of sacrum

PARTICULAR FEATURES

Pelvic (anterior) Sacral Foramina

Transmits

i. Ventral rami of upper four pairs of sacral nerves

ii. Lateral sacral arteries.

Pelvic surface (Fig. 5.19)

Origin of piriformis: From bony bars between first and second, second and third, third and fourth foramina.

Dorsal surface

  i. Dorsal sacral foramina

    Transmits: Dorsal rami of upper four pairs of sacral nerves.

  ii. Origin of:

    a. Erector spinae: U-shaped origin over the spinous and transverse tubercles.

    b. Multifidus: Area within the U-shaped origin of erector spinae (Fig. 5.20).

Lateral surface: Behind the auricular surface, the rough pitted area gives attachment interosseous sacroiliac ligament.

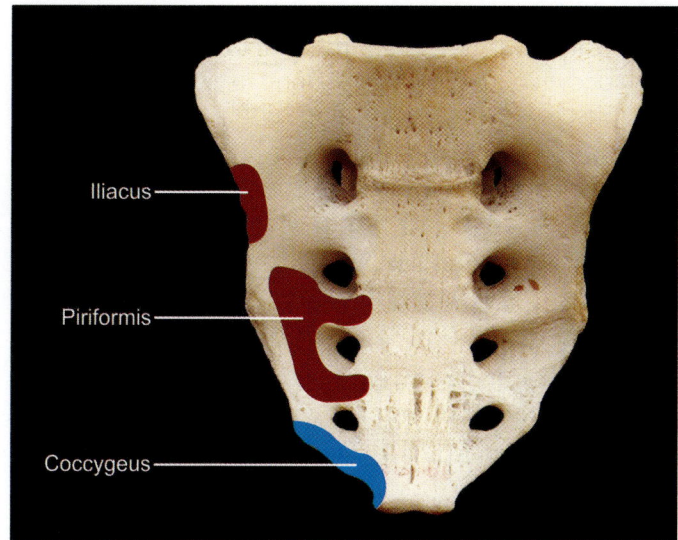

Fig. 5.19: Pelvic surface of sacrum, showing attachments

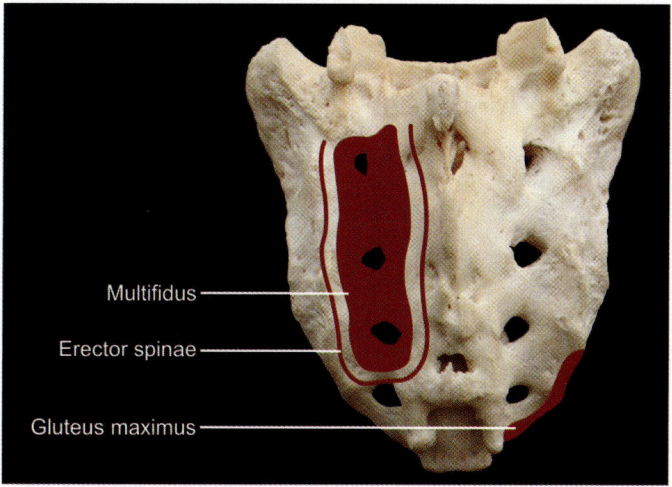

Fig. 5.20: Dorsal surface of sacrum, showing attachments

Lower narrower part

Attachments: From anterior to posterior

  a. Origin of coccygeus

  b. Sacrospinous ligament

  c. Sacrotuberous ligament

  d. Origin of gluteus maximus

Structures related to ala of the sacrum: From medial to lateral (Fig. 5.21)

  a. Sympathetic trunk

  b. Lumbosacral trunk

  c. Iliolumbar artery

  d. Obturator nerve.

Area in front of ala covered by psoas major muscle.

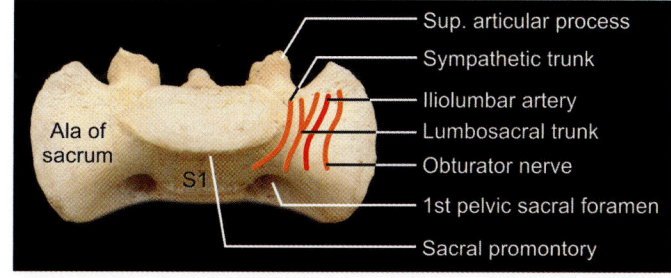

Fig. 5.21: Structures related to the smooth medial part of the ala of sacrum

Contents of sacral canal

  a. Cauda equina

  b. Filum terminale

  c. Spinal meninges

  d. Subdural and subarachnoid spaces, which ends at the level of second sacral vertebra.

Structures transmitted through the sacral hiatus:

  a. Filum terminale invested by dura, arachnoid and pia maters

  b. Fifth pair of sacral nerves

  c. The coccygeal nerves.

OSSIFICATION

  i. Ossification centers appears in upper segment in 3rd month

  ii. 5 sacral vertebrae are separated by cartilage until puberty

  iii. The sacrum becomes a single bone at about 30 years

  iv. A gap may be seen between S1 and S2 until 32 years due to 'Lapsed union'

  v. After mid-adult life the coccyx fuses with the sacrum.

The formers help in age determination.

Table 5.1 shows difference between the male sacrum and female sacrum

Table 5.1	Difference between the male and female sacrum
In male sacrum	In female sacrum
i. It is long and narrow ii. Sacral index is about 105 iii. The body of first sacral forms the larger part of the base iv. Curvature of the pelvic surface is uniformly concave v. The auricular surface contributes upper half of the third sacral vertebra vi. Coccyx becomes immobile early, due to sacralisation of first coccygeal vertebra. vii. Weight heavier viii. Muscular impression—more marked.	i. It is short and wide ii. Sacral index is about 115 iii. The ala of sacrum forms the larger part of the base iv. The lower part is abruptly concave forward. v. The auricular surface extends up to second sacral vertebra vi. Coccyx is more movable, and this permits its backward displacement especially during child birth.

CLINICAL ANATOMY

i. **Backache**
   a. As the cervical and lumbar regions of the vertebral column having free movements, therefore, these regions are frequent sites of pain.
   b. Low back pain most commonly occurs typically from 3rd to 6th decades of life.
   c. Pain in back but unable to move the limbs indicating fracture of the vertebral column.

ii. **Variations in the vertebrae:** Variations in the number of vertebrae may be clinically important.
   a. Due to error of development the number of vertebrae may occur 32 to 34
   b. Number increased often in males and reduced in females

iii. **Caudal epidural anesthesia:** In this procedure the anesthetic agent is injected into epidural space of sacral canal through sacral hiatus or through the posterior sacral foramina to act on the sacral and coccygeal nerves. This is done to relax the perineal muscles for pain-less child birth.

iv. **Coccydynia:** Pain in the region of coccyx is known as coccydynia. In most of the cases, it results from injury to coccyx or fall in sitting position.

v. **Back strain and sprains**
   a. Back strain is common problem among the sportsmans
   b. It results from excessive movements of the vertebral column
   c. The sacrospinalis muscle is the cause of low back pain
   d. To prevent strains and sprains require sufficient warm up and stretching is required.

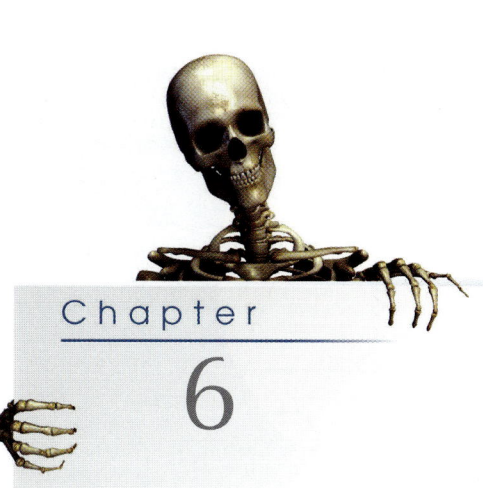

Skull

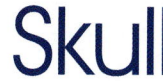

INTRODUCTION

a. The skeleton of the head is called the skull. It consists of several bones that are joined together to form cranium

b. The skull consists of 22 bones

c. The skull can be divided into two main parts.

I. BRAIN BOX OR CALVARIA

Upper part of cranium, which encloses the brain. Brain box composed of eight bones.

Paired

a. Parietal
b. Temporal

Unpaired

a. Frontal
b. Occipital
c. Sphenoid
d. Ethmoid

II. FACIAL SKELETON

The facial skeleton (splanchnocranium) constitutes rest of skull.

It is composed of 14 bones, which are following:

Paired

a. Maxillae
b. Zygomatic
c. Nasal
d. Lacrimal
e. Palatine
f. Inferior nasal concha.

Unpaired

a. Mandible
b. Vomer.

ANATOMICAL POSITION OF SKULL

Hold the skull in such a way that the inferior margin of the orbit and the superior margin of the external acoustic meatus of both sides lie in the same horizontal plane (Frankfurt's horizontal plane).

SKULL JOINTS

Joints of the skull are immovable and fibrous in type known as sutures only exception is temporomandibular (synovial type) joint.

SUTURES

Articulation between cranial bones firmly interlocked each other by thin layer of fibrous tissue, called sutural ligament.

Classification of Sutures

i. **Sutura serrata:** Articulation between two parietal bones along the sagittal suture.

ii. **Sutura denticulata:** Articulated with each other by tooth like process.
Example: Mastoid part of temporal bone with occipital bone.

iii. **Sutura squamosa:** Two bones articulate each other by bevelled margins which overlapped each other, e.g. squamous part of temporal bone with the parietal bone.

iv. **Sutura limbosa:** Serrated sutura where margins overlapped each other.

v. **Sutura plana:** It is a plane suture of two bones, e.g. horizontal plate of palatine bone with the palatal process of the maxilla.

vi. **Schindylesis:** A joint between a wedge and a groove, e.g. rostrum of sphenoid bone with the alae of vomer.

THE STUDY OF SKULL

i. Exterior of skull
ii. Interior of skull

EXTERIOR OF SKULL

NORMA

i. The exterior of skull may be examined from above, from the sides, from the front, from the below and from behind.

ii. Each of these aspects is called norma.
   Types:
   a. Norma verticalis
   b. Norma frontalis
   c. Norma lateralis
   d. Norma basalis
   e. Norma occipitalis.

NORMA VERTICALIS

Shape: When viewed from above, it is usually oval in shape, but wider posteriorly than anteriorly.

Bones Taking Part

Anteriorly: By the squamous part of the frontal bone.
Posteriorly: By the squamous part of the occipital bone.
On each side: By the two parietal bones.
They articulate with one another by sutures

Sutures

Coronal suture: Between the frontal and two parietal bones

Sagittal suture: It is placed in the median plane between the two parietal bones.

Lambdoid suture: It lies between the occipital bone and the two parietal bones. Sometimes, isolated sutural bone (*see* occipitial bone external surface) is seen in the lambdoid suture (Fig. 6.1)

Age of closure of cranial sutures

i. **Sagittal suture:** Starts—25 years. Closing age: Posterior 1/3rd—30 to 40 years; Anterior 1/3rd—40 to 50 years and Middle 1/3rd—50 to 60 years.

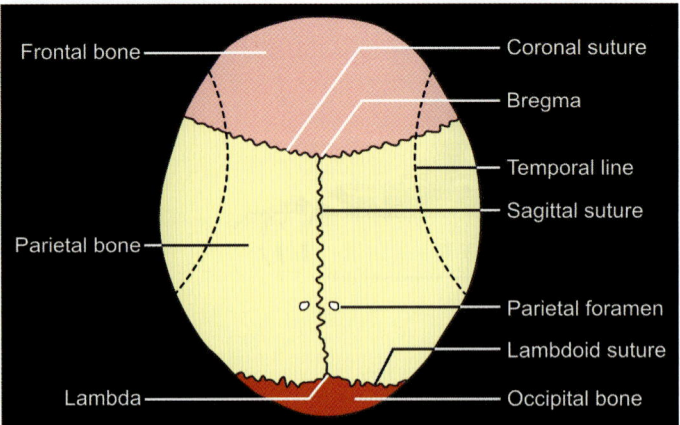

Fig. 6.1: Norma Verticalis

ii. **Coronal suture:** Starts—25 to 30 years. Closing age: Lower half—40 to 50 years. Upper half—50 to 60 years.

iii. **Lambdoid suture:** Starts—30 years. Closing age: Medial half—50 to 60 years; Lateral half—60 to 70 years.
   Suture closure begins from the bregma and involves successively sagittal, coronal and lambdoid sutures.
   Endocranial suture closure takes place about 10 years earlier to ectocranial suture closure.

Metopic suture

i. The metopic suture closes about 2nd—8th years.

ii. This is occasionally present in the frontal bone about 9% individuals, lies on the lower part of the median plane.

Important Features

Vault: It is the arched roof or the dome of the skull.
Vertex: It is the highest point on the sagittal suture.

Bregma

i. It is the meeting point between the coronal and sagittal sutures

ii. It is the meeting point between frontal and two parietal bones.

iii. In the fetal and infant skull there is a thin site of membranous gap, called the anterior fontanelle, which, closes between the eighteenth month and two years of age.

Lambda

i. It is the meeting point between the sagittal and lambdoid sutures

ii. It is the meeting point between occipital and two parietal bones.

iii. In the fetal and infant skull it is the site of posterior fontanelle, which is unossified membrane, closes at third month of age.

Parietal eminences/tubers: Area of maximum convexity of the each parietal bone.

Parietal foramen: One on each side of the parietal bone near its upper border about 3 cm in front of lambda.

Transmits: Emissary vein from veins of scalp into the sagittal sinus.

Obelion: It is the point on the sagittal suture between the two parietal foramina.

Temporal lines

i. Begins as a single line from zygomatic process of frontal bone and run upwards and backwards.

ii. It divides over the parietal bone into superior and inferior temporal lines (Fig. 6.1).

CLINICAL ANATOMY

Anterior fontanelle and its clinical importance: It is diamond shaped area situated at the junction of sagittal, coronal and frontal sutures, corresponds to the bregma.

Measurements: Length about 4 cm and 2.5 cm in breadth.

Relation: Deep to it lies superior sagittal sinus (Fig. 6.2).

Closure of anterior fontanelle: Between the age of 18th month and 2 years.

Clinical importance

i. It helps determination of age in child, because the anterior fontanelle is closed after the 2 years.

ii. If the fontanelle does not closed after the age of 2 to 3 years indicating there is disturbance of calcium metabolism due to vit D deficiency.

iii. Bulging of anterior fontanelle indicate increased intracranial tension and depression of it dehydration.

iv. The superior sagittal sinus is readily accessible for collecting of blood or for intravenous transfusion of fluid or drug.

v. Allows postnatal growth of the brain.

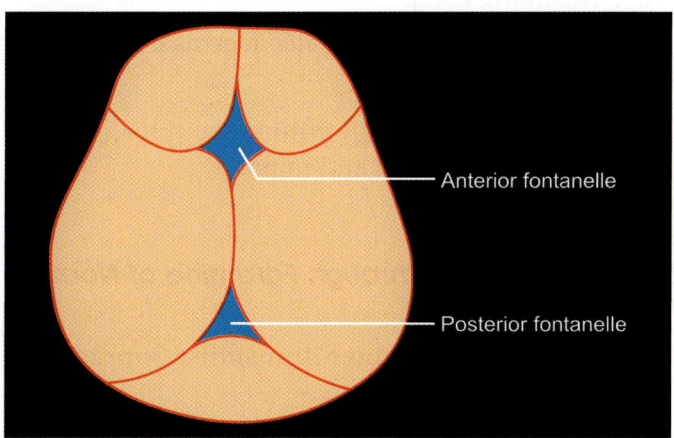

Fig. 6.2: Fontanellae

NORMA FRONTALIS

The anterior aspect of the skull forms the facial skeleton or splanchno-cranium (Fig. 6.3).

Shape

When seen from the front:

i. The norma frontalis is roughly oval in outline.

ii. It is wider above than below.

Bones Forming the Norma Frontalis

i. Frontal bone (squamous part)

ii. Nasal bones (two)

iii. Zygomatic bones (two)

iv. Maxillae (two)

v. Mandible

Important Features

In upper part of the face

i. Frontal eminences or tuberosities: One on either side, above the superciliary arches.

ii. Superciliary arches: Curved elevations above the supraorbital margins.

iii. Supraorbital margins: Below the superciliary arch present the curved supraorbital margin which forms a part of circumference of the orbit.

iv. Glabella: It is a median elevation between the two superciliary arches.

v. Nasion: It is a median point at the root of the nose, where the internasal suture meets with frontonasal suture (Fig. 6.3).

vi. Orbits: The orbits are pair of bony cavities which contain the eyeballs and their associated muscles, vessels, nerves and connective tissues.

vii. Supraorbital notch: On each supraorbital margin presents supraorbital foramen or notch transmits supraorbital vessels and nerves.

viii. Infraorbital margin: It is formed by the zygomatic bone laterally and maxilla medially.

Infraorbital groove or notch

i. It presents near the center of the posterior border of the orbital surface of maxilla.

ii. It leads to infraorbital canal which ends in infraorbital foramen on the anterior surface of maxilla. Transmitting infraorbital vessels and nerve

ix. Medial orbital margin

i. It is ill defined.

ii. It is formed by the frontal maxilla and lacrimal bones.

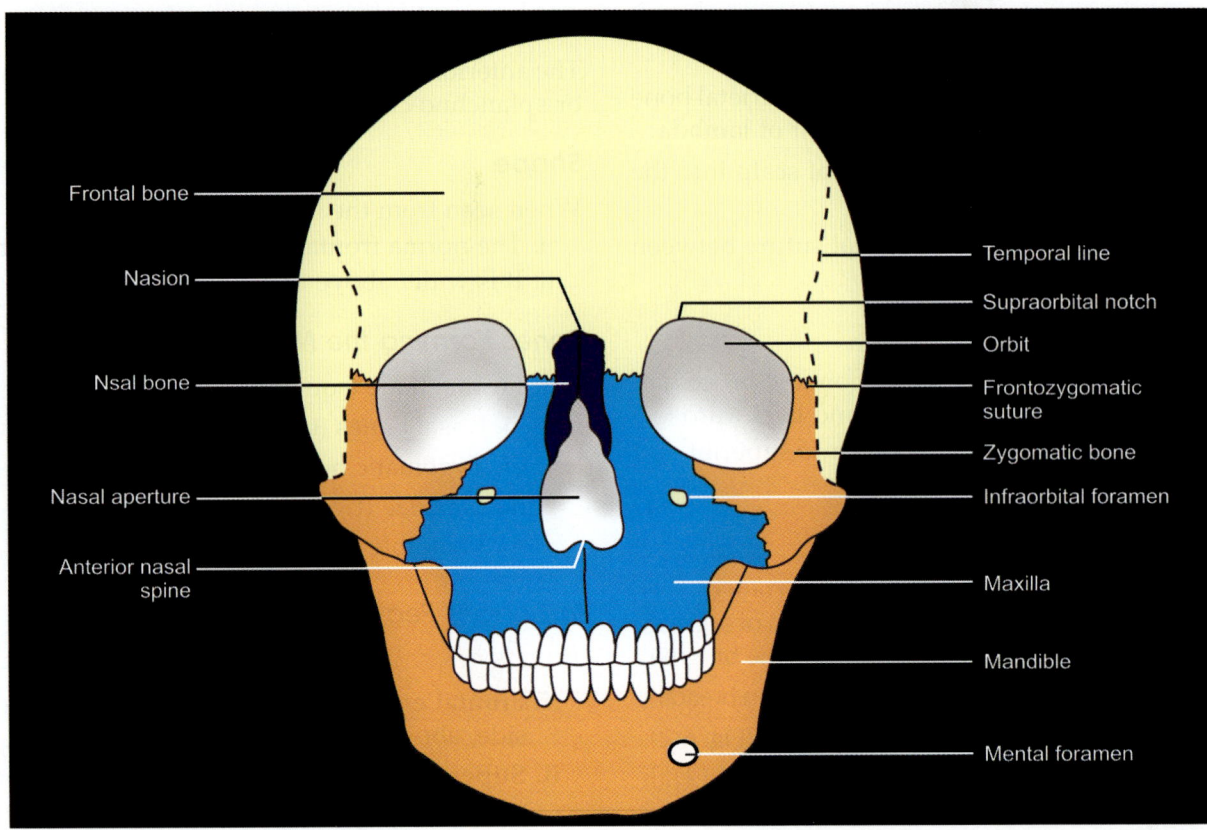

Fig. 6.3: Norma frontalis

x. Lateral orbital margin
   a. It is formed by zygomatic and frontal bones.
   b. Frontozygomatic suture lies at their union.
xi. Anterior bony aperture of the nose
   i. It is pear shaped being wide below and narrow above.
   ii. The lower border of nasal bones above, and below by the nasal notch of the body of maxilla on each side.

Bones Forming the Lower Part of the Face

i. Following processes of maxillae
   a. The frontal process of maxilla
   b. Zygomatic process of maxilla
   c. Alveolar process of maxilla
ii. Zygomatic bone
   a. It forms the prominence of check
   b. Zygomaticofacial foramen is seen on its surface
iii. Anterior surface of body of mandible presents
   a. Symphysis menti
   b. Mental protuberance
   c. Mental tubercles.

Sutures of the Norma Frontalis

i. Internasal
ii. Frontonasal
iii. Nasomaxillary
iv. Lacrimomaxillary
v. Frontomaxillary
vi. Intermaxillary
vii. Zygomaticomaxillary
viii. Zygomaticofrontal.

Important Muscles Presents in Norma Frontalis

i. Corrugator supercilii
ii. Procerus
iii. Orbicularis oculi
iv. Levator labii superioris alaequae nasi
v. Levator anguli oris
vi. Nasalis and depressor septi
vii. Zygomaticus major and minor
viii. Buccinator

Structures Passing through Foramina of Norma Frontalis

i. **Supraorbital foramen transmits:** Supraorbital vessels and nerve.
ii. **Infraorbital foramen transmits:** The infraorbital vessels and nerve.

iii. **Zygomatico-facial foramen transmits:** Zygomaticofacial nerve a branch of maxillary nerve.

iv. **Mental foramen transmits:** Mental nerve and vessels.

NORMA LATERALIS

Bones Taking Part

i. Frontal (Fig. 6.4)

ii. Parietal

iii. Temporal

iv. Occipital

v. Greater wing of sphenoid

vi. Zygomatic

vii. Mandible

viii. Maxilla

iv. Nasal.

Some Important Features

i. **Temporal lines:** Begins from zygomatic process of frontal bone runs upwards and backwards and divides over parietal bone into superior and inferior temporal lines.

ii. **Zygomatic arch:** A bar of bone situated horizontally in front and little above the ear (Fig. 6.4).

iii. **External acoustic meatus:** Situated below the posterior root of zygomatic process.

iv. **Suprameatal triangle:** Triangular depression situated posterosuperior to meatus.

v. **Mastoid part:** Situated behind the meatus.

vi. **Pterion:** It is the meeting point between following bones:

a. Frontal

b. Parietal

c. Greater wing of sphenoid

d. Squamous part of temporal bone.

vii. **Asterion:** Meeting point of three bones, namely parietal, mastoid part of temporal and occipital bones.

viii. **Mastoid process:** Projected part of mastoid portion, behind and below the external acoustic meatus.

ix. **Styloid process:** A bony projection from anteromedial part of mastoid process.

x. **Temporal fossa:** A bony fossa situated on the lateral aspect of skull.

Contents of temporal fossa

i. Temporalis muscle

ii. Deep temporal nerve

iii. Middle temporal vessels

iv. Zygomaticotemporal nerve

v. It communicates with infratemporal fossa through the gap between zygomatic arch and the side of the skull. Structures transmitting through the gap:

a. Tendon of temporalis

b. Deep temporal vessels

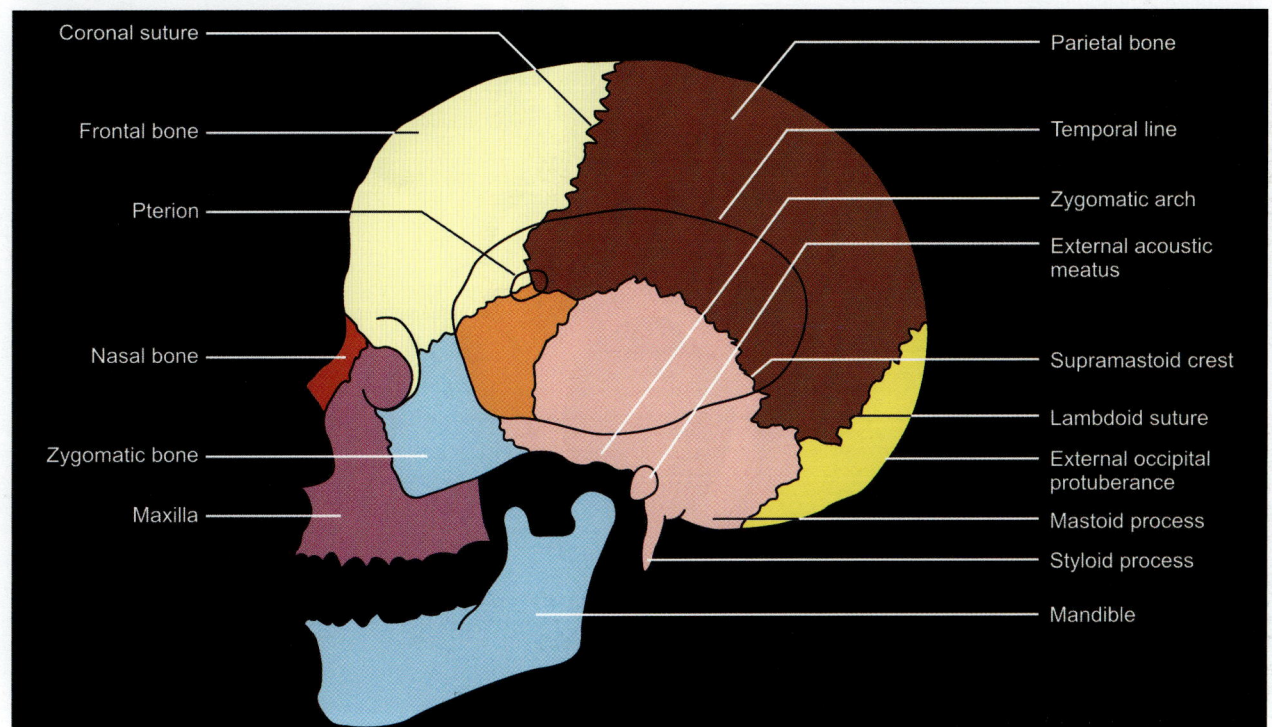

Fig. 6.4: Norma lateralis

c. Deep temporal nerve

d. Zygomaticotemporal vessels and nerve

xi. Infratemporal fossa: An irregular bony space situated below the middle cranial fossa of skull, behind the body of maxilla and lateral to lateral pterygoid plate.

Contents of infratemporal fossa

Muscles

a. Medial pterygoid

b. Lateral pterygoid

c. Buccinator

d. Temporalis.

Nerves

a. Mandibular nerve and its branches

b. Chorda tympani

c. Small part of maxillary nerve.

Ligament: Sphenomandibular ligament.

xii. Pterygopalatine Fossa: A small bony space situated deep to pterygomaxillary fissure.

Contents

a. Third part of maxillary artery and its branches.

b. Maxillary nerve with three branches.

c. Pterygopalatine ganglion with its root and branches.

CLINICAL ANATOMY

Fracture or blow at pterion may rupture the middle meningeal vessels and produce extradural hematoma.

NORMA BASALIS

It is subdivided into three parts—anterior, middle and posterior (Fig. 6.5 and also *see* Fig. 7.2).

Formation

Anterior part is formed by hard palate and the alveolar arches, middle and posterior parts are separated by an imaginary transverse line passing through the anterior margin of the foramen magnum.

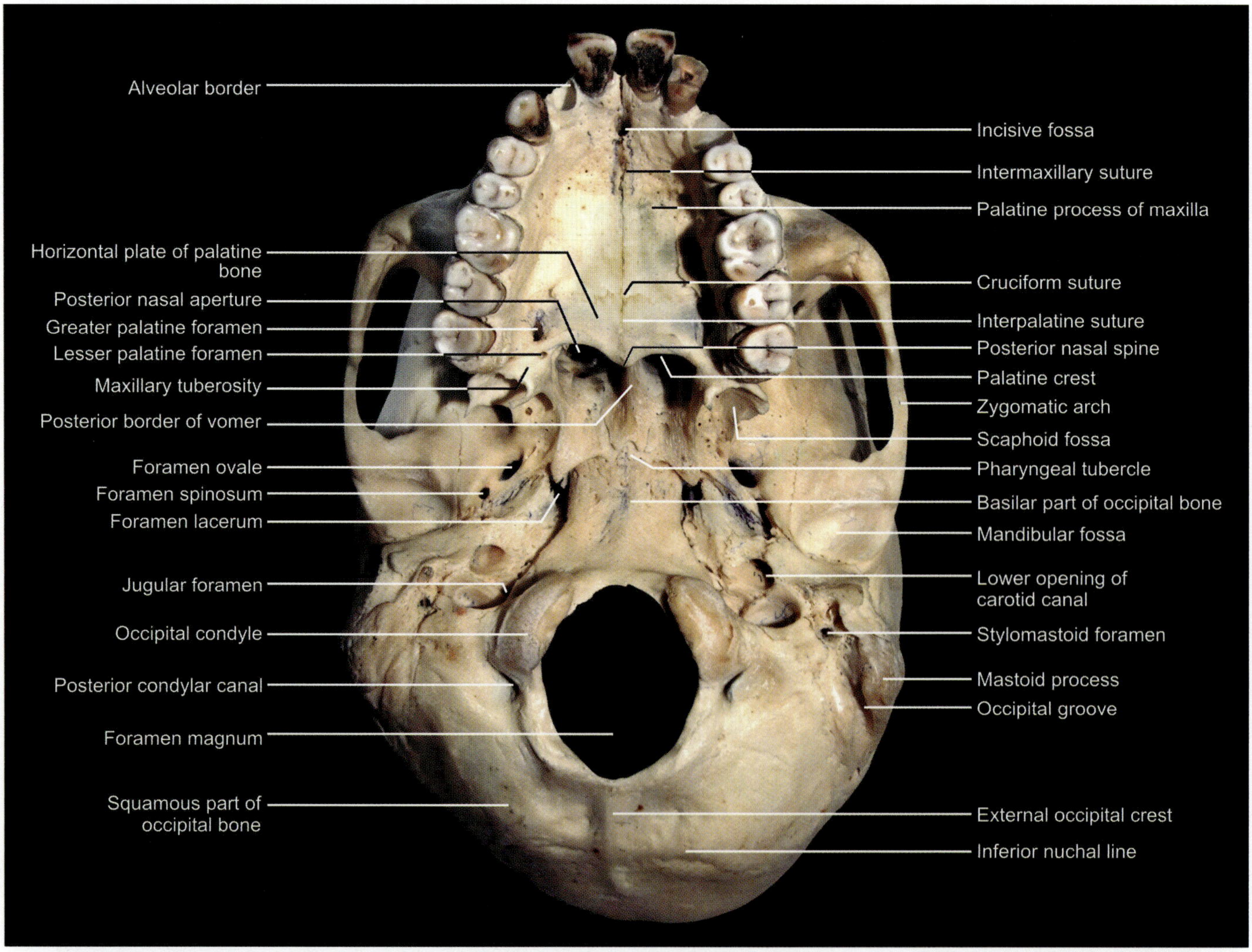

Alveolar border

Incisive fossa

Intermaxillary suture

Palatine process of maxilla

Horizontal plate of palatine bone

Posterior nasal aperture

Greater palatine foramen

Lesser palatine foramen

Maxillary tuberosity

Posterior border of vomer

Cruciform suture

Interpalatine suture

Posterior nasal spine

Palatine crest

Zygomatic arch

Scaphoid fossa

Foramen ovale

Foramen spinosum

Foramen lacerum

Pharyngeal tubercle

Basilar part of occipital bone

Mandibular fossa

Jugular foramen

Occipital condyle

Posterior condylar canal

Foramen magnum

Squamous part of occipital bone

Lower opening of carotid canal

Stylomastoid foramen

Mastoid process

Occipital groove

External occipital crest

Inferior nuchal line

Fig. 6.5: Norma basalis

Features of Anterior Part of Norma Basalis

i. **Alveolar arch:** It bears sockets for the roots of the upper teeth.
ii. Hard palate:
  a. Anterior two-thirds by the palatine processes of maxillae.
  b. Posterior one-third by the horizontal plates of palatine bones (Fig. 6.5).
  c. Sutures:
    – Intermaxillary
    – Interpalatine
    – Palatomaxillary
  d. **Shape:** Arched in all directions and shows pits for palatine glands.
iii. **Incisive fossa:** It is a deep fossa situated anteriorly in the median plane.
iv. **Greater palatine foramen:** It is situated on the posterolateral part.
v. **Lesser palatine foramen:** Number may variable on each side situated behind the greater palatine foramen.
vi. **Posterior nasal spine:** Situated in the median plane of posterior free border of hard palate.
vii. **Palatine crest:** Situated near the posterior border of hard palate.

Features of Middle Part of Norma Basalis: Features of this part may be divided under two headings
i. In the median area
ii. In the lateral areas.

In the median area

i. Posterior border of vomer separating two posterior nasal apertures
ii. Superior border of vomer splits into two alae articulating with rostrum of sphenoid
iii. Palatinovaginal canal formed by vaginal process of medial pterygoid plate with sphenoidal process of palatine bone.
iv. Vomerovaginal canal formed by alae of vomer and vaginal process of medial pterygoid plate
v. Broad bar of bone formed by union of body of sphenoid and basilar part of occipital bones on which present pharyngeal tubercle.

In the lateral area (on each side): It presents following:
i. Pterygoid process and greater wing of sphenoid.
ii. Three parts of temporal bone—Petrous, tympanic and squamous.

Features of pterygoid process
a. Medial and lateral pterygoid plates
b. Pterygoid fossa
c. Pterygoid fissure.

Foramina present in the part of greater wing
a. Foramen ovale
b. Foramen spinosum
c. Emissary sphenoidal foramen or foramen of Vesalius
d. Sometimes canaliculus innominatus

Inferior surface of petrous part of temporal bone
i Foramen lacerum lies behind near the apex of petrous part
ii Carotid canal the apex, transmits
  a. Internal carotid artery
  b. Vein and sympathetic plexus around artery.
iii. Rough anterior part—**origin of** levator palatini.
iv. Squamo-tympanic fissure with projected tegmen tympani within it.

Inferior surface of tympanic part
i. It forms a sheath of styloid process (Fig. 6.15).
ii. Its upper curved part forms anterior wall, floor and lower part of posterior wall of the external acoustic meatus.
iii. It forms non-articular part of mandibular fossa containing a part of the parotid gland.

Features of Posterior Part of Norma Basalis
Median area presents from before backwards
i. Foramen magnum (Fig. 6.5)
ii. External occipital crest
iii. External occipital protuberance

Lateral area on each side presents
i. Condylar part of occipital bone
ii. Squamous part of occipital bone
iii. Jugular foramen
iv. Styloid process of temporal bones
v. Mastoid part of temporal bones
vi. Alar ligament which is attached on the medial sides of tubercles of occipital condyles by which foramen magnum is divided into two compartments.
  a. Anterior compartment or osseoligamentous compartment.
  b. Posterior compartment or neurovascular compartment.
vi. The middle part of the anterior margin of the foramen magnum is known as basion.

NORMA OCCIPITALIS
Formation
i. Posterior part of parietal bones above
ii. Upper part of squamous part of occipital bone below (Fig. 6.6)
iii. Mastoid part of the temporal bones on each side

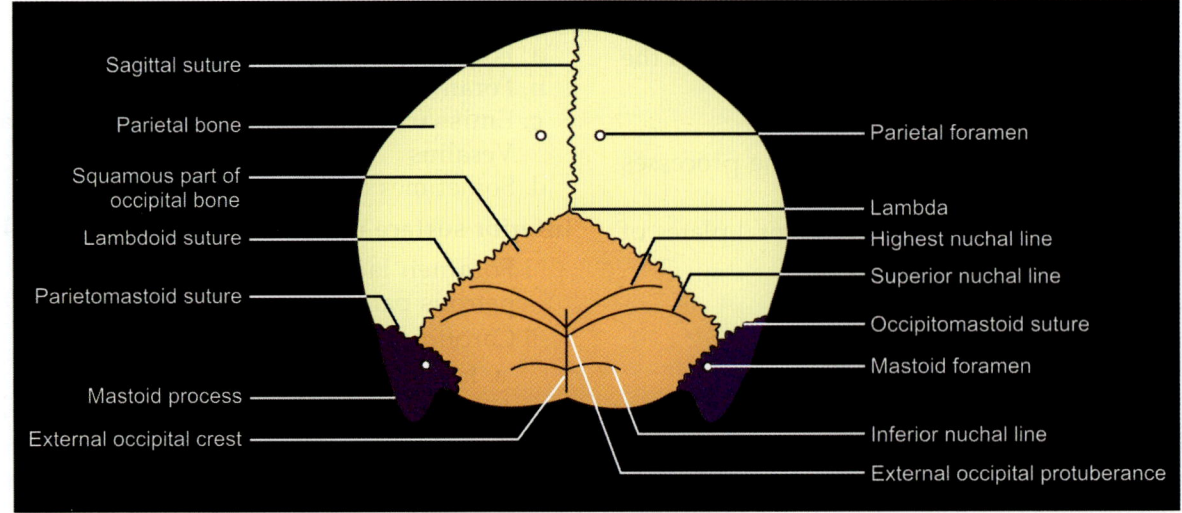

Fig. 6.6: Norma occipitalis

Sutures

i. **Lambdoid suture:** The lambdoid suture lies between the occipital bone and the parietal bones.

ii. **Posterior part of sagittal suture:** Between the two parietal bones.

iii. **Occipitomastoid suture:** It lies between the occipital bone and the mastoid part of temporal bone.

iv. **Parietomastoid suture:** It lies between the parietal bone and mastoid part of temporal bone.

Important Features (Fig. 6.6)

i. **External occipital protuberance**

   a. It is a median prominence at the junction between the lambda and the foramen magnum.

   b. The most prominent point on this protuberance is called the inion

ii. **Highest nuchal lines:** They are curved bony ridges situated about 1 cm above the superior nuchal lines.

iii. **Superior nuchal lines:** These are the curved bony ridges passing laterally from the external occipital protuberance to lateral angle of occipital bone.

iv. **Inferior nuchal lines:** They are curved bony lines running laterally from the middle of the external occipital crest to jugular process of occipital bone.

Muscles and ligaments attached

i. To external occipital protuberance: Ligamentum nuchae.

ii. To the superior nuchal line

   a. **Origin of** trapezius (medial one-third).

   b. **Insertion of** sternocleidomastoid (lateral two-thirds).

iii. To the highest nasal line.

Attachments: Epicranial aponeurosis or galea aponeurotica.

CLINICAL ANATOMY

i. **Fractures of the skull:** Fractures of the skull are common in the adult but much less in young.

   a. **In adult:** A severe localized blow produced a local indentation often accompanied by splintering of the bone.

   Blows to the vault often result in a series of linear fractures.

   b. **Pond fracture (in young):** It is like a table tennis ball. A localized blow produced a depression without splintering.

ii. **Common sites of fracture of skull**

   a. In the vault—parietal area

   b. In the base of the skull the bones forming the middle cranial fossa due to presence of numerous foramina and canals weaken the bones.

   c. Inner table of the skull bones are more commonly fractured because it is more brittle than the outer table.

   d. The most common facial fractures involve the nasal bones, then zygomatic bone and then the mandible.

iii. **Depressed fracture**

   a. It is caused by hard blows to the head in thin area of the cranium

   b. In this fracture a fragment of bone is depressed inward to compress or injure the brain

iv. **Linear skull fractures:** It is the most common type of skull fracture, but fracture line often radiates away from it in two or more directions.

v. **Comminuted fractures**

a. In this type of fracture the bone is broken into several pieces.

b. Although, a fracture may result some distance from the site of direct trauma where the calvaria is thinner.

vi. **Counterblow fracture:** In this fracture no fracture occurs at the point of impact but fracture occurs on the opposite side of the skull.

INNER SURFACE OF THE SKULL

The inner surface of the skull is divided into two broad surfaces by an imaginary horizontal plane at the level of glabella.

i. Roof is formed by inner surface of vault of the skull or calvaria

ii. Floor is formed by inner aspect of base of skull, known as cranial fossae.

These two surfaces are continuous each other anteriorly, posteriorly and laterally.

CALVARIA

Internal surface of cranial vault is formed by only squamous part four bones.

i. Anteriorly: Squamous part of frontal bone

ii. In the middle: Squamous part of two parietal bones.

iii. Posteriorly: Squamous part of occipital bone

iv. On all sides: The outer margin of the vault is ill defined and continuous with the cranial fossa.

Inner aspect of vault presents following features

i. Coronal suture

ii. Sagittal suture

iii. Lambdoid suture

iv. Cerebral grooves and impressions for cerebral gyri.

v. Many vascular impressions including most prominently visible impression for meningeal vessels.

vi. Anteromedian frontal creast—it is formed by attachment of falx cerebri.

vii. Granular fovea situated on the either side of sagittal suture

viii. Parietal foramina situated on either side of the sagittal suture to transmit emissary vein.

CRANIAL FOSSAE

It is further divided into three fossae:

i. **Anterior cranial fossa:** It is at the highest horizontal level (Fig. 6.7).

ii. **Middle cranial fossa:** It is at a mid-plane between anterior and posterior cranial fossae.

iii. **Posterior cranial fossa:** It is at the lowest horizontal plane among the three.

ANTERIOR CRANIAL FOSSA

Boundaries

Anteriorly: Squamous part of the frontal bone including frontal air sinuses (Fig. 6.8).

Posteriorly: Medial to lateral

i. Aanterior margin of sulcus chiasmaticus

ii. Anterior clinoid process

iii. Posterior border of lesser wings of sphenoid bone.

Bones Forming Anterior Cranial Fossa

i. **Frontal bone**

a. **Anterior aspect** formed by orbital plate of the frontal bone.

b. **Sides and front wall** formed by squamous part of the frontal bone.

Table 6.1 shows difference between male and female skulls

Table 6.1	Difference between male and female skulls	
Male skull	**Female skull**
i. **Bones**—thicker	i. **Bones**—thinner and lighter
ii. **Cranial cavity**—more	ii. **Cranial cavity**—less
iii. **Muscular impressions and ridges**—more prominent	iii. **Muscular impressions and ridges**—less prominent
iv. **Superciliary arches**—prominent	iv. **Superciliary arches**—less prominent
v. **Mastoid process**—prominent	v. **Mastoid process**—less prominent
vi. **Frontal and parietal tubers**—less prominent	vi. **Frontal and parietal tubers**—prominent.

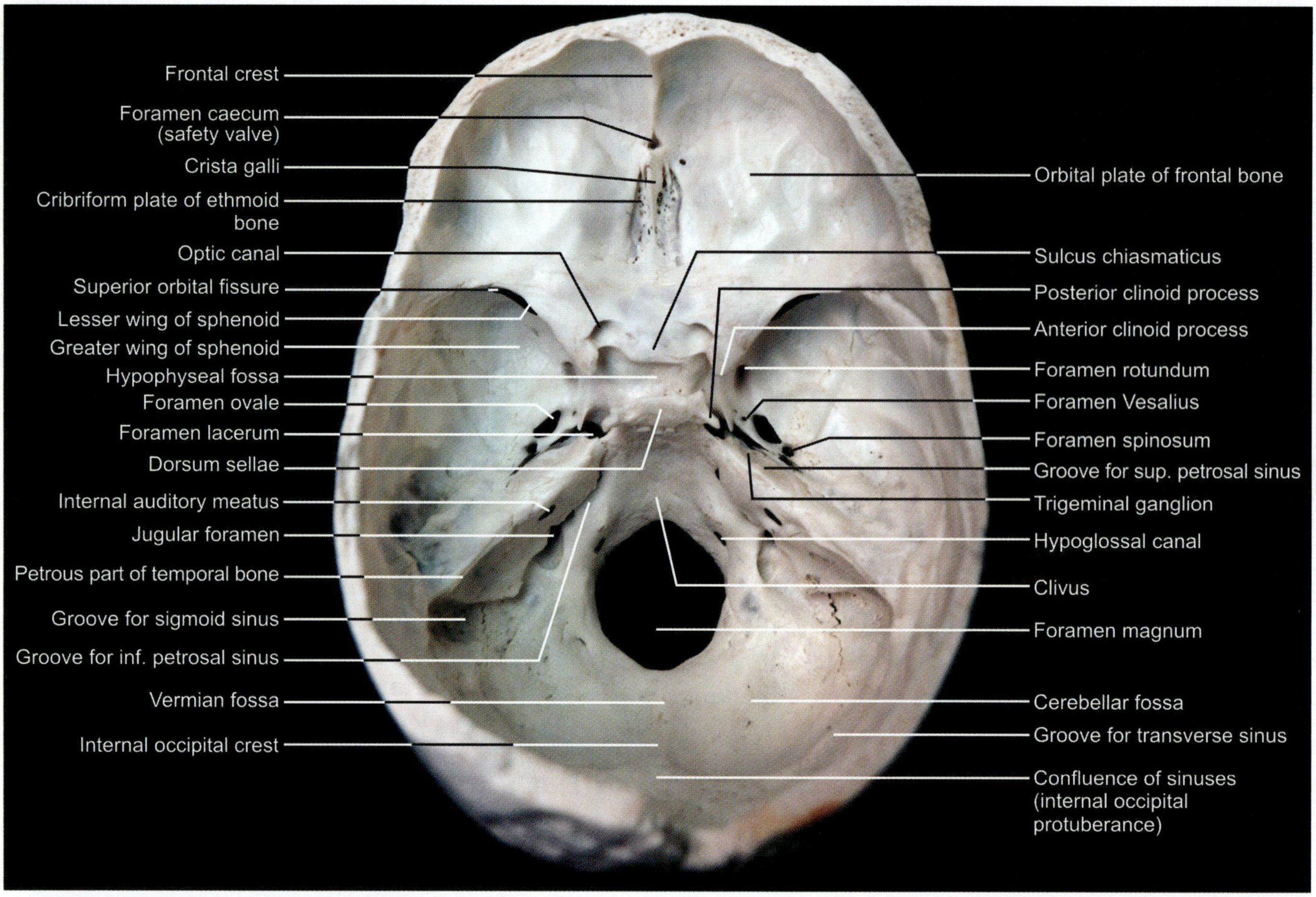

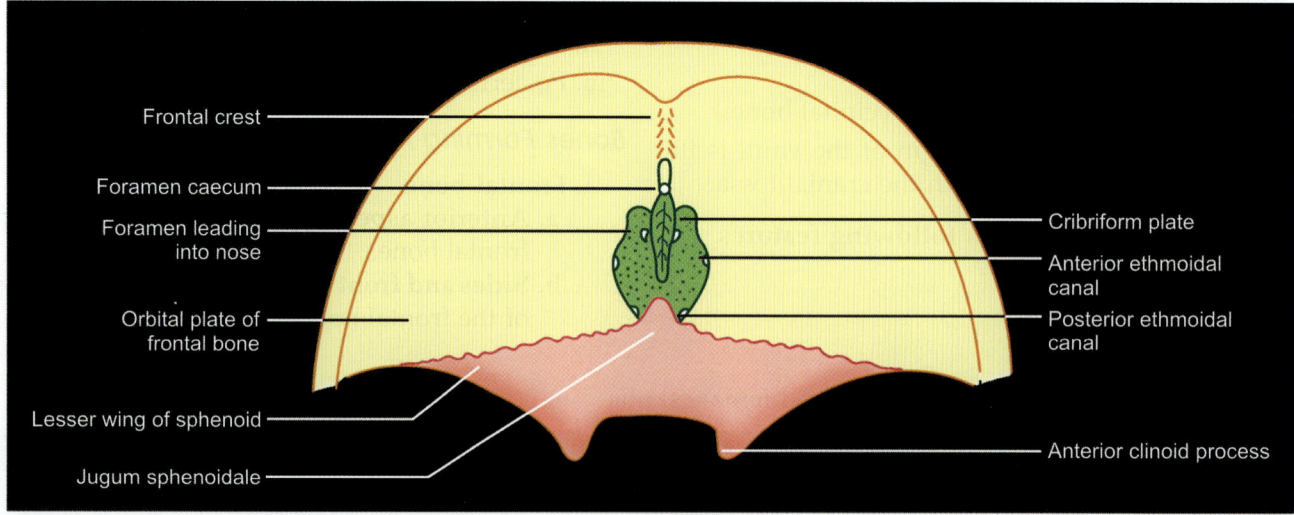

Frontal crest

Foramen caecum (safety valve)

Crista galli

Cribriform plate of ethmoid bone

Optic canal

Superior orbital fissure

Lesser wing of sphenoid

Greater wing of sphenoid

Hypophyseal fossa

Foramen ovale

Foramen lacerum

Dorsum sellae

Internal auditory meatus

Jugular foramen

Petrous part of temporal bone

Groove for sigmoid sinus

Groove for inf. petrosal sinus

Vermian fossa

Internal occipital crest

Orbital plate of frontal bone

Sulcus chiasmaticus

Posterior clinoid process

Anterior clinoid process

Foramen rotundum

Foramen Vesalius

Foramen spinosum

Groove for sup. petrosal sinus

Trigeminal ganglion

Hypoglossal canal

Clivus

Foramen magnum

Cerebellar fossa

Groove for transverse sinus

Confluence of sinuses (internal occipital protuberance)

Fig. 6.7: Interior of the skull showing the cranial fossae

Frontal crest

Foramen caecum

Foramen leading into nose

Orbital plate of frontal bone

Lesser wing of sphenoid

Jugum sphenoidale

Cribriform plate

Anterior ethmoidal canal

Posterior ethmoidal canal

Anterior clinoid process

Fig. 6.8: Features on the anterior cranial fossa

ii. Ethmoid bone with two features: Cribriform plate of ethmoid bone forms roof of the nasal cavity. A median triangular process known as crista galli projects upwards from the cribriform plate.

Foramen caecum lies between the crista galli and the frontal crest.

iii. Sphenoid bone: Jugum sphenoidale forms the posterior aspect and lesser wings of sphenoid bone.

Fractures of the anterior cranial fossa may cause escape of CSF into the nasal cavity, resulting in CSF rhinorrhea or blood may collect into roof of the orbital cavity producing black eye.

MIDDLE CRANIAL FOSSA

Boundaries

i. **Anteriorly:** It is bounded by posterior border of lesser wings of sphenoid..
ii. **Posteriorly:** By dorsum sellae of sphenoid and petrous part of the temporal bone.
iii. **Laterally:** By squamous parts of temporal bones, parietal bones and greater wings of sphenoid bone.

Bones Forming Middle Cranial Fossa

Median part: By the body sphenoid bone.

Lateral parts: By the cranial surface of the greater wings of sphenoid, inner surface of squamus part and anterior surface of petrous part of temporal bones.

Body of the sphenoid: It has following features—

i. **Optic groove or sulcus chiasmaticus:** It lies posterior to the jugum sphenoidale which is a transverse groove.

   Lodges: Optic chiasma.
ii. **Optic canal:** It transmits the following structures
   a. optic nerve
   b. Meningeal sheath of optic nerve
   c. Ophthalmic artery.
iii. **Sella turcica:** From before backwords it is made up of following structures

a. Tuberculum sellae
b. Hypophyseal fossa
c. Dorsum sellae.

iv. **Carotid groove:** For internal carotid artery

Openings of the Middle Cranial Fossa (Fig. 6.9)

i. Foramen rotundrum transmits maxillary nerve
ii. Foramen ovale transmits mandibular nerve
iii. Foramen spinosum transmits middle meningeal artery and corresponding vein.
iv. Foramen lacerum internal carotid artery with accompanying sympathetic plexus.
v. Hiatus for greater petrosal nerve at tegmen tympani
vi. Hiatus for lesser petrosal nerve at tegmen tympani.

i. Due to close relationship of the middle ear and mastoid antrum to the middle cranial fossa. It is responsible for spread of infection to the cranial cavity in middle ear infection and mastoiditis.
ii. Fracture of the middle cranial fossa involving tegmen tympani (roof of the middle ear) may produce bleeding and escape of CSF through ear.
iii. The middle cranial fossa is commonly fractured because presence of numerous foramina and canals weaken the bones.

POSTERIOR CRANIAL FOSSA

It is situated at the lowest level among the three fossae. It is the largest (Fig. 6.10).

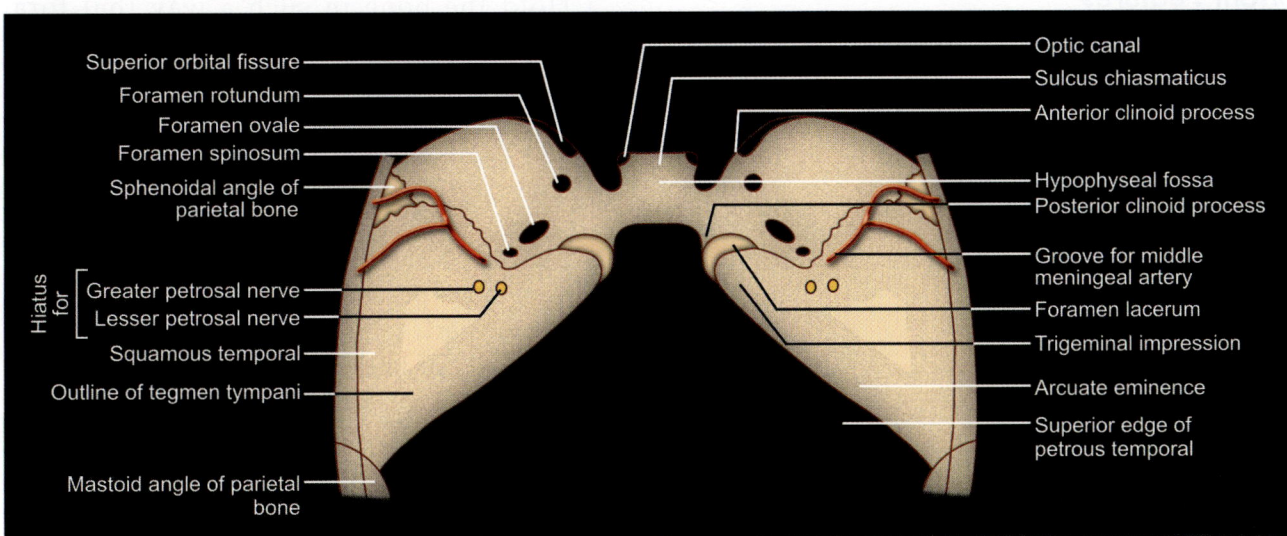

Fig. 6.9: Features on the middle cranial fossa

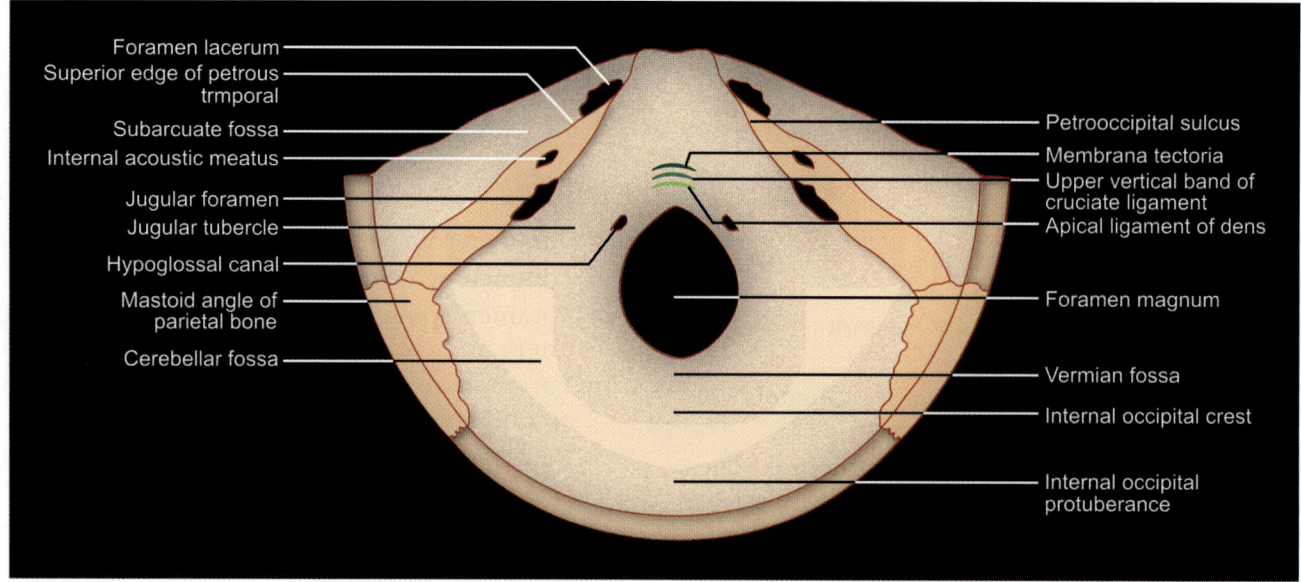

Fig. 6.10: Features on the posterior cranial fossa

Boundaries

Anteriorly

i. Upper border of petrous parts of the temporal bone on either side.

ii. Dorsum sellae of sphenoid bone.

Posteriorly: Squamous part of the occipital bone.

Laterally

i. Mastoid part of the temporal bone

ii. Mastoid angle of the parietal bone.

BONES FORMING MIDDLE CRANIAL FOSSA

Sphenoid, occipital, temporal and posteroinferior angles of parietal bones.

Important Features

i. Internal acuoustic meatus

ii. Foramen magnum

iii. Jugular foramen

iv. Facial canal—it transmits facial nerve through petrous part of temporal bone.

v. Tractus spiralis foraminosus

vi. Transverse creast

vii. Inferior vestibular area

viii. Foramen singular.

ix. Internal occipital protuberance

x. Internal occipital crest

xi. Transverse sulcus

xii. Sigmoid sulcus

xiii. Hypoglossal canal

xiv. Condylar canal.

CLINICAL ANATOMY

Fracture of the posterior cranial fossa causes extravasation of blood in the suboccipital region and a swelling appears at the upper part of the back of the neck.

OCCIPITAL BONE

INTRODUCTION

It is situated at the posteroinferior part of the skull

Shape: Trapezoid in shape.

ANATOMICAL POSITION

i. Hold the bone in such a way that foramen magnum in horizontal plane.

ii. The basilar part of the bone is directed forward and upward.

iii. The squamous part will be behind and above with convexity backwards and concavity forwards.

PARTS

i. Squamous part

ii. Basilar part

iii. Condylar or lateral parts.

SQUAMOUS PART

a. **Surfaces:** External and internal.

b. **Angles:** Superior and two lateral angels.

c. **Borders:** Lambdoid and mastoid.

External Surface

Following features present (Fig. 6.11):

i. **External occipital protuberance and inion:** It presents a prominence known as external occipital protuberance and forms an important bony landmark known as inion.
  Attachment: Ligamentum nuchae.

ii. **External occipital crest:** From external occipital protuberance it descends downwards along the median plane up to the posterior margin of foramen magnum.
  Attachment: Ligamentum nuchae.

iii. **Highest nuchal line:** It is arched less prominent line extends lateralward from external occipital protuberance.
  Attachment: Galea aponeurotica or epicranial aponeurosis.

iv. **Superior nuchal line:** From the external occipital protuberance extends lateralward below the highest nuchal line (more marked).
  Attachments
  Medially: Origin of trapezius.
  Laterally (Fig. 6.12)
  a. Origin of: Occipital belly of occipitofrontalis.
  b. Below, it insertions of: Sternocleidomastoid and splenius capitis.

v. The area in between superior and inferior nuchal lines.
  Insertion of (Fig. 6.12)
  a. Obliquus capitis superior: Laterally.
  b. Semispinalis capitis: Medially.

vi. **Inferior nuchal line:** It is another arched line extends laterally from the middle of external occipital crest.

vii. The inferior nuchal line and area below it:
  Laterally: Insertion of rectus capitis posterior major.
  Medially: Insertion of rectus capitis posterior minor.

viii. **Planum occipitale:** The portion above the external occipital protuberance and highest nuchal lines is smooth called planum occipitale which is covered by galea aponeurotica (epicranial aponeurosis).

ix. **Planum nuchale:** Remaining portion of the external surface is rough for muscular attachments.

x. Posterolateral margins of the foramen magnum
  Attachment: Posterior atlanto-occipital membrane.

Internal Surface

Following features present (Fig. 6.13):

i. **Internal occipital protuberance:** The internal surface is deeply concave and is divided into four fossae by a cruciate eminence known as internal occipital protuberance.
  a. Upper fossae: The upper two fossae are triangular for the lodgments of posterior lobes of cerebral hemispheres.
  b. Lower fossae: The lower two fossae are quadrilateral in shape, occupied by cerebellum.

ii. **Sagittal sulcus:** This sulcus extends upwards from internal occipital protuberance.
  Lodges: Superior sagittal sinus and margins of the sulcus gives attachment falx cerebri.

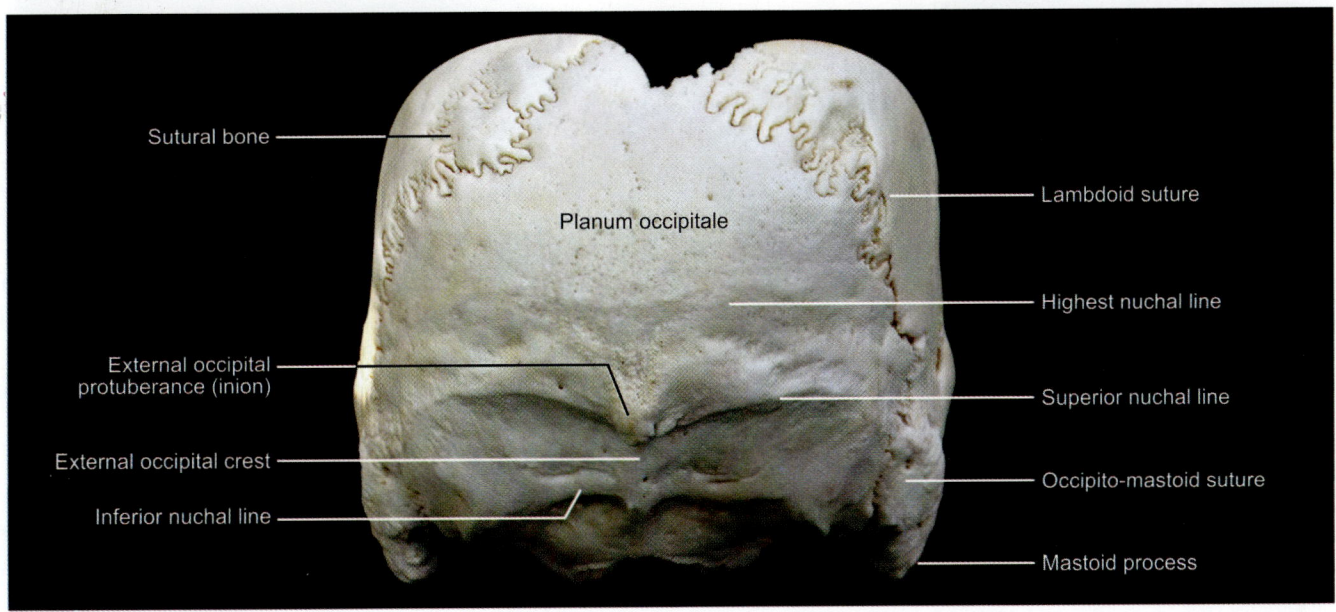

Fig. 6.11: Occipital bone external surface

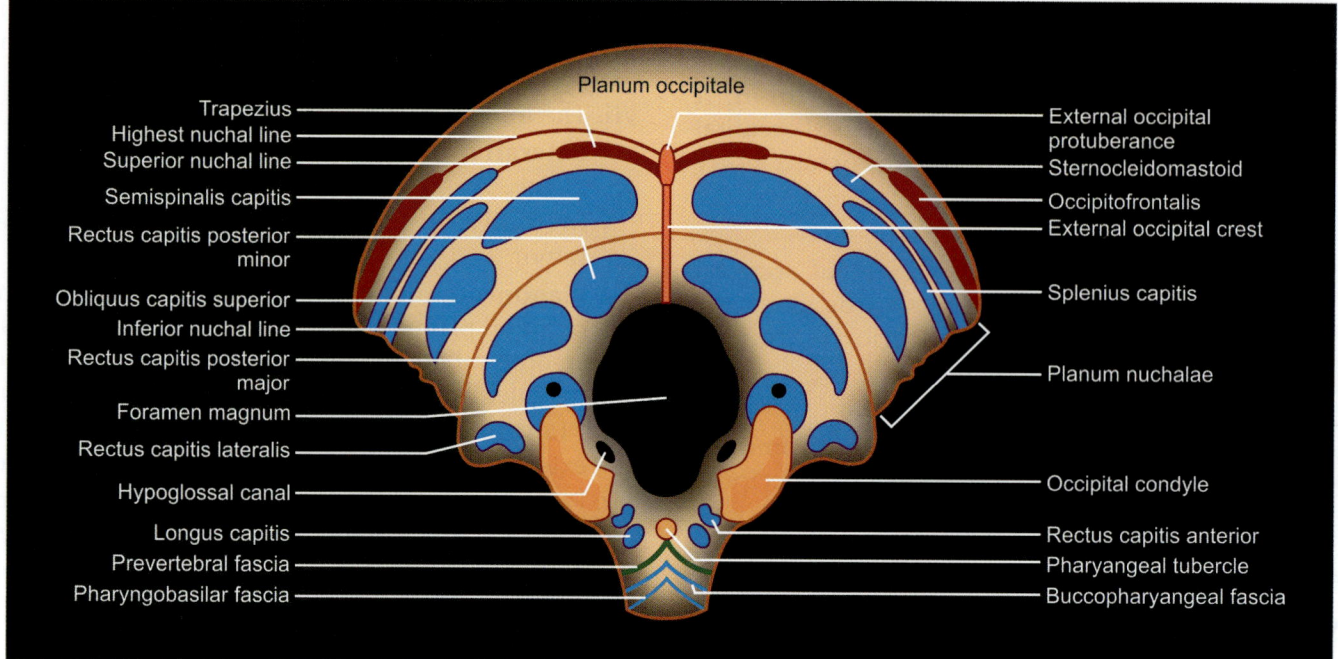

Fig. 6.12: Attachments of external surface of occipital bone

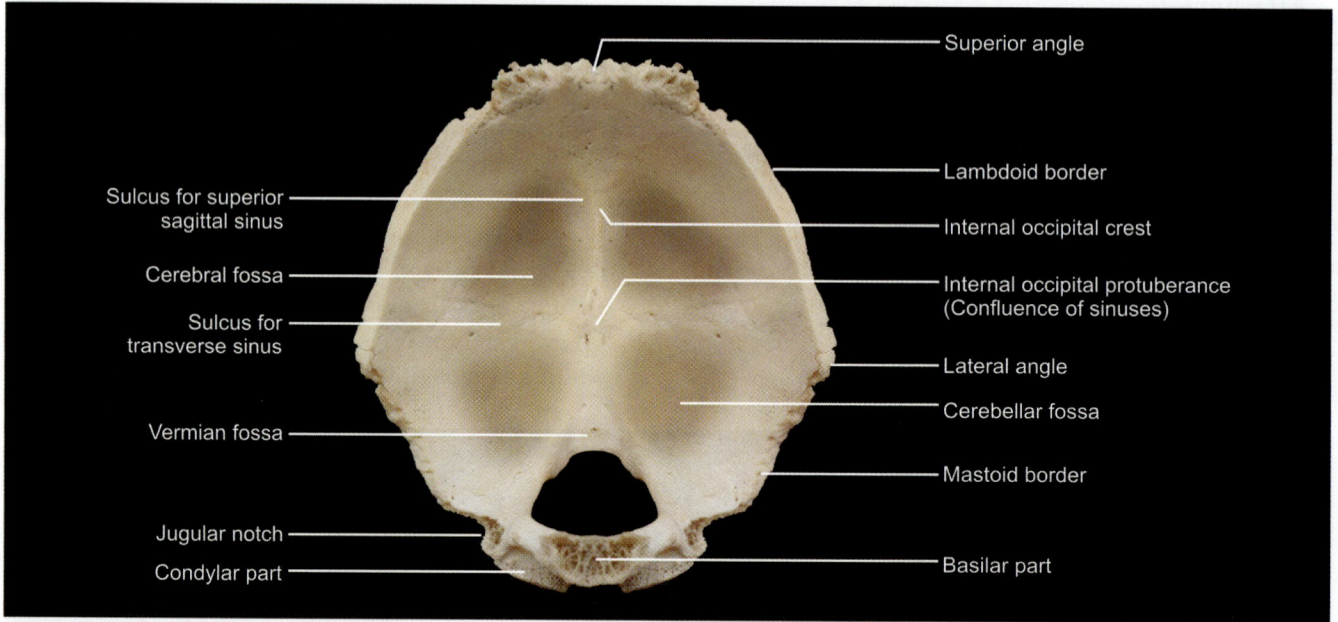

Fig. 6.13: Occipital bone internal surface

iii. Internal occipital crest: A ridge from the internal occipital protuberance runs downwards and forwards, towards foramen magnum.

Attachments

Falx cerebelli: In between the two layers of falx cerebelli lodges occipital sinus.

iv. Vermian fossa: Near the posterior margin of foramen magnum, there is a depression at the lower part of the internal occipital crest, called vermian fossa.

Lodges: Inferior vermis of cerebellum.

v. Transverse sulcus: Extends from the internal occipital protuberance runs lateralward horizontally.

Lodges: Transverse sinus.

Attachments: Margins of the groove-tentorium cerebelli.

vi. Confluence of sinuses

Situation: The right transverse sulcus is continuous with the superior sagittal sulcus and the point of union between the two presents a depression.

Lodges: Confluence of sinuses

vii. Formation confluences of sinuses: It is formed by the union of sagittal sinus and right transverse sinus, the occipital sinus and straight sinus opens into the confluence of sinuses here.

viii. Superior angle: It is the summit of squamous part by the union of two lambdoid borders.
Articulation: With the posterosuperior angles of parietal bones.

ix. Lateral angles: Placed at the lateral ends of transverse sulci.

x. Lambdoid border: It extends from superior angle to lateral angle.
Articulation: With the occipital border of parietal bone.

xi. Mastoid border: It extends from lateral angle to the jugular process.
Articulation: Mastoid part of temporal bone

BASILAR PART

It projects upwards and forwards from the foramen magnum.
Surfaces: Anterior, superior and inferior.
Borders: Lateral and posterior.

Anterior Surface

i. Rough, quadrilateral in shape
ii. Articulates with the body of sphenoid by a plate-like cartilage
iii. Become ossified with sphenoid bone at twentyfifth year of life

Superior surface: Smooth and hollowed out called clivus.

Lodges

i. Lower part of the pons and the medulla oblongata
ii. On either side close to the lateral margin sulcus for inferior petrosal sinus
iii. Two inferior petrosal sinuses unites on the superior surface of basilar part by the basilar sinus

Attachments

The posterior part of surface close to the margin of foramen magnum gives attachment to the following structures from above downwards and backwards.

i. Membrana tectoria—it is the continuation of the posterior longitudinal ligament of vertebral column
ii. Upper band of cruciate ligament of Atlas
iii. Apical ligament
iv. Anterior atlanto-occipital membrane

Inferior surface: It is rough, on the median plane presence of pharyngeal tubercle.

Attachments

i. Fibrous raphe of the pharynx to the pharyngeal tubercle.
ii. **Insertion of longus capitis:** On either side of the tubercle (Fig. 6.12).
iii. **insertion of rectus capitis anterior:** In front of the condyle.

Lateral borders

Articulation: With the petrous part of temporal bone.

Posterior border: Its posterior margin is formed the anterior margin of foramen magnum.
Attachment: Anterior atlanto-occipital membrane.

CONDYLAR OR LATERAL PART

Situation: On either side of the foramen magnum connects squamous part with basilar part.

Following features present

i. **Articular surface:** Inferiorly each condyle presents a convex articular surface.
Articulation: With superior articular facet of Atlas forming atlanto-occipital joint.

ii. **Hypoglossal canal:** Immediately above the anterior end of each condyle presents the anterior opening of hypoglossal canal.
Structures transmit: *See* foramina of skull.

iii. **Condylar fossa**
i. Behind the posterior end of each condyle on inferior surface presents of a depression called condylar fossa to receives the superior facet of atlas when the head is bent backwards
ii. Sometimes condylar fossa is perforated by condylar canal.
Structures transmit: *See* foramina of skull

iv. **Tuberculum jugulare:** It is a rounded eminence on the superior surface of the condylar part which bridges across the hypoglossal canal.

v. **Groove on the posterior part of the tuberculum jugulare**
Lodges
a. Glossopharyngeal, vagus and accessory nerves.
b. Medial aspect of the condyles presents a rough area or a tubercle attachment to alar ligament.

vi. **Jugular process**
a. At the junction of the condylar and squamous parts there is a short process projects laterally known as jugular process.

b. It consists of superior, inferior, anterior and lateral surfaces.

c. **Superior surface:** Presents a curved groove, lodges the terminal part of sigmoid sinus.

d. **Inferior surface:** It is rough and receives insertion of rectus capitis lateralis.

e. **Anterior surface:** The anterior surface of jugular process presents a notch known as jugular notch, which articulates with the petrous part of temporal bone forming the jugular foramen.

f. **Lateral surface:** It articulates with the inferior aspect of the petrous part of the temporal bone.

vii. **Jugular foramen:** It is divided into anterior, posterior, and intermediate compartments by two bony spicules known as intrajugular processes.

Structures transmit: *See* foramina of skull

viii. **Foramen magnum**

a. It is bounded anteriorly by the basilar part, posteriorly by the squamous part and laterally by the condylar part.

b. The alar ligament divides the foramen into smaller anterior and larger posterior compartments.

Structures transmit: *See* **foramina of skull**

OSSIFICATION

i. The condylar portion of occipital bone fuses with the squamous part at 3rd year and with basi-occipital at 5th year.

ii. The basioccipital fuses with the besisphenoid at about 20th–25th years, helps in age determination.

CLINICAL ANATOMY

Fractures occur in the squamous part of occipital bone may produce bleeding in the back of the neck muscles.

TEMPORAL BONE

INTRODUCTION

i. It lies at the sides and base of the skull.

ii. The organ of hearing is situated within the petrous part of the bone.

Type: Pneumatic irregular bone.

ANATOMICAL POSITION

i. Expanded and thin squamus part of the bone directed anterosuperiorly.

ii. Zygomatic process looks forward.

iii. Petrous part is directed upward, forward and medially.

iv. Thick mastoid part occupies the posterior part of the bone.

v. External auditory meatus lies on the lateral aspect of the bone.

SIDE DETERMINATIONS

After holding the bone in anatomical position the external auditory meatus will determine the side of the bone.

PARTS (Fig. 6.14)

i. **Anatomically**

a. Squamous

b. Mastoid

c. Petrous part and styloid process.

d. Tympanic

ii. **Morphologically**

a. Petromastoid (ossified in membrane)

b. Rest of the parts (ossified in cartilage).

SQUAMOUS PART

It is a thin plate of bone projects upward and forward, and forms the side of skull

Surfaces: External and internal.

Borders: Superior and anteroinferior.

External Surface (Fig. 6.15)

i. It forms the greater part of the temporal fossa which gives origin to temporalis muscle.

ii. A vertical groove runs upward just above the external auditory meatus for the middle temporal artery.

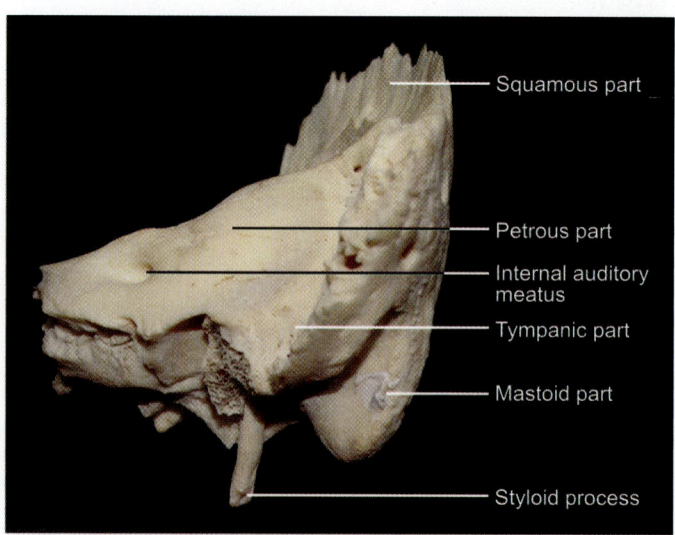

Fig. 6.14: Parts of the right temporal bone

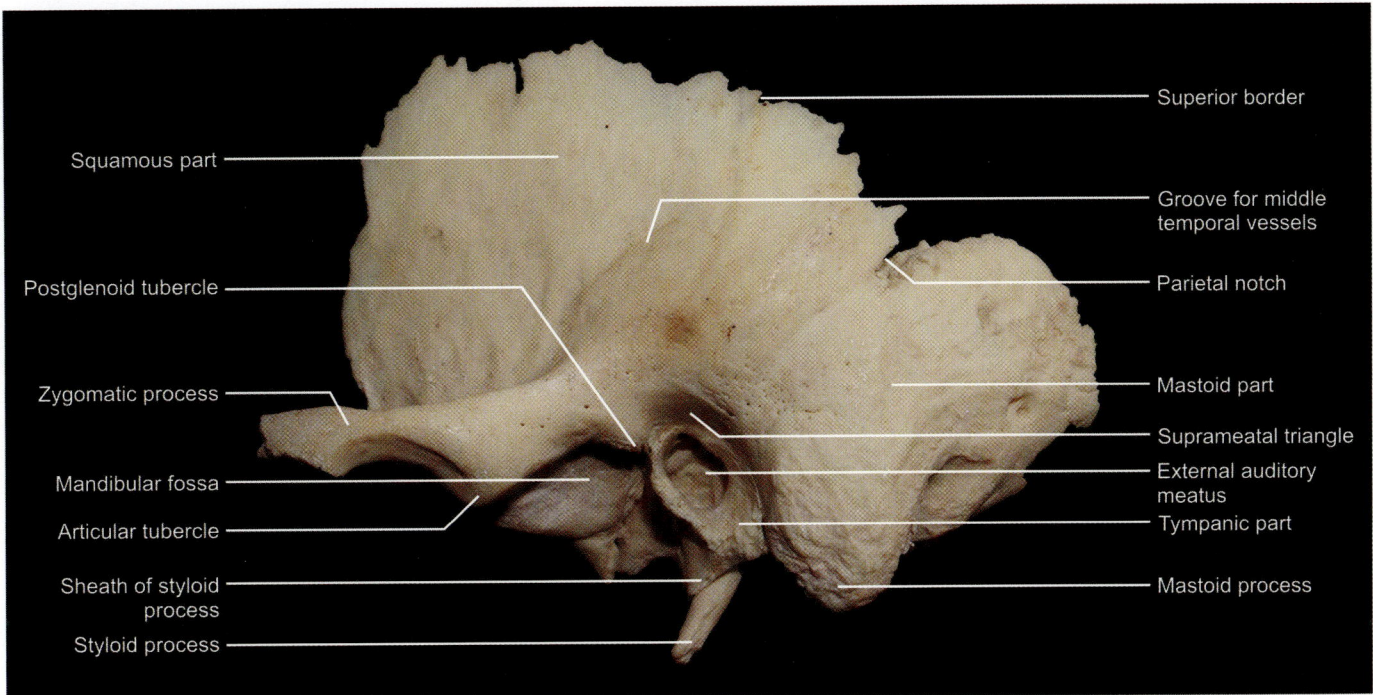

Squamous part

Postglenoid tubercle

Zygomatic process

Mandibular fossa

Articular tubercle

Sheath of styloid process

Styloid process

Superior border

Groove for middle temporal vessels

Parietal notch

Mastoid part

Suprameatal triangle

External auditory meatus

Tympanic part

Mastoid process

Fig. 6.15: Left temporal bone, external aspect

Features of external surface

i. **Supramastoid crest:** It is a curved ridge, passes backwards, and upwards which limits the lower boundary of the temporal surface.
Attachment: Temporal fascia.

ii. **Suprameatal triangle:** A triangular depression at the posterosuperior part of external auditory meatus.

iii. **Suprameatal spine:** A bony projection in front of the suprameatal triangle.

iv. **External auditory meatus:** It is present on the most anterior part of the squamous part.

v. **Zygomatic process**
a. It is an elongated bony process from the lower and anterior parts of temporal surface.
b. It consists of two roots, anterior and posterior and an elongated anterior part.
Articulation: Anterior end of the zygomatic process articulates with temporal process of zygomatic bone to complete the zygomatic arch.

vi. **Roots (anterior and posterior):** Two roots unite to form a tubercle known as tubercle of the root of zygoma attachment of lateral temporomandibular ligament.

vii. **Anterior portion of the zygomatic process:** It consists of two surfaces two borders and anterior extremity.
Lateral surface: Convex and subcutaneous.
Medial surface: Concave with origin of masseter.

Superior border
Attachment: Temporal fascia and galea aponeurotica.
Inferior border: It is rough with origin of masseter muscle.
Anterior extremity: It is serrated, articulates with the temporal process of zygomatic bone.

viii. **Mandibular fossa:** It is a depression formed in front by the squamous part which is articular and behind by the tympanic part which is non-articular.
Articular part: It is deeply concave.
Articulation: Condyle (head) of mandible with an intervening articular disc forming temporo-mandibular joint.
Nonarticular part: Occupied by a portion of parotid gland.

ix. **Postglenoid tubercle:** Laterally articular part is separated from the non-articular part by a small conical eminence, called postglenoid tubercle.

x. **Squamotympanic fissure:** It is present between the squamous part in front and tympanic part behind.

Internal Surface/cerebal Surface

It is concave and marked by irregular impressions caused by gyri of the cerebrum and presents grooves for the anterior and posterior divisions of middle meningeal artery (Fig. 6.16).

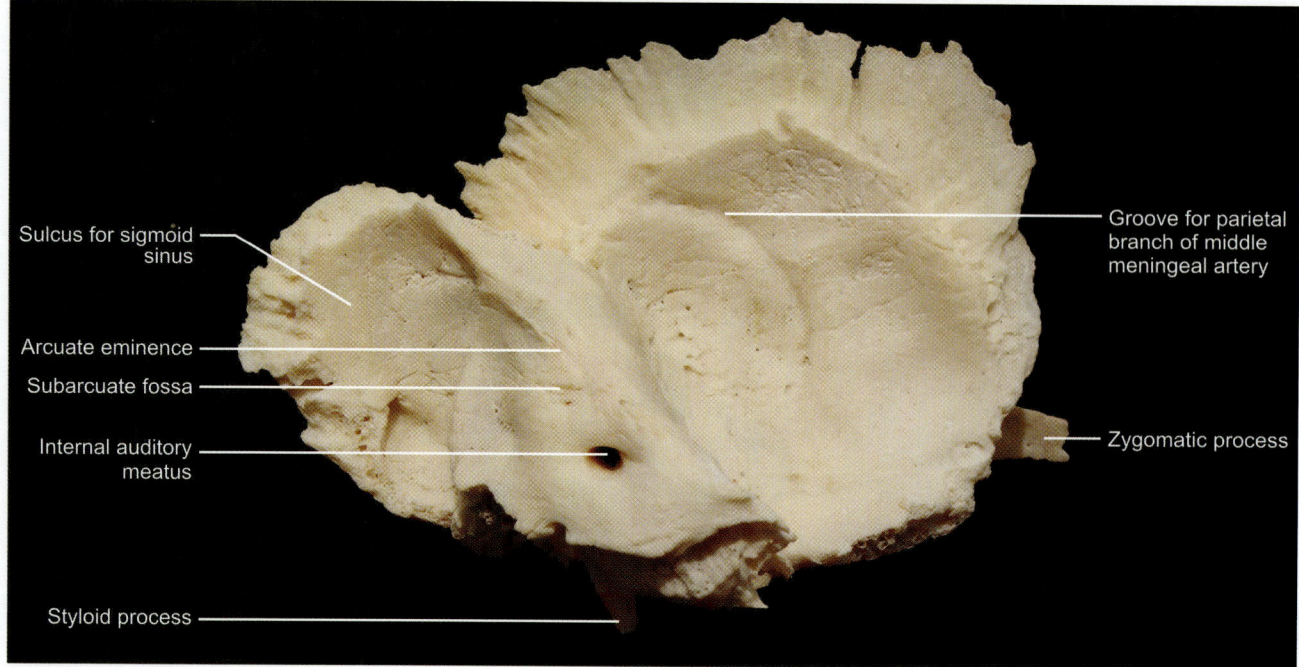

Fig. 6.16: Left temporal bone, internal aspect

Superior border: This border is convex, bevelled internally for articulates with the middle one-thid or more of the inferior (squamosal) border of the parietal bone.

Anteroinferior border: This border articulates with the squamosal border of the greater wing of the sphenoid bone.

MASTOID PART

It is more thick lies below and behind the squamous part.

It consists of:
i. Surfaces: External and internal/cerebral surfaces.
ii. Borders: Posterior and superior borders
iii. Mastoid process and mastoid air cells.

External Surface: It is rough and convex.

Attachments

i. **Origin of** auricularis posterior and occipital belly of occipitofrontalis close to the squamo-mastoid junction.

ii. **Insertion of the following muscles:** From above downwards and forwards
   a. Sternocleidomastoid
   b. Splenius capitis
   c. Longissimus capitis.

iii. **Mastoid foramen:** May or may not present close to the squamo-mastoid suture.

Structures transmit: *See* foramina of skull

Internal or Cerebral Surface

a. Sigmoid sulcus: For sigmoid sinus.
b. Mastoid foramen: Occasionally presents in the floor of the sigmoid sulcus.

Superior border: Articulates with posterior one-third of inferior border of the parietal bone, where it takes part in the formation of asterion.

Posterior border: It articulates with squamous part of occipital bone.

Mastoid process: It is an extension of the mastoid part as a conical downward projection.
   a. **Origin of** posterior belly of digastric from the mastoid notch.
   b. Below the mastoid notch presents a groove transmits-occipital artery.

Mastoid air cells: A section of mastoid bone presents number of small irregular spaces called mastoid air cells and a large irregular space called mastoid or tympanic antrum.

PETROUS PART AND STYLOID PROCESS

i. It is pyramidal in shape and the most important part of the bone.

ii. This part contains the labyrinth of the internal ear, tympanic cavity (middle ear), mastoid antrum, bony part of auditory tube and traversed by internal carotid artery and facial nerve through their bony canals.

iii. It consists of:
- a. Base
- b. An apex
- c. Surfaces: Anterior, posterior and inferior.
- d. Borders: Superior, posterior and anterior

Base: It is fused with the inner surfaces of squamous and mastoid parts.

Apex

i. It projects forwards and medially with an upward tilt, articulates with petrosal process of sphenoid bone.

ii. It bears the anterior opening of the carotid canal.

SURFACES

Anterior Surface

i. It is continuous with the cerebral surface of squamous part.

ii. Marked by irregular impressions for temporal lobe of the cerebrum.

Features of anterior surface

i. **Trigeminal impression:** Immediately behind the apex there is a depression known as trigeminal impression.
Lodges: Semilunar ganglion of the trigeminal nerve.

ii. **Arcuate eminence**
- a. It is an irregular eminence behind the trigeminal impression.
- b. It is formed by the upward bulging of the superior (anterior) semicircular canal of internal ear.

iii. **Tegmen tympani**
- a. Between arcuate eminence and squamous part on the lateral side there is a thin plate of bone called tegmen tympani, which forms a common roof from behind forward—mastoid antrum, tympanic cavity and the bony part of the auditory tube.
- b. Tegmen tympani present two foramina, lateral and medial.
- c. Lateral foramen transmits lesser petrosal nerve.
- d. The medial foramen transmits greater petrosal nerve.

Posterior surface: It faces backwards and upwards.

Features of posterior surface

i. **Internal acoustic meatus/internal auditory meatus**
- a. Opposite the middle of the posterior surface a circular aperture which leads into internal acoustic (auditory) meatus.
- b. It is a short canal 1 cm length and 3 to 5 mm diameter.

Structures transmit: *See* **foramina of skull**

ii. **Opening of aqueduct of the vestibule:** An oblique slit under cover of a thin plate of bone behind the internal acoustic meatus.
Lodges: Saccus and ductus endolymphaticus filled with endolymph and a small artery and vein.

iii. **Subarcuate fossa:** An irregular depressed area above and between the openings of internal auditory meatus and opening of aqueduct of vestibule.
- a. Lodges a process of dura mater.
- b. Transmits a small vein.

Inferior surface

i. It is rough and irregular forms the part of the exterior of the base of skull.

ii. It lies between the greater wing of sphenoid and basilar part of occipital bones.

Features of inferior surface

From before backwards

i. **Quadrilateral area:** Below the apex origin of levator veli palatini muscle, lateral part of the area forms the sulcus tubae and is related to cartilaginous part of the auditory tube.

ii. **Lower opening of the carotid canal:** Lower opening: Circular opening behind the quadrilateral area.
Structures transmit: Internal carotid artery and a plexus of sympathetic nerves.

iii. **Jugular fossa:** A deep depression behind the carotid canal.
Lodges: Superior bulb of internal jugular vein.

iv. **Tympanic canaliculus:** An aperture on the ridge between the opening of carotid canal and the jugular fossa.
Structure transmits: Tympanic branch of glosso-pharyngeal nerve.

v. **A triangular depression:** It is situated in front of jugular fossa and medial to the carotid canal, lodges inferior ganglion of glossopharyngeal nerve.

vi. **Mastoid canaliculus:** Minute foramen on the jugular fossa.
Structure transmits: Auricular branch of vagus nerve.

vii. **Jugular surface:** It is situated behind the jugular fossa, articulates with the jugular process of occipital bone.

vii. **Styloid process**
- i. It is thin long-pointed process directed downward and forward, developed from the second branchial arch (Fig. 6.15).
- ii. Length: 2.54 cm which is gradually narrows from its base to apex.

Attachments

Origin of

i. **Styloglossus:** From anterior aspect close to its tip.

ii. **Stylohyoid:** From middle of its posterior aspect.

iii. **Stylopharyngeus:** From medial aspect close to its base.

Ligaments

i. **Stylomandibular:** from lateral aspect.

ii. **Stylohyoid:** From the tip.

Relations

Laterally: Parotid gland through which facial nerve and external carotid artery traverses.

Medially: Internal jugular vein behind, internal carotid artery in front and 9th, 10th, 11th, and 12th cranial nerves lies between them.

ix. **Stylomastoid foramen:** It lies between the styloid and mastoid processes.

Transmits: Exit of facial nerve and entry of stylomastoid branch of posterior auricular artery.

Borders

Superior border

i. It lies between the floor of middle and posterior cranial fossae between the anterior and posterior surfaces, presents a narrow groove.

ii. Margins of the groove give attachments tentorium cerebelli.

Lodges: Superior petrosal sinus in the groove.

Posterior border

i. The medial part articulates with the basilar part of occipital bone and groove between them lodges inferior petrosal sinus.

ii. The lateral part forms the superolateral boundary of jugular foramen.

iii. A notch is present on this border for the lodgement of inferior ganglion of glossopharyngeal nerve

Anterior border: Divided into two parts.

Lateral part: Joins with squamous part of the same bone and presents two bony canals, upper and lower. The upper canal transmits tensor tympani muscle and lower canal forms the bony part of the auditory tube.

Medial part: Articulates with posterior margin of the greater wing of sphenoid bone.

TYMPANIC PART

i. It is a curved plate of bone.

ii. It lies between the squamous and mastoid parts.

iii. It consists of two surfaces anterior and posterior and three borders superior, inferior and lateral.

Surfaces

Anterior surface: It forms the posterior nonarticular part of the mandibular fossa.

Relation: A part of the parotid gland.

Posterior surface

i. It is concave and forms the anterior wall and lower part of the posterior wall and floor of the bony part of the external auditory meatus.

ii. The medial end of the posterior surface is marked by the tympanic sulcus.

Attachment: Tympanic membrane.

Borders

Lateral border: It forms the circumferential margin of the bony external auditory meatus.

Attachment: Cartilaginous part of external auditory meatus.

Superior border: Meets with squamous part separated by squamo-tympanic fissure.

Inferior border

i. It is sharp and thin, extends from carotid canal to styloid process.

ii. The lateral part of this border splits to enclose the root of the styloid process to form the sheath of the styloid process (Fig. 6.15).

CLINICAL ANATOMY

i. Infection from the middle ear may spread into cranial cavity to involve the structures related to it like temporal lobe of the cerebrum, cerebellum and sigmoid sinus.

ii. Fracture of the middle cranial fossa breaks the roof (tegmen tympani) of the middle ear leading to leakage CSF into the middle ear. If ruptures the tympanic membrane resulting in discharge of CSF through the external auditory meatus (CSF otorrhea).

iii. Infection from the middle ear leads to infections of mastoid antrum and mastoid air cells.

iv. Suprameatal triangle is clinically very important because it helps in localizing the mastoid antrum, which lies depp to it.

v. Fracture of petrous part may damage the facial nerve and produce paralysis of it.

vi. Involvement of vestibulocochlear nerve in fracture of petrous part may produce loss of hearing, vertigo and nystagmus.

vii. Discolouration and edema of the overlying tissue of the mastoid process is indication of damage of the sigmoid sinus.

MANDIBLE

INTRODUCTION

It is the largest, strongest and lowest bone in the face and the only movable bone among the facial bones (Fig. 6.17).

ANATOMICAL POSITION

i. Curved body will be horizontally and convexity forwards.
ii. A pair of flattened plate of bone called ramus projected vertically upward from the posterior ends of the body.

PARTS

i. Body
ii. Two rami
iii. Processes

BODY

Flattened arch, convexity outwards and horseshoe shaped.
Surfaces: External and internal.

Borders: Superior (alveolar) and inferior.

External Surface

Following features present

i. **Symphysis menti:** It is the line of fusion between two halves of mandible inbetween two incisor teeth.
ii. **Mental protuberance:** It is a triangular elevation at the lower part of symphysis menti (Fig. 6.17).

iii. **Mental tubercle**
a. Lies oposite the angles of the base of the mental protuberance.
b. An oblique ridge ascends upwards and backwards from the mental tubercle across the body which is continuous behind with anterior border of the ramus.
c. Posterior part of the ridge is more distinct.
Attachment: Origin of
a. **Depressor anguli oris:** Posterior part of the ridge.
b. **Depressor labii inferioris:** Anterior part of the ridge.
iv. **Mental fossa:** On either side of median ridge small depression.
Attachments: Origin of mentalis and part of orbicularis oris.
v. **Mental foramen:** The mental foramen situated on the external surface of the body in the interval between the premolar teeth (Fig. 6.18).
Structures transmit: Mental vessels and nerve.
Attachment: Origin of buccinator muscle.

Internal Surface

It is concave.

Following features present

i. **Mylohyoid line:** It extends from opposite the level of last molar tooth, ends in the lower part of the symphysis menti, below the genial tubercle.

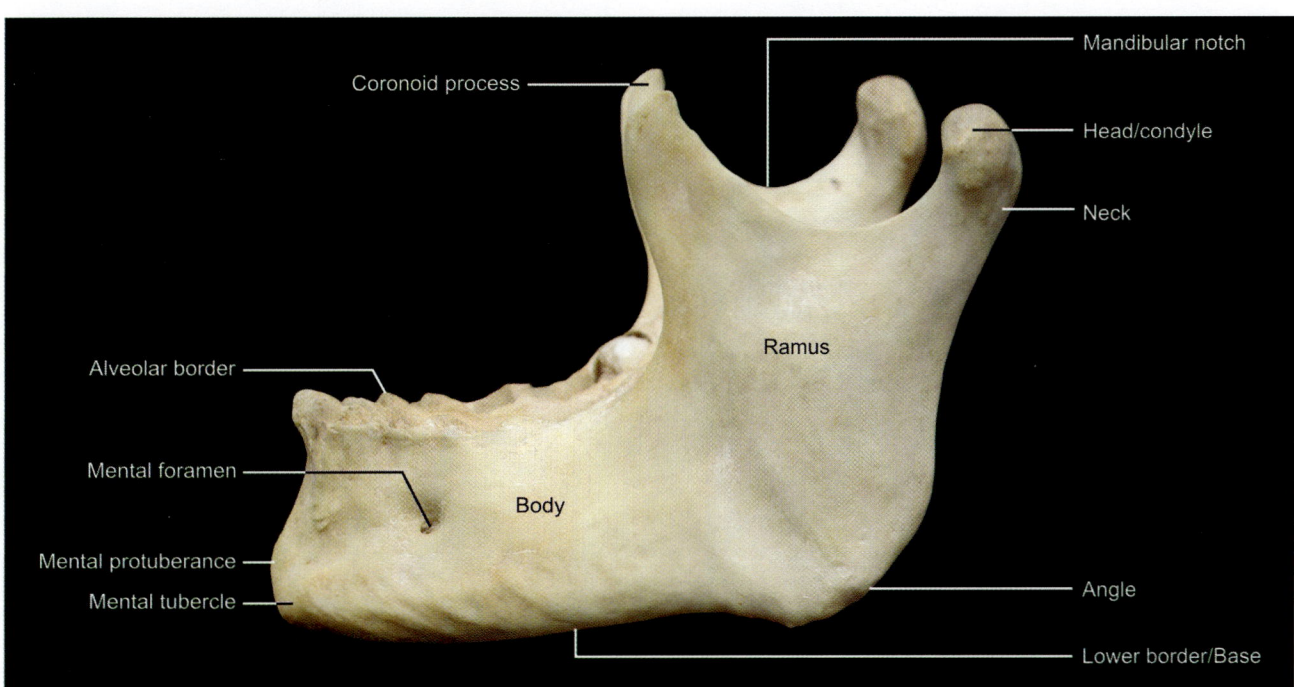

Fig. 6.17: External surface of mandible, showing lateral view

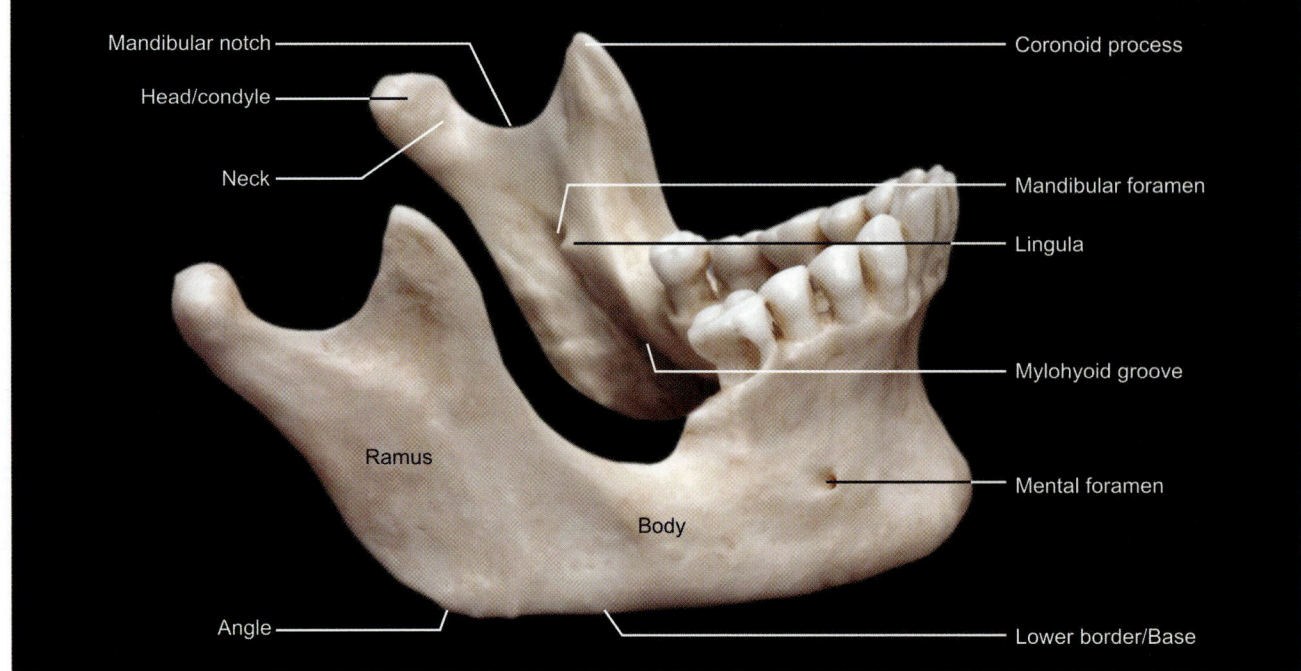

Fig. 6.18: External surface of mandible, showing lateral view and internal surface of ramus

Attachments

　　i. Origin of: Mylohyoid muscle.

　ii. Origin to superior constrictor muscle: From the posterior end of mylohyoid line.

　iii. Pterygomandibular ligament: Behind the last molar tooth.

ii. Mylohyoid groove: Below the mylohyoid line an oblique groove known as mylohyoid groove.

Lodges: Mylohyoid vessels and nerve (Fig. 6.19). Mylohyoid line divides the internal surface into two triangular areas: Upper and lower.

iii. Submandibular fossa: The base of the lower triangular area hollowed out known as submandibular fossa.

Lodges: Submandibular salivary gland and submandibular lymph nodes.

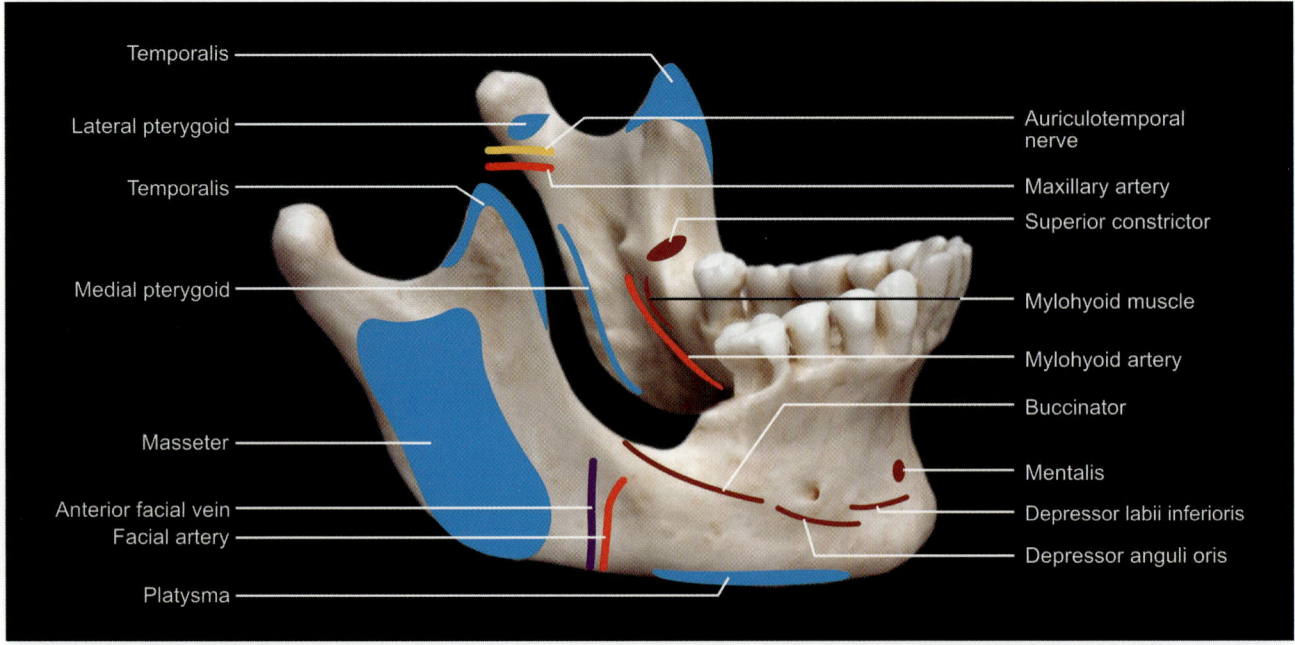

Fig. 6.19: Attachments of mandible, showing external and internal surfaces

iv. **Sublingual fossa:** The base of the upper triangular area also hollowed out known as sublingual fossa.
Lodges: Sublingual salivary gland.

v. **Genial tubercles:** These are small tubercles placed above the anterior ends of mylohyoid line in the median plane and divided into four tubercles.
Attachments (Fig. 6.20):
Upper two—**origin of** genioglossus.
Lower two—**origin of** geniohyoid.

vii. **Digastric fossa:** Below the anterior end of mylohyoid line on either side there is a shallow depression called digastric fossa.
Attachment: Origin of anterior belly of digastric muscle.
Superior border: Each half of superior border is excavated into eight sockets for the teeth. From before backwards:

i. Medial incisor
ii. Lateral incisor
iii. Canine
iv. First premolar
v. Second premolar
vi. First molar
vii. Second molar
viii. Third molar.

Inferior border: It is rounded, called base of the mandible.
Attachment: Platysma is inserted into lower border which extends anteriorly over external surface, where it forms the risorius muscle.

RAMUS OF MANDIBLE

It projects upwards from the posterior end of the body and forms the square shaped flattened bone.

An imaginary vertical line extends from behind the third molar teeth. Anterior to imaginary line is body and posterior to imaginary line is ramus.

Surfaces: internal and external.

Borders: Anterior, posterior, supereior and inferior.

Processes: Coronoid and condylar.

Internal Surface

Following features present (Fig. 6.20):

i. **Mandibular foramen:** It presents at its middle which leads into mandibular canal.
Transmits: Inferior alveolar (dental) vessels and nerve.

ii. **Lingula:** Anteromedial margin of mandibular foramen there is a tongue-like bony projection called lingula.
Attachment: Sphenomandibular ligament.

iii. **Mylohyoid groove:** Behind the mandibular foramen and lingula, presents a vertical groove which marks the beginning of mylohyoid groove.
Transmits: Mylohyoid vessels and nerve.

iv. Below and behind the mylohyoid groove presents rough area.
Attachment: Insertion of medial pterygoid muscle.

External Surface

It is almost rough except the upper and posterior smooth area covered by parotid gland.

Attachment: Insertion of masseter muscle (Fig. 6.19).

Anterior border: It is sharp and prominent.

Attachment: Insertion of some fibers of temporalis.

Posterior border: It is rounded with middle concavity.

Relation: Parotid gland.

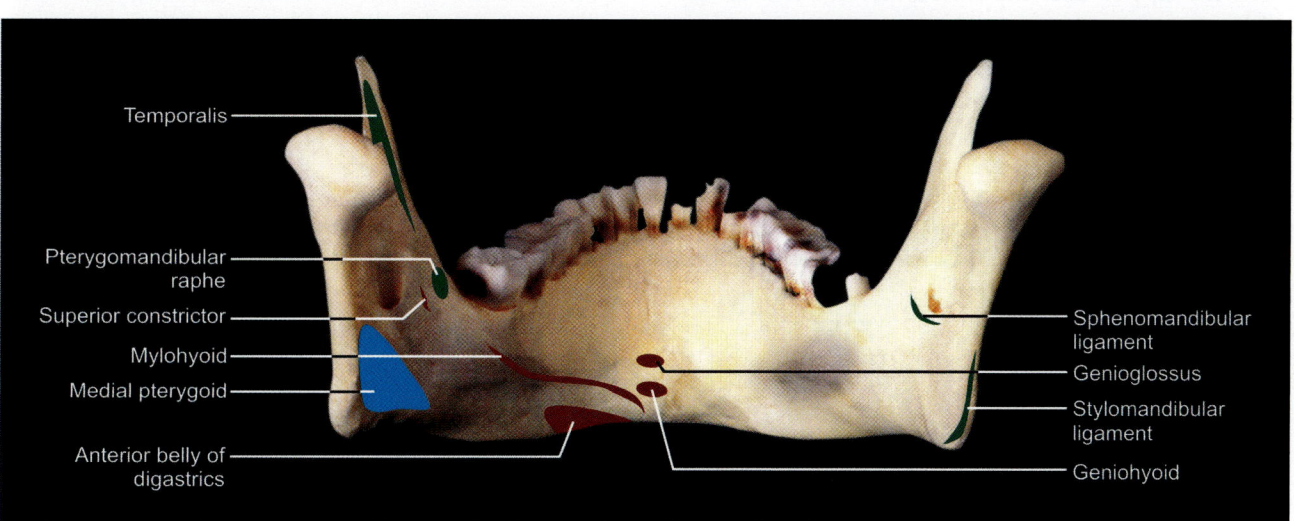

Fig. 6.20: Internal surface of mandible, showing attachments

Superior border: It forms a concave notch known as mandibular notch or incisure.

Transmits: Masseteric vessels and nerve.

Inferior border: Very short, joins with posterior border at an angle, called angle of mandible.

Attachment: Stylomandibular ligament.

Neck : Below the head the narrow part of the bone is called neck.

Attachment

i. Capsular ligament of temporomandibular joint.

ii. Temporomandibular ligament at the lateral and posterior aspects of neck.

Pterygoid fovea: Immediately below the anterior part of the head there is a depressed area.

Attachment: Insertion of lateral pterygoid muscle.

Mandibular canal: It begins in the mandibular foramen at first runs through the ramus then through the body below the sockets of the teeth and finally ends by dividing into mental and incisive canals (between the first and second premolars).

Transmits: Inferior alveolar (dental) vessels and nerve.

Processes

Coronoid process: It is a triangular piece of bone projected upwards from the anterior aspect of the upper part of the ramus.

Attachment: Insertion of temporalis muscle.

Condylar process or head: It ascends upwards from the upper and posterior part of the ramus.

Where the upper end expanded called head of the mandible.

Articulation: Mandibular fossa of the temporal bone forming temporomandibular joint.

CLINICAL ANATOMY

It has some medicolegal importance and age determination.

  i. In infants and children

    a. The two halves of the mandible fuse during the first year of life.

    b. The mandibular canal runs near the lower border.

    c. The mental foramen presents close to the lower border of the body.

    d. The angle of mandible is about 140°

    e. The coronoid process lies higher than the condylar process.

  ii. In adults

    a. Angle of mandible reduces to 110 to 120°.

    b. Alveolar border are well developed and teeth are erupted.

    c. Mental foramen opens midway between upper and lower borders of the body.

    d. The mandibular canal runs parallel with mylohyoid line.

    e. Condylar process is at higher level than the coronoid process.

  iii. In old age

    a. Teeth fall out and the alveolar border is absorbed.

    b. The mental foramen presents close to the alveolar border.

    c. The mandibular canal runs close to the alveolar border.

    d. The angle of mandible again becomes about 140°.

    e. The coronoid process lies higher than the condylar process.

  iv. Fracture of the mandible: Mandibular fracture is common by direct blows during fights.

    a. Weaker part of mandible is canine socket where it is commonly fractured.

Table 6.2	Difference between male and female mandibles	
Male		**Female**
i. Size—Larger and thicker		i. Size—Smaller and thinner
ii. Hight of the body—Greater		ii. Hight of the body—Lesser
iii. Angle of mandible—Everted		iii. Angle of mandible—Inverted
iv. Chin—Quadrilateral		iv. Chin—Rounded
v. Lower border of body of mandible—Irregular		v. Lower border of body of mandible—Smooth
vi. Condyles or head—Larger		vi. Condyles or head—Smaller.

b. Involvement of the inferior alveolar (dental) nerve in such causes neuralgia and pain may referred to the areas along the distribution of buccal and auriculotemporal nerves.

c. The second most common site of fracture at the angle of mandible.

d. Removal of the mandibular teeth causes alveolar process of the mandible to resorb which results in mental foramen comes in close to the superior border of the body of the mandible.

e. In extreme cases due to disappearance of the mental foramina causes exposing the mental nerves which are injured by dental prosthesis (artificial denture) due to pressure and may produce pain during chewing.

f. Indications of the fracture of mandible
  • Occlusal deformity
  • Excruciating or dull aching pain
  • Restriction of movements
  • Inability to masticate
  • Trismus
  • Gingival laceration
  • Ecchymosis
  • Drooping of salivation
  • Halitosis or foul smell.

v. **Mandibular nerve block**: In the extraoral approach the injecting anesthetic agent the needle passes through the mandibular notch of the ramus of the mandible about 4 cm deep into the infratemporal fossa.

Nerves anesthetize: The auriculotemporal, inferior alveolar, lingual and buccal branches.

vi. **Inferior alveolar nerve block:** The Inferior alveolar nerve enter the mandibular foramen which is situated in the middle of the inner surface of the mandibular ramus, which leads into mandibular canal transmitting the inferior alveolar nerve, artery and vein.

  • Injecting anesthetic agent the needle introduced around the mandibular foramen.
  • **Areas anesthetized:** In this block all the mandibular teeth are anesthetized.
  • **Other areas are also to be anesthetized:** The skin and mucous membrane of the lower lip, the labial alveolar mucosa, and skin of the chin because they are supplied by the mental branch of inferior alveolar nerve.
  • **Complication:** If the needle passes too posteriorly, it may penetrate the parotid gland and produce temporary paralysis of branches of facial nerve.

vii. **Mental and incisive nerve blocks:** Inject the anesthetic agent into the mental foramen situated on the external surface of the body of mandible between alveolar and lower borders in the interval between the premolar teeth, will block the mental nerve.

Areas anesthetized: Skin and mucous membrane of the lower lip from mental foramen to the midline.

viii. **Toothache of lower jaw pain referred to external auditory meatus:** The teeth of lower jaw are supplied by inferior alveolar nerve and external auditory meatus is supplied by auriculotemporal nerve as both nerves are branches of mandibular nerve, therefore, pain is referred to external auditory meatus.

SPHENOID BONE

The sphenoid bone is an unpaired, pneumatic irregular bone (Fig. 6.21).

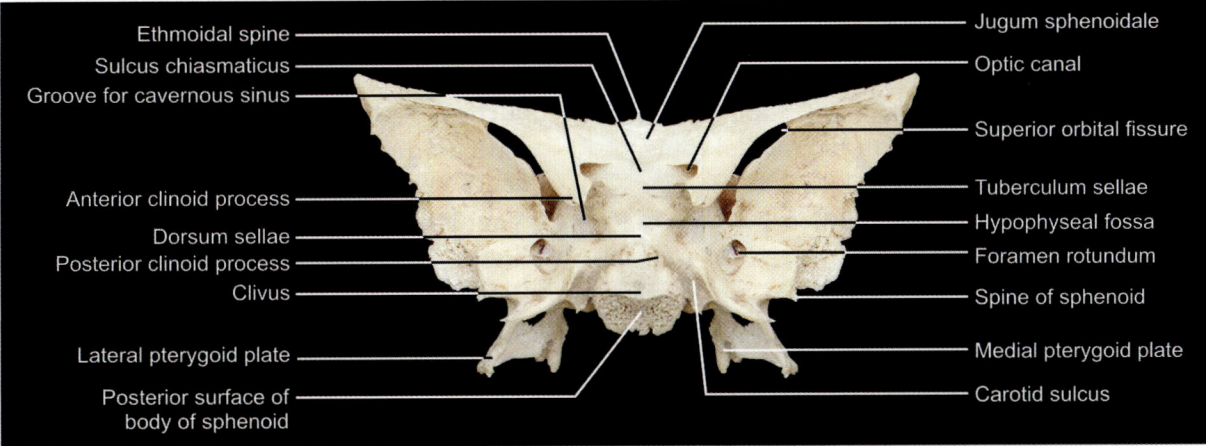

Fig. 6.21: Superior view of sphenoid bone

ANATOMICAL POSITION

i. Pterygoid processes is vertically downwards from the junction of body and greater wings,
ii. Lesser wings anteriorly and greater wings posteriorly
iii. Anterior surface presenting opening of air sinus
iv. Anterior surface with sphenoidal crest looks vertically.

SITUATION

At the base of skull.

Behind: Basilar part of occipital bone and petrous part of temporal bone.

In Front: Frontal and ethmoid bones.

Sides: Squamous part of temporal bones.

PARTS

i. Body
ii. Two greater wings
iii. Two lesser wings
iv. Two pterygoid processes.

BODY

It is cuboidal in shape and contains a pair of sphenoidal air sinuses.

Surfaces

i. Superior/cerebral
ii. Inferior/nasal
iii. Anterior
iv. Posterior
v. Two lateral surfaces.

Superior or Cerebral Surface

Features present on the superior surface:

i. **Ethmoidal spine**
   a. It is a triangular projection between two lesser wings
   b. It articulates with the posterior border of cribriform plate of ethmoid bone.
ii. **Jugum sphenoidale:** It is the smooth anterior part of superior surface lies behind the ethmoidal spine.
iii. **Sulcus chiasmaticus (optic groove):** It lies posterior to the jugum sphenoidale which is a transverse groove.
   Lodges: Optic chiasma.
iv. **Optic canal:** The sulcus chiasmaticus ends laterally into optic canal.
   Transmits: The optic nerve, ophthalmic artery and the cerebral meninges.

v. **Sella turcica:** It resembles a Turkish saddle consisting of following parts: From before backwards—tuberculum sellae, hypophyseal fossa and dorsum sellae.
   Relations:
   a. **The anterior margin of sella turcica:** The anterior intercavernous sinus.
   b. **Posterior margin of sella turcica:** Posterior intercavernous sinus.
vi. **Tuberculum sellae:** Behind the optic groove, there is a rounded elevation called the tuberculum sellae.
   Attachment: Anterior attachment of the diaphragm sellae.
vii. **Middle clinoid process:** The lateral sides of tuberculum sellae present a projection, called middle clinoid process.
viii. **Hypophyseal fossa:** It is a deep depression on the superior surface of body of sphenoid bone
   Lodges: Pituitary gland or hypophysis cerebri
ix. **Dorsum sellae:** The sella turcica posteriorly overhung by a square shaped plate of bone called dorsum sellae.
x. **Posterior clinoid process:** The superior angle of dorsum sellae projected upward called posterior clinoid process.
   Attachment: Tentorium cerebelli.
xi. **Petrosal process:** The posterior part of the dorsum sellae at its lateral angles is projected laterally, which articulate with the apex of the petrous part of the temporal bone called petrosal process.
xii. **Clivus:** The smooth concave sloping downward and backward part on the posterior part of the dorsum sellae.
   Relations: Upper part of the pons.
   Nasal or inferior surface: It forms the roof of the nasal cavity (posterior part).

Features present on the inferior surface

i. **Sphenoidal rostrum:** It is a ridge projected downwards on median plane of the inferior surface.
   Articulation: With grooved superior border of the ala of vomer.
ii. **Vaginal process:** It is a narrow triangular plate of bone projected downwards and medially from the base of the medial pterygoid plate.
iii. **Sphenoidal concha:** It is a thin triangular plate of bone extends between vaginal process and sphenoidal rostrum.
   Articulation: Ala of the vomer.

Anterior surface

Feature present on the anterior surface:

Sphenoidal crest

a. It is a crest opposite the median plane on the anterior surface.
b. It articulates with the posterior border of the perpendicular plate of ethmoid bone.
c. It forms a small part of nasal septum.
d. On either side of the crest inferiorly there is a rounded opening which leads into sphenoidal air sinus within the body of the sphenoid bone.

Lateral surface

i. The lateral surface of the body is fused with the two greater wings.
ii. At the junction of body and greater wing superiorly there is shallow anteroposterior groove knows as carotid sulcus for the internal carotid artery surrounded by sympathetic plexus of nerves.

Relations: Cavernous sinus with its contents

Posterior surface

i. It is rough and quadrilateral.
ii. It articulates with the basilar part of occipital bone by a plate of hyaline cartilage forming a primary cartilaginous joint.
iii. It undergoes ossification at the twenty-fifth year, which helps in determination of age.

Greater Wings

i. These are two strong processes that projects laterally then upward from the side of the body.
ii. Surfaces
a. Superior or cerebral
b. External or lateral
c. Anterior or orbital.

iii. **Borders**
a. Posterior
b. Squamosal.
iv. **An apex**
v. A rough triangular articular area medial to the apex articulates with the frontal bone.
vi. Spine of sphenoid.

Cerebral surface: It is concave and marked by depressions for the temporal lobe of cerebrum.

Following foramina present: From before backward arranged in a crescentic line.

i. **Foramen rotundum:** At the anteromedial part of the superior surface (Fig. 6.22).
   Transmits: Maxillary nerve.
ii. **Foramen ovale:** An oval aperture behind and lateral to foramen.
   Structures transmit: *See* **foramina of skull**
iii. **Foramen spinosum:** It lies posterolateral to foramen ovale.
   Structures transmit: *See* foramina of skull
iv. **Canaliculus innominatus:** Occasionally presents in the bony bar between the foramina spinosum and ovale.
   Transmits: Lesser petrosal nerve (when it does not pass through the foramen ovale).
v. **Emissary sphenoidal foramen** (foramen of Vesalius), medial to foramen ovale sometimes present.
   Transmits: Emissary vein that connects the cavernous sinus with pterygoid venous plexus.

Lateral surface

It is convex and is divided into upper and lower areas by a transverse crest known as infratemporal crest into:

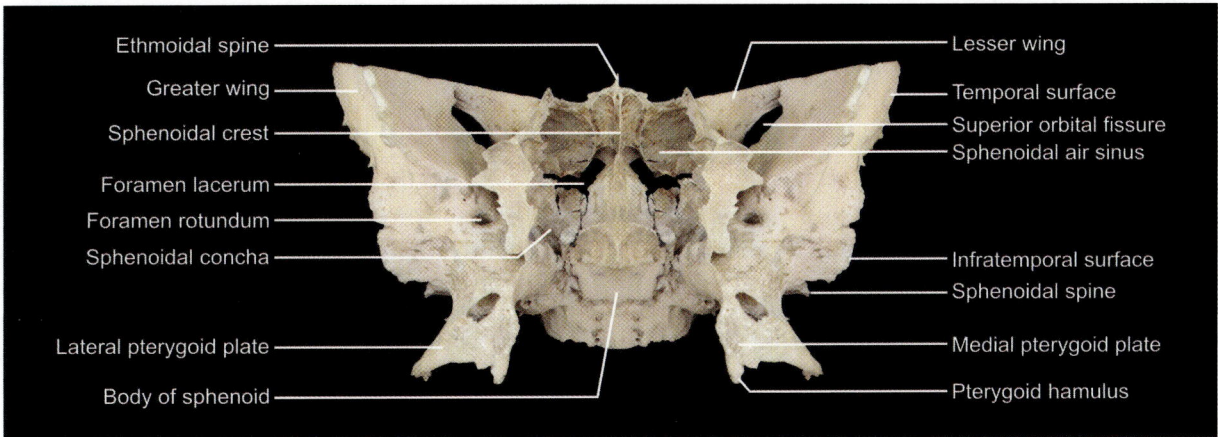

Fig. 6.22: Inferior view of sphenoid bone

Ethmoidal spine
Greater wing
Sphenoidal crest
Foramen lacerum
Foramen rotundum
Sphenoidal concha
Lateral pterygoid plate
Body of sphenoid

Lesser wing
Temporal surface
Superior orbital fissure
Sphenoidal air sinus
Infratemporal surface
Sphenoidal spine
Medial pterygoid plate
Pterygoid hamulus

i. Upper area or temporal fossa gives origin temporalis muscle.

ii. Lower area including infratemporal crest gives origin upper head of lateral pterygoid muscle.

Orbital surface

i. It is quadrilateral in shape, directed forwards and medially.

It consists of:

ii. Borders
   a. Upper
   b. Lower
   c. Lateral
   d. Medial.

Upper border: Its upper border articulates with the lateral part of orbital plate of frontal bone.

Lower border: It is smooth and forms the posterolateral boundary of the inferior orbital fissure.

Lateral border: It is serrated, articulates with superior part of posteromedial margin of the zygomatic bone.

Medial border

i. It is sharp and presents a tubercle in its middle.

ii. In articulated skull it forms the inferolateral margin of superior orbital fissure.

Attachment: Annulus tendinous communis to the tubercle.

Borders of greater wing

Posterior border

i. Its medial half forms the anterior boundary of foramen lacerum in articulated skull.

ii. Its lateral half articulates with the petrous part of temporal bone.

iii. Presents a groove called sulcus tubae below the lateral half in articulated skull for the cartilaginous part of the auditory tube.

Squamosal border: It articulates with the squamous part of temporal bone.

Apex

i. It is thin and directed upwards.

ii. Apex is bevelled on the inner aspect for articulation with the sphenoidal angle of the parietal bone forming the pterion.

Spine of sphenoid

It is a small pointed process projecting downward from the junction of posterior and squamosal borders of greater wing.

Attachments

Ligaments

i. Sphenomandibular
ii. Anterior ligament of malleus
iii. Pterygospinous.

Muscles

i. Tensor veli palatini
ii. Tensor tympani.

Relations

Medially: Chorda tympani nerve and auditory tube.
Laterally: Auriculotemporal nerve.

Lesser Wings

i. Two triangular plates which project laterally on each side from the upper and anterior parts of the side of the body.

ii. It is connected with the body by the anterior and posterior roots, between the roots and the body forming the optic canal.

iii. **Surfaces**
   a. Superior or cerebral
   b. Inferior or orbital surface.

iv. **Borders**
   a. Anterior
   b. Posterior.

Superior or cerebral surface: It is smooth and is continuous with jugum sphenoidale of the body.

Lodges: The orbital surface of the frontal lobe of the cerebrum.

Inferior or orbital surface: It forms the posterior part of the orbital roof.

Attachments

i. **Origin of** superior oblique muscle of eyeball medially
ii. **Origin of** levator palpebrae superioris laterally.
iii. Common tendinous ring.

Anterior border: It is serrated and articulates with the posterior border of the orbital plate of frontal bone.

Posterior border

i. It is concave and free, forms the junction of the floor of the anterior and middle cranial fossae.

ii. It ends medially into a bony process called anterior clinoid process

Attachment

i. Free border of the tentorium cerebelli.
ii. Carotido-clenoid ligament
iii. Interclenoid ligament.

Superior orbital fissure: It is an oblique cleft between the lesser and greater wings.

Boundaries

Above: By the under surface of lesser wing.

Below: By medial margin of orbital surface of greater wing.

Laterally: By frontal bone.

Medially: By body of sphenoid.

　ii. It is divided into three compartments by the attachment of annulus tendinous communis.
　　a. The portion lateral to annulus
　　b. The portion through the annulus
　　c. The portion medial to annulus.

Structures transmit: *See* foramina of skull

Pterygoid Processes

　i. The two pterygoid processes represent the legs of the bat (as sphenoid bone resembles a bat).
　ii. They descend downwards from the junction of body with the greater wings.
　iii. Each consists of two plates of bone:
　　a. Lateral pterygoid lamina/plate.
　　b. Medial pterygoid lamina/plate.

Some features of the pterygoid processes

　i. Pterygoid fossa
　　a. Posteriorly, the pterygoid plates diverge each other and forms pterygoid fossa.
　　b. It is divided into upper and lower areas.
　　c. The lower area is deeper.
　　d. The upper area form a shallow depression known as scaphoid fossa.
　Attachment: Origin of tensor veli palatini muscle from the scaphoid fossa.

　ii. Pterygopalatine fossa
　　a. Anteriorly, both plates are continuous and form the posterior boundary of pterygopalatine fossa in articulated skull.
　　b. In the upper part of the pterygopalatine fossa presents three foramina: From lateral to medial
　　　– Foramen rotundum,
　　　– Anterior opening of pterygoid canal
　　　– Palatinovaginal or pharyngeal canal.

　iii. Pterygoid fissure
　　a. Inferiorly, anterior borders of two pterygoid plates are separated and form a triangular gap called pterygoid fissure.
　　b. Which articulates with the margins of the pyramidal processes of palatine bones.

　iv. Lateral pterygoid plate or lamina: It is a quadrilateral plate of bone.
　　i. Borders: Anterior and posterior.
　　ii. Surfaces: Medial and lateral.
　Anterior border
　Upper part: Non-articular forms the posterior boundary of pterygopalatine fissure in articulated skull.
　Lower part: Articulates with tubercle of the palatine bone.
　Posterior border: It is also free
　Attachment: Pterygospinous ligament.
　Lateral surface: Origin of lower head of lateral pterygoid muscle.
　Medial surface: Origin of medial pterygoid muscle.

　v. Medial pterygoid plate or lamina: It is longer than lateral pterygoid plate.
　Borders: Anterior and posterior borders.
　Surfaces: Lateral and medial surfaces.
　Anterior border: Whole border articulates with the posterior border of the perpendicular plate of palatine bone.

Posterior border

Attachments

　i. To pharyngobasilar fascia (whole extent).
　ii. Lower part—**origin of** superior constrictor muscle of pharynx.

Medial surface: It forms the lateral boundary of the posterior nasal aperture.

Lateral surface: It forms the medial aspect of pterygoid fossa and related to tensor veli palatini muscle.

Features produced by medial pterygoid plate:

　i. Pterygoid hamulus: Lower end of medial pterygoid plate curves laterally to form a hook-shaped process known as pterygoid hamulus.
　Attachment: Pterygomandibular raphe.
　ii. Processus tubarius: A projection in the midpoint of the posterior border supports the pharyngeal end of pharyngotympanic (auditory) tube.
　iii. Vaginal process
　　i. It is the upward prolongation of medial surface of medial pterygoid plate pass to the under surface of the body of sphenoid as thin lamina.
　iv. Articulations
　　a. Anteriorly with the sphenoidal process of the palatine bone.
　　b. Medially with the ala of the vomer.

c. Anteriorly, the inferior aspect of the vaginal process presents a groove, which is converted into palatinovaginal canal after articulating with the sphenoidal process of the palatine bone.

d. **Transmits:** Pharyngeal nerve and pharyngeal branch of maxillary artery.

e. Superior aspect of the vaginal process with the ala of the vomer forms the vomerovaginal canal.

Sphenoidal concha (bone of Bertin)

i. It covers the anterior and inferior aspects of the sphenoidal air sinuses.

ii. It consists of:

  a. Anterior, vertical and quadrilateral parts.

  b. Posterior, horizontal and triangular parts.

CLINICAL ANATOMY

i. Fracture of the sphenoidal spine

  a. The spine of sphenoid is related laterally with auriculotemporal nerve and medially with chorda tympani nerve.

  b. Injury of the auriculotemporal nerve result in dry mouth due failure of secretion of parotid gland because the postganglionic fibers from the otic ganglion are carried through the auriculotemporal nerve which are secretomotor to the parotid glands

  c. Injury to the chorda tympani nerve causes loss of taste sensation from the anterior two-thirds of tongue as taste sensation from the anterior two-thirds of tongue is carried through the chorda tympani nerve.

ii. Depression of the nasal bridge: It occurs due to union between pre- and post-sphenoidal parts of the sphenoid bone.

iii. Hypertelorism and a broad nasal bridge: It is caused by abnormal growth of the presphenoidal part produces abnormal wide separation of orbital cavities.

iv. Surgical approach of the pituitary gland: Surgery of the pituitary gland is approached through the transnasal and trans-sphenoidal routes through the roof of the nasal cavity, by removing the rostrum of the sphenoid bone, then passing through the sphenoidal air sinus or by transorbital–transethmosphenoidal approach to reach the ethmoidal sinuses and break the ethmoidal air cells to access the pituitary gland.

v. Medicolegal importance: The basisphenoid joint is of medicolegal importance to age determination of the individual. Body of sphenoid unites with basilar part of occipital bone at the age of 25 years where the cartilaginous plate is completely replaced by the bone.

PARIETAL BONES

▌ INTRODUCTION

The parietal bones are two in number and by their union form the greater part of the vault and sides of the cranium. Each is irregularly quadrilateral in shape (Fig. 6.23).

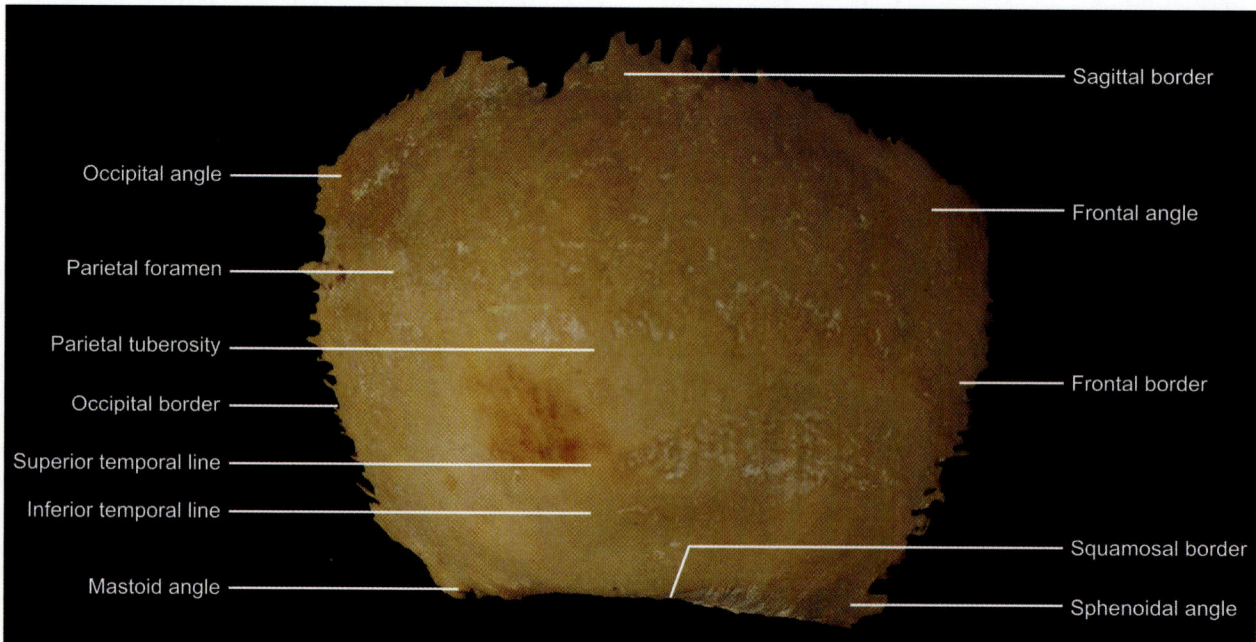

Fig. 6.23: External surface of parietal bone

ANATOMICAL POSITION

i. The longest serrated border lies above and to the median plane.

ii. Pointed anteroinferior angle which is internally marked by groove for anterior division of middle marginal antery directed downward and forward.

SIDE DETERMINATION

After holding the bone in anatomical position the convex external surface determines the side of the bone.

GENERAL FEATURES

i. **Two surfaces:** External and internal.

ii. **Four borders:** Sagittal, squamousal, frontal and occipital.

iii. **Four angles:** Frontal, sphenoidal, occipital and mastoid.

External Surface

Following features present (Fig. 6.23)

i. **Parietal tuber:** It is convex, near its center presents a rounded eminence known as parietal tuber.

Importance of parietal tuber or eminence:

a. It forms an important bony landmark

b. The maximum transverse diameter of the skull corresponds to these eminences

c. First center of ossification starts at this point

d. It corresponds to the posterior upterned end of the posterior limb of the lateral sulcus of the cerebral hemisphere at the angular gyrus where the areas of writing and printed words lie.

ii. **Superior temporal line:** Arched line passes from before backwards.

Attachment: Temporal fascia.

iii. **Inferior temporal line:** Arched line below the superior temporal line.

Attachment: Highest fibers of temporalis muscle.

iv. **Parietal foramen:** It is about 5 cm in front of occipital angle, close to the superior border.

Transmits

a. A branch of occipital artery

b. An emissary vein connects superior sagittal sinus with occipital vein.

Internal Surface

i. The internal surface is deeply concave (Fig. 6.24)

ii. It is marked by impressions of the cerebral gyri and branches from the middle meningeal vessels.

Following features present

i. **Sagittal sulcus:** Opposite the sagittal border, it presents a longitudinal shallow groove, which with a similar groove on the opposite side forms sagittal sulcus.

Lodges: Superior sagittal sinus.

ii. **Margin of the groove:** Attachment of falx cerebri and close to the sagittal sulcus there are numerous granular foveolae (pits) lodges arachnoid granulations.

iii. **Groove for anterior division of middle meningeal artery:** It begins from the inner surface of anteroinferior angle and soon divides into two (Fig. 6.24).

iv. **Groove for the posterior division of middle meningeal artery:**

a. It runs upwards and backwards near the posteroinferior angle.

b. Opposite the posteroinferior angle, presents an arched groove for end of transverse sinus and commencement of sigmoid sinus.

Sagittal/superior border: It is longest, thickest, serrated and straight.

Articulation: With the fellow of its opposite side to form sagittal suture.

Squamosal/inferior border

It is arched and divided into three portions:

i. Anterior

ii. Intermediate

iii. Posterior.

Anterior portion: Bevelled outwardly, articulates with greater wing of sphenoid bone.

Intermediate portion: It is arched and bevelled outwardly, articulates with squamous part of temporal bone.

Posterior portion: It is straight and thickly serrated, articulates with mastoid part of temporal bone.

Frontal or anterior border: It is serrated and bevelled inwardly above and outwardly below and forms half of coronal suture.

Articulation: With posterior border of frontal bone.

Occipital or posterior border

i. It is also thick, serrated and articulates with lambdoid border of the squamous part of the occipital bone.

ii. It forms the half of the lambdoid suture.

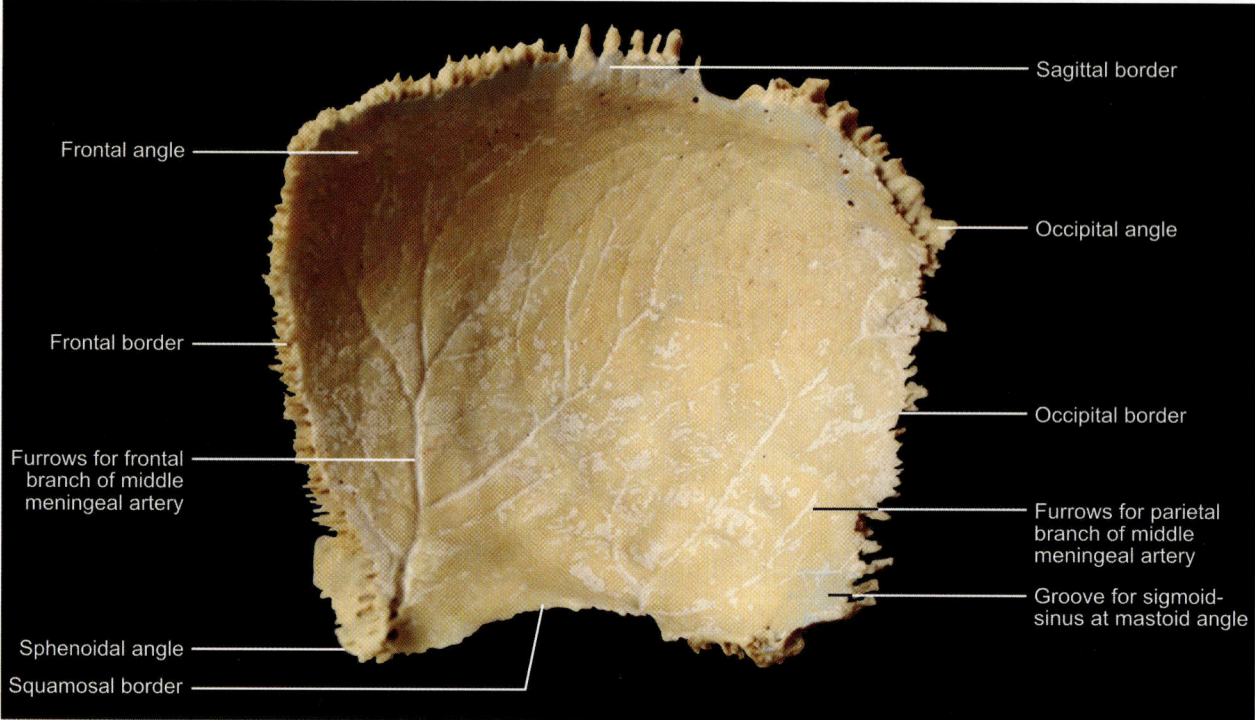

Fig. 6.24: Internal surface of parietal bone

Frontal or anterosuperior angle

i. It is formed by the union of the sagittal and frontal borders.

ii. It forms a point of union on the skull, called bregma.

Sphenoidal or anteroinferior angle

i. In articulated skull it meets with four bones and the area is known as pterion.
The four bones are:
  a. Frontal
  b. Parietal
  c. Greater wing of sphenoid
  d. Squamous part of temporal bone.

Occipital or posterosuperior angle

i. It corresponds to lambda in articulated skull.

ii. It is the union between the sagittal and lambdoid sutures.

Mastoid or posteroinferior angle

i. It corresponds to the asterion or meeting points of three bones on the skull.

ii. The three bones are:
  a. Posteroinferior angle of parietal bone
  b. Lateral angle of occipital bone
  c. Mastoid part of temporal bone.

CLINICAL ANATOMY

Epidural Hematoma

i. A blow to the side of the head may fracture the bones forming the pterion which causes rupture of the anterior division of middle meningeal artery resulting epidural hematoma, and symptoms of brain compression generally appear within three hours.

ii. This is a surgical emergency, in this case the cranial cavity should be explored immediately to arrest bleeding and remove the clot.

iii. In an undiagnosed epidural haematoma there is transient loss of consciousness, followed by recovery from initial concussion only to die hours later. This is known as 'talk and die' syndrome.

iv. Clinically the four angles of each parietal bone has great importaence, because the bregma and lambda are related with sagittal sinus, pterion with anterior division of middle meningeal vessels and asterion with sigmoid sinus. Therefore trephining (perforating the skull) of skull at its any angle produces hemorrhage.

v. **Moulding of calvaria:** Parietal bones are loosely attached to the surrounding bones along the sutures during intrauterine life, which allow moulding (change in shape of calvaria) at the time when passing through the birth canal. Calvaria returns to normal shape within few days after birth.

FRONTAL BONE

INTRODUCTION

Frontal bone forms the forehead, superior orbital plate and a major part of anterior cranial fossa (Fig. 6.25).

ANATOMICAL POSITION

  i. Squmous part is vertical and convex forwards.

  ii. Orbital plates will project horizontally backward.

  iii. Nasal spine will be directed downwards.

GENERAL FEATURES

Surfaces: External, internal and temporal

Plates: Orbital plates.

External/Frontal Surface

Following features present

  i. Frontal tuber or eminence

    a. It is situated one on each side of median plane about 3 cm above the supraorbital margin.

    b. It is more prominent in female.

  ii. Superciliary arches

    a. Two arched eminences, immediately above the supraorbital margins, one on each side called superciliary arches.

    b. They meet in the median plane in an elevation called **Glabella.**

  iii. Supraorbital margin

    a. It is the lower or orbital border of squamous part and presents two notches or foramena.

    b. It forms the upper circumferential margin of the orbit.

  iv. Supraorbital foramen or notch: Situated at the junction of medial one-third and lateral two-thirds of the supraorbital margin.

    Transmits: Supraorbital nerve, vessels and frontal diploic vein.

  v. Supratrochlear notch or foramen: Situated medial to the supraorbital notch or foramen.

    Transmits: Supratrochlear vessels and nerve.

  vi. Zygomatic process: Situated laterally where supraorbital margin ends in a thick process.

    Articulation: With frontal process of zygomatic bone.

  vii. Nasal part: Below the glabella and between the supraorbital margins the portion of the bone projecting downwards, called nasal part of frontal bone.

  viii. Nasal notch: It presents an irregular articular notch called nasal notch.

    Articulations: From medial to lateral

    a. Nasal bone

    b. Frontal process of maxilla

    c. Lacrimal bone

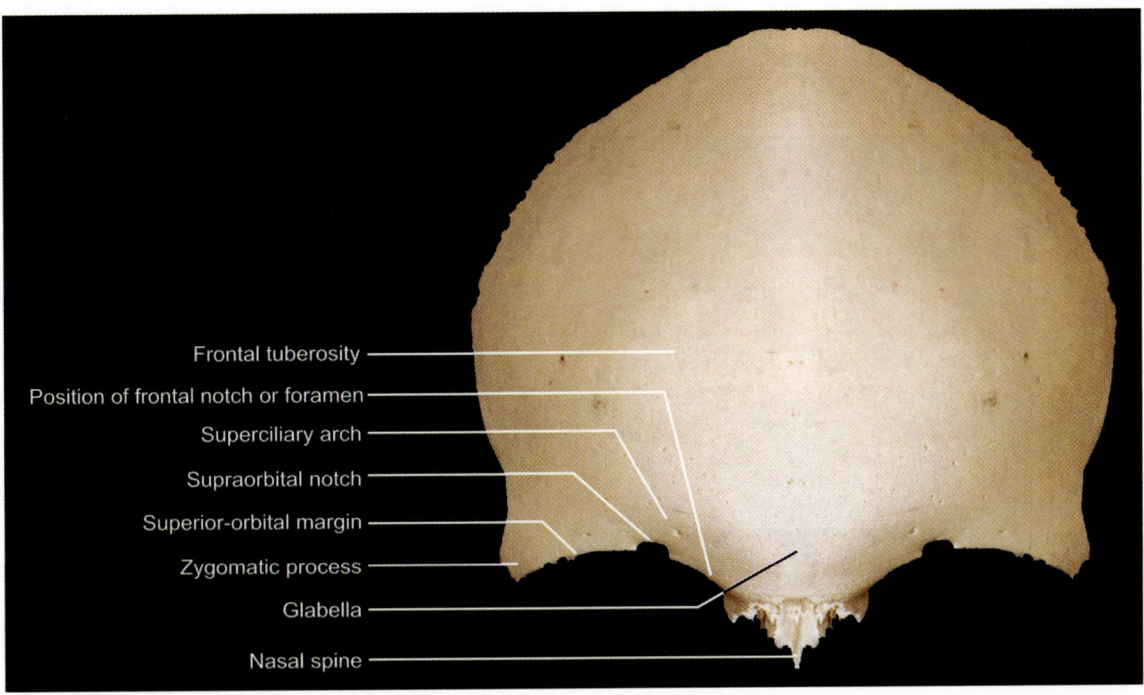

Fig. 6.25: Frontal bone (external surface)

ix. Nasal spine It is a pointed process projects downwards from the lower part of nasal notch, opposite median plane. The nasal spine forms a part of nasal septum.

Internal/Cerebral Surface

It is deeply concave and is occupied by the frontal lobe of the cerebral hemisphere (Fig. 6.26).

Following features present

i. Sagittal sulcus

a. Opposite the median plane, this surface presents a shallow groove, called sagittal sulcus.

b. Margins of the groove gives attachment to falx cerebri.

Lodges: Superior sagittal sinus.

ii. Frontal crest: The margins of the sagittal sulcus as they descend downwards converge together and are joined to form frontal crest.

Attachment: Falx cerebri.

iii. Granular foveolae (pits): Close to the sagittal sulcus there are numerous granular foveolae.

Lodges: Arachnoid granulations.

iv. Foramen cecum

a. The frontal crest ends below into a notch.

b. Which articulates with the alae of the crista galli of the ethmoid bone where a foramen is present called foramen cecum.

Structure transmits: *See* **foramina of skull**

Temporal Surface: It forms a part of temporal fossa, limited above by superior temporal line.

Following features present

i. Temporal lines

a. It begins from the zygomatic process and divides into superior and inferior temporal lines.

b. It separates external (frontal) from temporal surface.

ii. Superior temporal line
Attachment: Temporal fascia.

iii. Inferior temporal line together with temporal fossa and the surface below it:
Attachment: Origin of temporalis muscle.

Borders of temporal surface: Upper and lower
Upper or parietal

a. Articulates with parietal bone forming coronal suture.

b. The rough triangular articular area behind the zygomatic process in the lower part of this border articulates with greater wing of sphenoid bone.

Lower or orbital: Forms the supraorbital margin.

Orbital Plates: It consists of two triangular plates of bones which are separated from each other by ethmoidal notch.

ii. Ethmoidal notch

a. In articulated skull, it is covered by the cribriform plate of the ethmoid bone

b. Margins of the notch presents broken air cells, articulates with the upper surface of the labyrinth of the ethmoid bone to complete the ethmoidal air sinuses.

iii. Surfaces: Orbital and cerebral.

iv. Borders: Posterior and medial.

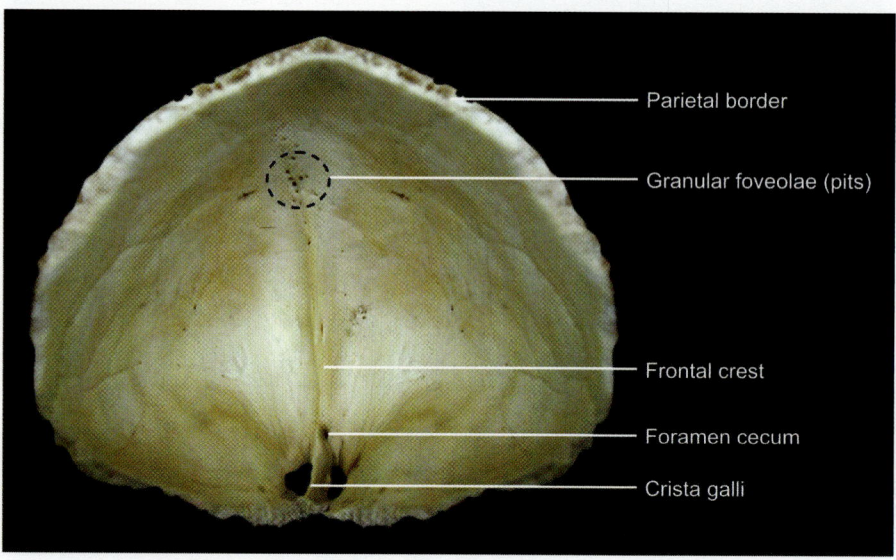

Fig. 6.26: Internal (cerebral) surface of the frontal bone

Orbital/Inferior surface

a. It forms the roof of the orbital cavity.

b. Its lateral part presents a deep depression called lacrimal fossa.

Lodges: Lacrimal gland

Trochlear fossa: Medial part of the orbital surface, below the medial end of supraorbital margin presents trochlear fossa.

Attachment: Fibrocartilaginous pulley of the superior oblique muscle of the eyeball.

Superior or cerebral surface: Impressions of cerebral gyri of the frontal lobe.

Posterior border: This border articulates with the anterior border of the lesser wing of sphenoid bone.

Medial border: It is irregular and forms the margin of the ethmoidal notch.

CLINICAL ANATOMY

i. **Safety valve:** Foramen cecum sometimes transmits an emissary vein, which communicates between the superior sagittal sinus with veins of nasal mucosa. In case of increased intracranial blood pressure the nasal bleeding (epistaxis) acts as safety valve and prevents vascular damage of the brain.

ii. **Exophthalmos:** If fracture occurs in the orbital plate of frontal bone result is collection of blood beneath the conjunctiva and in the orbital cavity producing exophthalmos.

iii. **Black eye:** A blow (during boxing match) to superciliary arches may cause profuse bleeding as a result blood accumulate surrounding the orbit and gravitate into upper eyelid producing black eye.

iv. **Metopic suture:** In most of the cases union between the two halves of frontal bone begins in the second year and union completed in the eighth year, which helps in age determination, but in 9% cases union does not take place properly and the condition called metopic suture.

In radiographic images this should not be mistaken for a fracture line.

MAXILLAE

INTRODUCTION

Maxilla is the second largest bone of the face. It forms the upper jaw by the union of two halves.

ANATOMICAL POSITION

i. The longest frontal process directed upward with backward tilt.

ii. The convex posterior surface faces postero-laterally.

iii. Alveolar border with sockets for the teeth of upper jaw downwards and its convexity outwards.

iv. The rough triangular zygomatic process projects laterally.

SIDE DETERMINATION

After holding the bone in anatomical position the zygomatic process on which side belongs will determine the same sided bone.

PARTS

i. A body
ii. Four processes
  a. Frontal
  b. Zygomatic
  c. Palatine
  d. Alveolar.

BODY

i. **Shape**—pyramidal
ii. Contain large air sinus known as maxillary air sinus.
iii. **Surfaces**
  a. Anterior
  b. Posterior (infratemporal)
  c. Superior (orbital)
  d. Medial (nasal).

Anterior surface

i. It looks forward and laterally.
ii. Lower part of this surface presence of ridges produced by the sockets of the upper teeth.

Following features present on the anterior surface (Fig. 6.27):

i. **Canine eminence:** It lies between the incisive and canine fossae caused by root of the canine tooth.
Attachment: Origin of levator anguli oris.

ii. **Incisive fossa:** Situated medial to canine eminence and above the sockets of the two incisor teeth.
Attachments
  a. Origin of depressor septi and part of orbicularis oris
  b. Origin of alar part of nasalis (dilator nares) muscle—above and lateral to incisive fossa.

iii. **Canine fossa:** Situated lateral to the canine eminence.
Attachment: Levator anguli oris.

iv. **Infraorbital foramen:** Situated above the canine fossa.

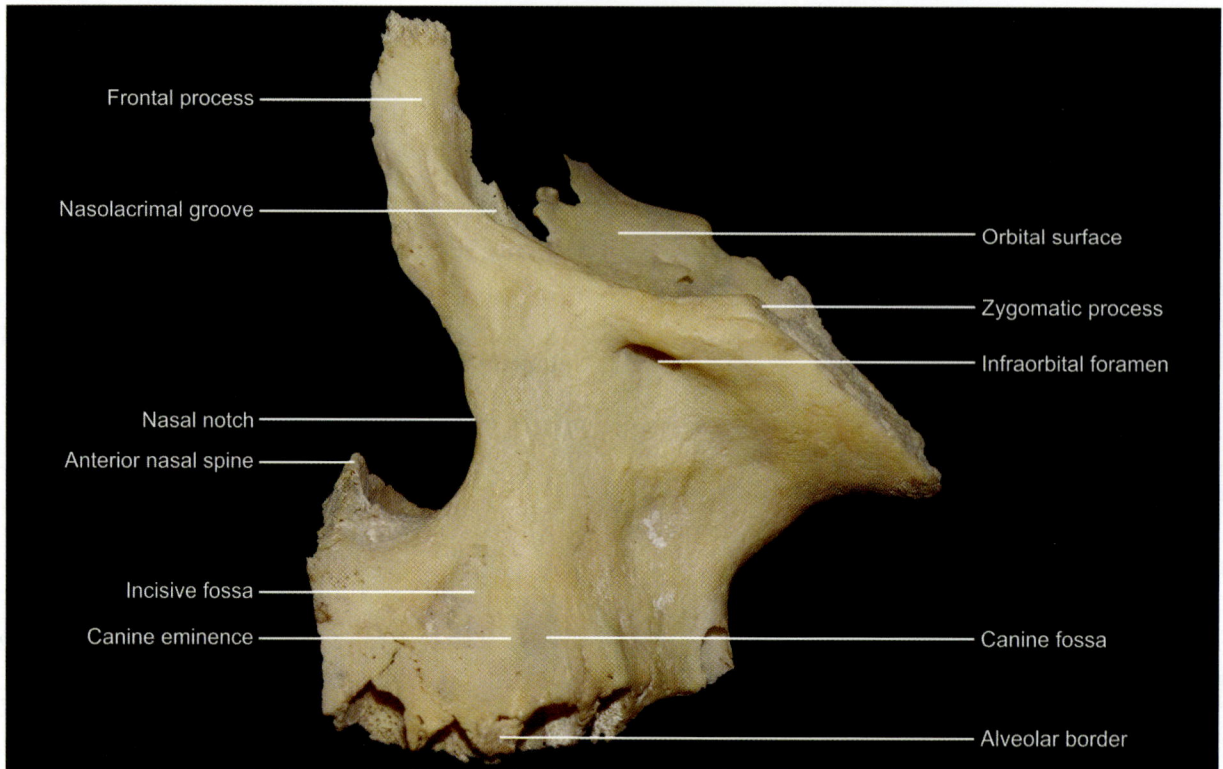

Fig. 6.27: Left maxilla (lateral aspect)

Structures transmits: Infraorbital nerve and vessels.

v. Area between the infraorbital foramen and infraorbital margin:

Attachment: Origin of levator labii superioris.

vi. **Nasal notch:** Anteromedially, the anterior surface separated from the medial surface by a thin concave margin called nasal notch.

Attachment: Origin of transverse part of nasalis (compressor naris).

vii. **Anterior nasal spine:** The pointed anterior bony projection of fellow of opposite side forms the anterior nasal spine.

Posterior surface (infratemporal)

i. It is convex, directed backwards and laterally.

ii. It is separated from the anterior surface by a ridge.

Fllowing features present on the posterior surface

i. **Alveolar canals:** Near the center this surface is perforated by two or three small foramina called alveolar canals.

Structures transmits: Posterior superior alveolar (dental) vessels and nerves.

ii. **Maxillary tuberosity**

a. Close to the posteroinferior angle this surface presents a rough articular area, called maxillary

tuberosity articulates with pyramidal process of palatine bone.

b. A little below, its posterosuperior angle, there is a shallow curved groove transmits maxillary nerve.

iii. Opposite the middle of the posterior border of the posterior surface is the upper end of the vertical groove known as greater palatine groove.

Structures transmits: Greater palatine vessels and nerves.

Orbital or superior surface

i. It is smooth and triangular in shape forms the greater part of the floor of the orbit.

ii. It is separated from the anterior surface by the infraorbital margin.

iii. It is separated from the posterior surface by a rounded margin.

Anterior margin: Anteriorly, limited by the lower margin of the orbit and medially, continuous with the lacrimal crest of the frontal process of maxilla.

Posterior margin

i. It presents a free posterior border, forms the lower boundary of the infraorbital fissure.

ii. It is marked near its center by the beginning of the infraorbital canal.

Medial margin

i. It separates the orbital surface from nasal surface.

ii. It articulates from before backwards.

a. Lacrimal bone

b. Orbital plate of ethmoid bone

c. Orbital process of palatine bone.

iii. The medial margin of the orbital surface anteriorly presents a notch the nasolacrimal notch, which is converted into the upper opening of the nasolacrimal canal by articulation with lacrimal bone.

Structure transmits: Nasolacrimal duct

Infraorbital groove or notch

i. It presents near the center of the posterior border of the orbital surface.

ii. It leads to infraorbital canal which ends in infraorbital foramen on the anterior surface.

Structures transmit: Infraorbital vessels and nerve.

iii. Just lateral to the nasolacrimal notch presents a small depression.

Attachment: Origin of inferior oblique muscle of eyeball.

Nasal surface: It forms a part of the lateral wall of the nose.

Following features present (Fig. 6.28)

i. **Maxillary hiatus:** On the upper and posterior part of this surface presents maxillary hiatus which leads into maxillary air sinus.

ii. **Broken air cells** (ethmoidal): Situated above the hiatus and completed by labyrinth of ethmoid and lacrimal bones.

iii. **Inferior meatus of nose**

a. It is situated below the maxillary hiatus.

b. Here nasolacrimal duct opens.

iv. **Nasolacrimal groove**

a. It is situated vertically in front of the hiatus.

b. It is converted into nasolacrimal canal by articulation with descending process of lacrimal bone above and inferior nasal concha below.

Structure transmits: Nasolacrimal duct to inferior meatus of nose.

v. In front of the nasolacrimal groove the nasal surface presents an oblique ridge known as conchal crest of the maxilla.

vi. Above, the conchal crest a shallow depressed area forms a part of the atrium, the middle meatus of the nose and below, it forms a part of the inferior meatus of nose

vii. Traversing this area there is a vertical groove, the greater palatine groove which is converted into greater palatine canal with a similar groove on the lateral surface of the perpendicular plate of palatine bone.

Structures transmit: Greater palatine nerves and vessels.

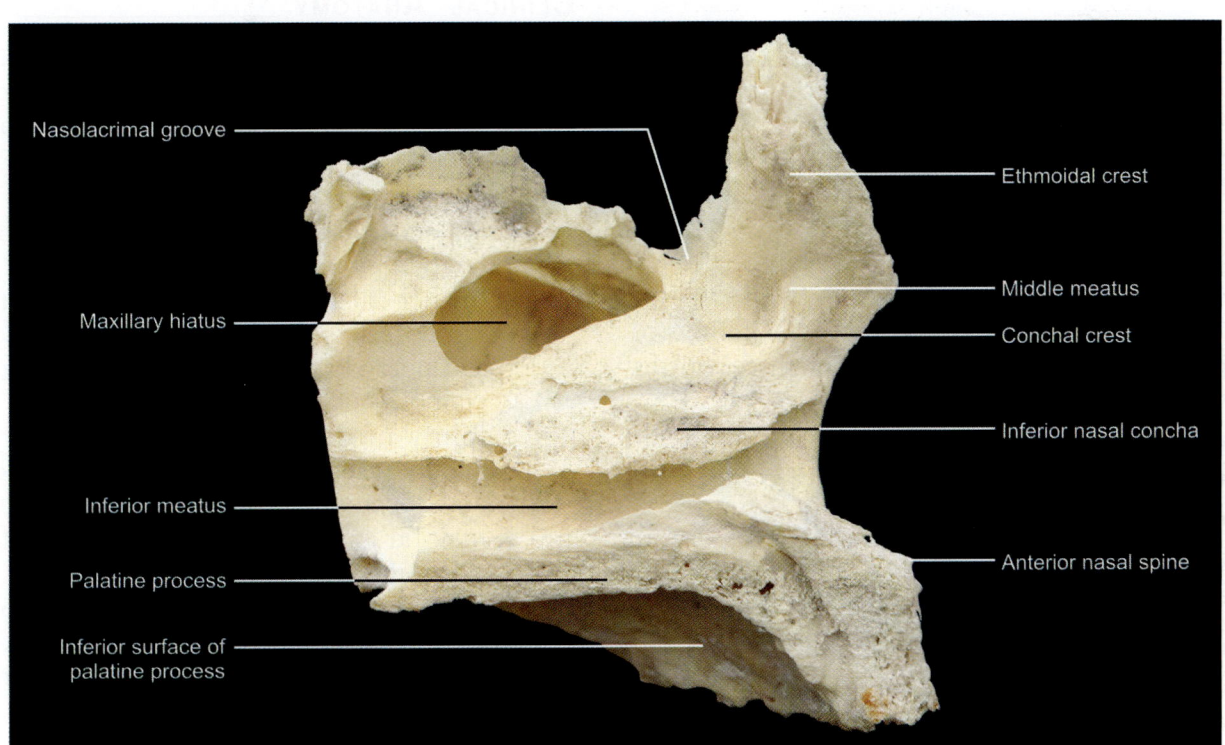

Fig. 6.28: Left maxilla (medial aspect)

PROCESSES

i. Frontal Process

a. It is a strong triangular process projects upwards with a backward tilt.

b. Its tip articulates above with the nasal notch of the frontal bone, in front with nasal bone and behind with lacrimal bone.

c. It consists of two surfaces lateral and medial.

Lateral surface: Divided into two areas by anterior lacrimal crest into anterior and posterior parts.

Anterior lacrimal crest

Attachments

a. Lacrimal fascia.

b. Medial palpebral ligament.

Anterior part

a. Origin of orbicularis oculi.

b. Levator labii superioris alaeque nasi.

Posterior part: Form lacrimal fossa for lodgment of lacrimal sac.

Medial surface

i. It forms the lateral wall of nose.

ii. Upper area is rough, articulates with ethmoid bone.

Ethmoidal crest: A transverse ridge in the middle.

Articulation: Posterior part articulates with middle nasal concha and anterior part forms the agger nasi.

II. Zygomatic process

a. It projects from the junction of anterior, posterior and orbital surfaces of the body.

b. Rough area articulates with the maxillary process of zygomatic bone.

iii. Palatine Process

a. It projects medially as a thick horizontal shelf.

b. It joins with the palatine process of fellow of opposite bone to form the anterior three-fourths of the hard palate.

c. Each process presents
- Superior and inferior surfaces.
- Medial, lateral and posterior borders.

Superior surface: It is smooth and concave and forms the major part of the floor of the nasal cavity.

Inferior surface

a. It is rough and uneven presents irregular pits for palatine glands

b. Posteriolaterally it presents a groove for greater palatine vessels and nerve.

c. Behind the central incisor teeth presents a small depression, which together with the fellow of its opposite side forms the incisive fossa.

iv. On each side of median plane of the incisive fossa there are incisive canals.

d. The incisive canal opens above into the corresponding nasal cavity.

Structures transmit: Long nasopalatine nerve and terminal branches of greater palatine vessels.

Medial border

a. It is raised into a crest called nasal crest.

b. It articulates with fellow on its opposite side forms a groove which receives the inferior border of the vomer.

Lateral border: The lateral margin is continuous with the alveolar processes.

Posterior border: It is serrated for articulation with the horizontal plate of the palatine bone.

iv. Alveolar processes

a. Thick arched border and presents sockets for the roots of upper teeth.

b. Unites with opposite process forming alveolar arch.

Attachment: Origin of buccinator from posterior part of outer surface up to the first molar tooth.

CLINICAL ANATOMY

i. **Fractures of the zygoma or zygomatic arch:** The zygoma or zygomatic arch can be fractured by a blow to the side of the face and in automobile accidents.

ii. **In maxillary fracture the result is**

a. Malocclusion of the teeth with anterior open bite.

b. Chance of leakage of cerebrospinal fluid through the nose (cerebrospinal rhinorrhea), which is secondary to fracture of the cribriform plate of ethmoid bone.

c. Injury of the infraorbital nerve results in anesthesia or paresthesia of the skin of the cheek and upper gum.

d. May be nasal bleeding and blood enters the maxillary air sinus.

iii. **Blowout fracture of maxilla:** A severe blow to the orbit may cause the contents of orbital cavity to burst downwards through the floor of the orbit into the maxillary air sinus.

iv. **Pain of maxillary sinusitis and its radiation:** The pain of maxillary sinusitis radiates to the upper teeth because of the close proximity of the anterior and posterior superior alveolar nerves.

v. **Surgical approach of the maxillary sinus**

  a. The level of maxillary hiatus is higher level than the floor of the sinus. This position is not favorable for natural drainage of sinus.

  b. Pus from frontal sinusitis tends to collect into the maxillary sinus by gravity because opening of frontal sinus being higher than that of maxillary hiatus.

  c. Therefore, surgical approach of the maxillary sinus is performed through the canine fossa in Caldwell-Luc operation or through the inferior meatus of nose.

VOMER

INTRODUCTION

It is a thin, flat and an irregularly quadrilateral-shaped bone forming the part of the bony nasal septum.

GENERAL FEATURES

Borders

  i. Superior border (Fig. 6.29)
  ii. Inferior border
  iii. Anterior border
  iv. Posterior border.

Surfaces

  i. It has two surfaces on each side of its surfaces forms the medial wall of the corresponding nasal cavities.

  ii. On each side of its surfaces marked by an antero-inferior groove for nasopalatine vessels and nerve.

Superior Border

  i. This border is broad and expanded and splits into two alae

  ii. Between the two alae, it articulates with the rostrum of the sphenoid bone.

Inferior Border

Articulates with the nasal crest formed by the two maxillae and two palatine bones.

Anterior Border

Articulates with the following

  i. Superiorly—with the perpendicular plate of the ethmoid bone,

  ii. Inferiorly—with the septal cartilage of the nose.

Posterior Border

It is short and non-articular and forms medial boundary of the posterior nasal apertures.

Tip of the vomer: It fits into the incisor crest of the maxillae and divides the incisive canal into two compartments.

NASAL BONES

Number: Two in number.

SITUATION

The bones are placed side by side between the frontal processes of the two maxillae and by their articulation form the bridge of the nose (Fig. 6.30).

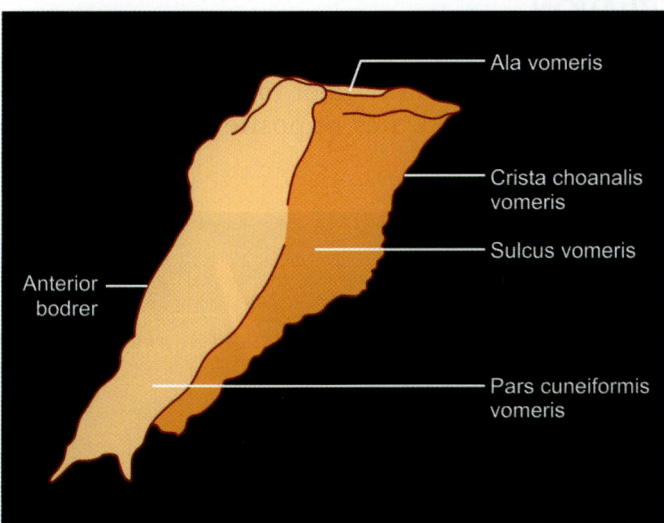

Fig. 6.29: Vomer (seen from left side)

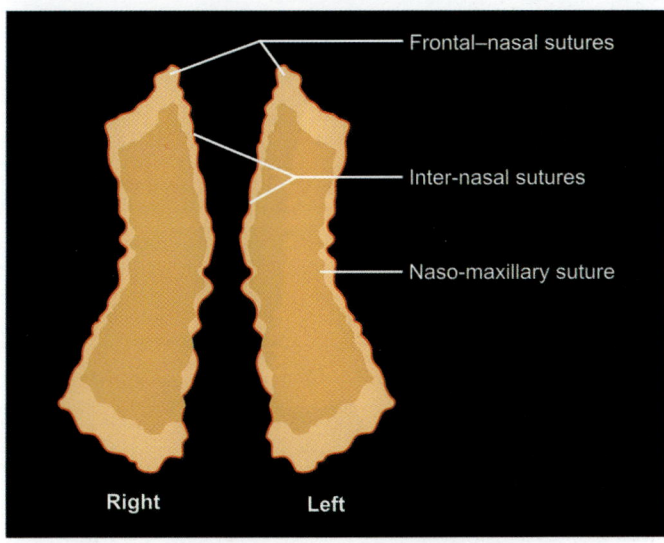

Fig. 6.30: Nasal bones

GENERAL FEATURES

Borders

Medial border: It articulates with the fellow of its opposite side

Lateral border: It articulates with the frontal process of the maxilla.

Superior border: It is thickest and serrated and articulates with the nasal notch of the frontal bone.

Inferior border: It is very thin and notched and articulates with the lateral cartilage of the nose.

Surfaces

External surface: It is convex from side to side.

Internal surface: It is concave and presents a groove directed above downwards

Lodges: The anterior ethmoidal nerve.

Clinical anatomy: Fracture of the nasal bones is more common by a blow on the nose.

LACRIMAL BONES

INTRODUCTION

This bone is the smallest and most fragile of all the cranial bones.

Situation: It is situated in the anterior part of the medial wall of the orbit.

GENERAL FEATURES

    i. Anterior border (Fig. 6.31)
   ii. Posterior border
  iii. Superior border
   iv. Inferior border.

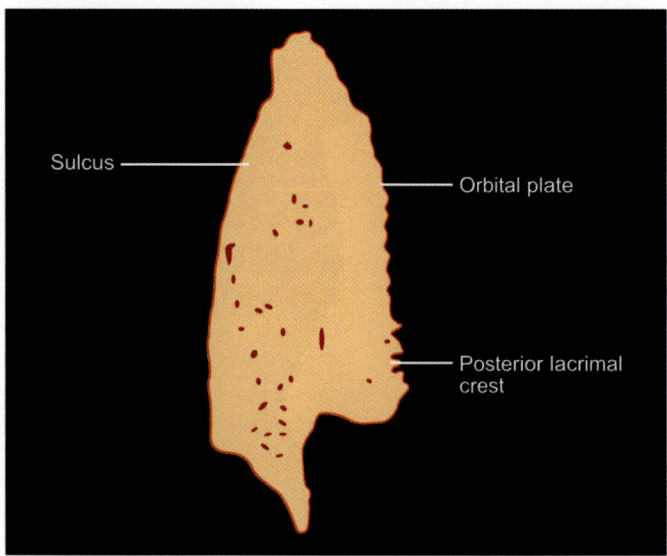

Fig. 6.31: Lacrimal bone

Surfaces

Medial or nasal surface: Forms a part of middle meatus of nose.

Lateral surface: Presents a ridge on this surface called posterior lacrimal crest which divides this surface into anterior and posterior parts.

Borders

   i. Anterior border: Articulates with the posterior border of the frontal process of the maxilla

 ii. Posterior border: Articulates with the anterior border of the orbital plate of the ethmoid bone

iii. Superior border: Articulates with the nasal notch of the frontal bone,

 iv. Inferior border: Articulates with the medial margin of the orbital surface of the maxilla,

  v. Descending process

     a. By its tip—articulates with the lacrimal process of the inferior nasal concha,

     b. By its margins—Articulates with the margins of the nasolacrimal groove.

 vi. The lacrimal hamulus—Articulates with the lacrimal tubercle on the orbital margin of the maxilla.

HYOID BONE

INTRODUCTION

It is a U-shaped bone the convexity of which is directed upwards and forwards and concavity directed downwards and backwards. It develops from the second and third branchial arches.

SITUATION

It is situated below and slightly below the symphysis menti at the junction of floor of the oral cavity and infront of the neck lies opposite the C3 vertebra (Fig. 6.32).

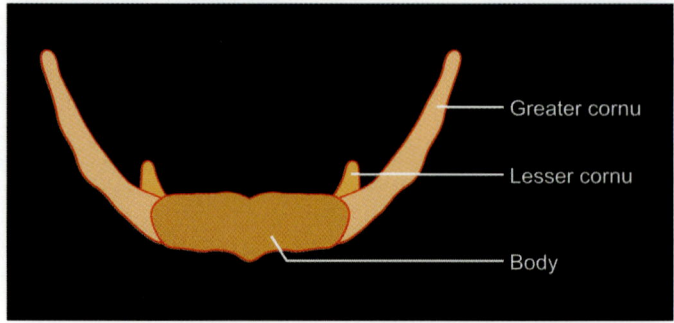

Fig. 6.32: Hyoid bone showing external features

ANATOMICAL POSITION

i. Convex and rough surface of the body in front
ii. Cocave and smooth surface of the body looks behind and downwards.

PARTS

Body: It is the broader central part of the bone.

Greater cornua: It is the narrow prolongation of the bone extends backward from the lateral ends of the bone ends in a tubercle.

Lesser cornua: It is a small conical bony process arises from the junction of the greater cornu and body which projects upwards.

Body: It is a flattened arch of the bone with the convexity upwards and forwards.

Surfaces: Anterior and posterior.

Borders: Superior and inferior.

Ends: Two lateral ends.

Anterior Surface

i. It is convex
ii. Presents a vertical ridge opposite the median plane which represents the line of fusion between the two halves of the body
iii. The anterior surface is divided into upper and lower areas by an arched transverse ridge.
iv. One each side of the median plane, the anterior surface is rough for muscular and ligamentous attachments
v. Insertion of geniohyoid muscle is attached over the rough impression which extends above and below the transverse ridge
vi. Hyoglossus muscle inserted lateral to the geniohyoid (Fig. 6.33)
vii. Mylohyoid inserted below the hyoglossus and geniohyoid muscles

viii. Sternohyoid (medially) and superior belly of omohyoid (laterally) muscles inserted below the mylohyoid
ix. Thyrohyoid is inserted lateral to the mylohyoid
x. Genioglossus (some fibers) muscle originates from above the geniohyoid muscle.

Posterior Surface

i. It is concave and directed downwards and backwards
ii. Relation of a bursa lies between the thyrohyoid membrane and the posterior surface.

Superior border

Attachments

i. Thyrohyoid membrane
ii. Hyoepiglottic ligament

Inferior border

Attachments

i. Sternohyoid
ii. Omohyoid
iii. Levator glandulae thyroideae (it presents occasionally, which is a band of muscular tissue connects the body of hyoid bone with isthmus or pyramidal lobe of thyroid gland).

CORNU

Greater cornu

It projects backwards from the lateral ends of the body.

Attachments

Upper surface

i. Hyoglossus originates from the upper surface
ii. Middle constrictor muscle of pharynx originates from above the origin of hyoglossus
iii. Insertion of stylohyoid and attachment of fibrous loop which anchors the central tendon of the digastric muscle below the hyoglossus muscle.

Inferior surface: It is oblique in direction.

Medial border: Attachment to the thyrohyoid membrane.

Lateral border

i. Insertion of thyrohyoid muscle from anteriorly
ii. Stylohyoid muscle attached close to the junction of greater cornu with the body.

Lesser cornu

i. It projects upwards from the junction of body and greater cornu.

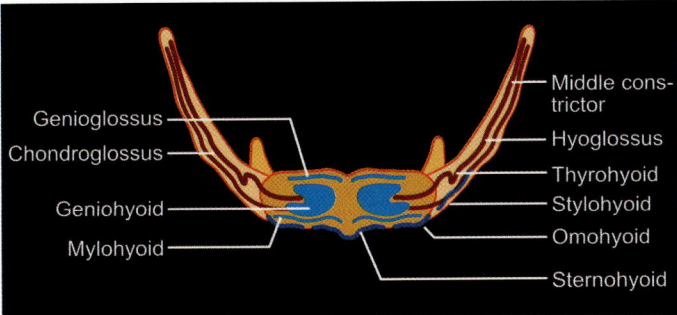

Fig. 6.33: Hyoid bone showing attachments

ii. Stylohyoid ligament attached to it.

iii. Middle constrictor of pharynx arises from the posterolateral aspect.

iv. Chondroglossus muscle arises from the medial aspect of its base.

CLINICAL ANATOMY

Medicolegal importance: In a suspected case of a death, fracture of hyoid bone causes death occurs by strangulation or throttling.

PALATINE BONES

SITUATION

It is a 'L' shaped bone situated on each side in between the pterygoid process of the sphenoid bone behind and the maxilla infront (Fig. 6.34).

GENERAL FEATURES

Parts

Vertical or perpendicular plate: It is oblong in shape, ascends upwards between the orbital process in front and the sphenoidal process behind

Surfaces: Medial/lateral or maxillary.

Borders: Anterior, posterior, superior and inferior.

Horizontal plate: This part forms the posterior one-fourth part of the bony palate.

i. This part directed medially from the lower margin of the perpendicular plate

ii. **Surfaces:** Superior and inferior.

iii. **Borders:** Anterior, posterior, medial and lateral,

Processes

Orbital process

i. It is projected upwards and laterally from the upper border of the perpendicular plate and contains an air cell with broken margins.

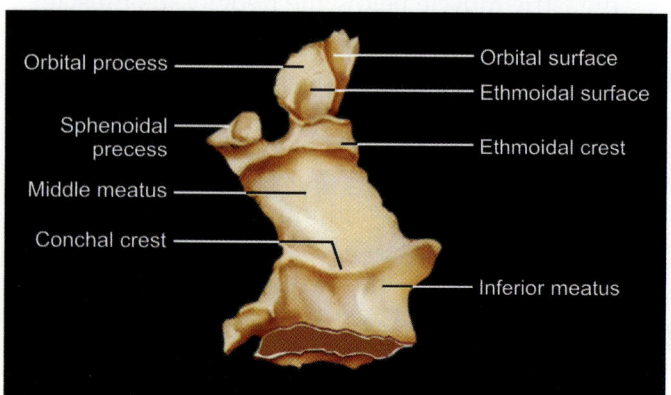

Orbital process — Orbital surface
— Ethmoidal surface
Sphenoidal precess —
— Ethmoidal crest
Middle meatus —
Conchal crest —
— Inferior meatus

Fig. 6.34: Palatine bone

Sphenoidal process

i. Directed upwards and medially from the superior border of perpendicular plate.

ii. It is in lower level than the orbital process

iii. **Surfaces:** Superior, inferomedial and lateral,

iv. **Borders:** Anterior, posterior and medial.

Pyramidal Process or Tubercle

i. It is projected downwards, backwards and laterally from the junction of horizontal and perpendicular plates

ii. **Surfaces:** Posterior, lateral and inferior.

INFERIOR NASAL CONCHAE

Definition: These are two curved laminae of bones.

Situation: In the lower parts on the lateral walls of the nose between the concha and floor of the nose lies the inferior meatus of the nose.

Borders

Superior border: It is irregular and articulates with maxilla, lacrimal, ethmoid and palatine bones

Inferior border: It is free, thick and spongy.

Surfaces

Medial surface: It is convex and presents numerous vascular foramina.

Lateral surface: It forms the medial wall of the inferior meatus of the nose.

Ends: The posterior end is more pointed than the anterior end.

ZYGOMATIC BONES (MALAR BONE)

ANATOMICAL POSITION

i. Thick and long process looks upwards.

ii. The non-articular (posterosuperior) border resembling letter 'f' will directed upwards and backwards (Fig. 6.35).

SIDE DETERMINATION

After holding the bone in anatomical positions the convex lateral surface determines the side of the bone.

SITUATION

Zygomatic bone is two in number situated in the infero-lateral aspect of the orbit and it forms the prominence of cheek.

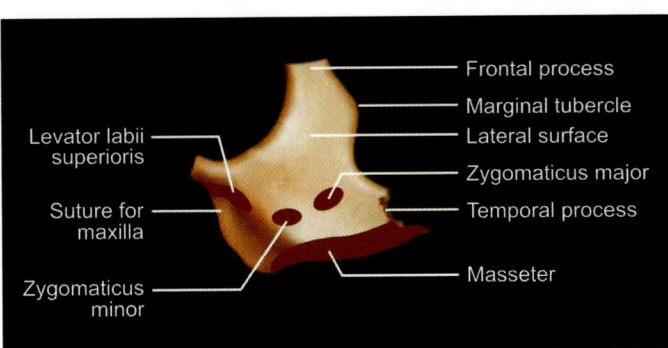

Levator labii superioris

Suture for maxilla

Zygomaticus minor

Frontal process

Marginal tubercle

Lateral surface

Zygomaticus major

Temporal process

Masseter

Fig. 6.35: Zygomatic bone

Contributions

i. It forms the floor and lateral wall of the orbit.

ii. Walls of the temporal and infraorbital fossae.

GENERAL FEATURES

Surfaces

Lateral or malar surface

i. It is convex, looks laterally and forwards.

ii. It presents a foramen near the orbital margin, called zygomaticofacial foramen.

   Transmits

   a. Zygomaticofacial nerve

   b. Zygomaticofacial vessels.

iii. Below the foramen an elevation which gives origin to zygomaticus minor muscle.

iv. Area posterior to the elevation gives origin to zygomaticus major muscle

v. Close to the posteroinferior margin, gives origin to some fibers of masseter.

Medial or temporal surface

i. It is smooth and concave and forms a part of the infratemporal fossa.

ii. Near the base of frontal process presents a foramen called zygomaticotemporal foramen.

Transmits—zygomaticotemporal vessels and nerves.

Orbital Surface

i. Expanded plate of bone projects medially and backward.

ii. It is smooth and gently concave and forms a part of the floor and lateral wall of the orbit.

Borders

i. **Anterosuperior/orbital border:** It forms the infero-lateral margin of the orbit.

ii. **Anteroinferior or maxillary border:** Articulates with the maxilla.

iii. **Posterosuperior or temporal border:** It forms an italic 'f'' shaped sharp border.

iv. **Posteroinferior border:** Attachment to masseter.

v. **Posteromedial border:** It articulates with the lateral border of orbital surface of greater wing of sphenoid bone in the upper part and with the maxilla in lower part.

Processes

i. **Frontal process:** It projects upwards.

ii. **Temporal process:** It is directed backwards

OSSIFICATION

Each of the zygomatic bone develops in membrane and usually ossifies from one center during 8th week of intrauterine life.

CLINICAL ANATOMY

i. **Japonicum:** Sometimes the bone is dividing into upper and lower parts by a fissure making the malar prominence flat, which is usual feature of the Mongolian race and this is known as Japonicum.

ii. **Depressed fracture**

   a. It occurs usually caused by hard blows to the head in thin area of the cranium,

   b. In this fracture a fragment of bone is depressed inward to compress or injure the brain

iii. **Linear skull fractures**

   It is the most common type of skull fracture, but fracture line often radiate away from it in two or more direction.

iv. **Comminuted fractures**

   a. In this type of fracture it is broken into several pieces,

   b. If the bone is at the site of impact, the bone usually bends inward without fracturing,

   c. Although a fracture may result some distance from the site of direct trauma where the calvaria is thinner.

v. **Contrecoup or counterblow fracture**

   In this case no fracture occurs at the point of impact but fracture occurs on the opposite side of the skull

vi. **Fracture of the pterion**

   a. It may occurs due to blow on the side of the head where thin bones forming the pterion

   b. Due to fracture of the pterion, the anterior branch of the middle meningeal artery rupture which lies deep to the pterion.

   c. As a result hematoma occur which exert pressure on the underlying cerebral cortex

   d. In a untreated case of rupture of middle meningeal artery may cause death in a few hours.

ETHMOID BONE

SITUATION

In the part of the cranium below the ethmoidal notch of the frontal bone.

CONSISTENCY

Light and fragile (Fig. 6.36).

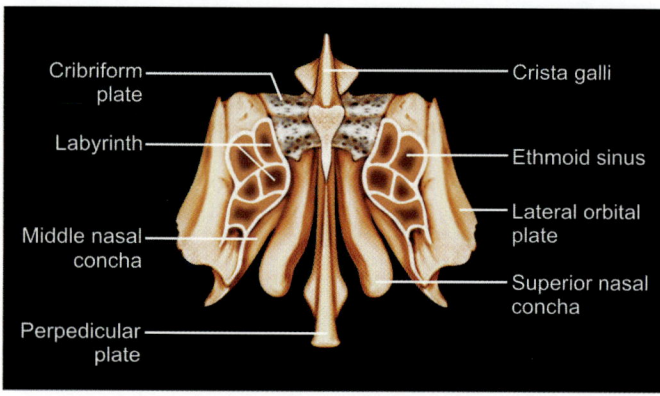

Fig. 6.36: Ethmoid bone

Contribution (in Articulated Skull)

It forms the following
  i. Roof and medial wall of the orbit.
  ii. Roof and lateral wall of the nasal cavity
  iii. Part of the nasal septum.

Parts

  i. Horizontal cribriform plate.
  ii. A pair of labyrinths.
  iii. Perpendicular plate.

Horizontal Part of Cribriform Plate

Features

  i. It is perforated by numerous foramina for the olfactory nerve rootlets.
  ii. Occupying the ethmoidal notch of frontal bone.

Crista Galli

  i. It is a smooth triangular process directed upwards from the anterior part of the floor of the anterior cranial fossa.

  ii. Posteriorly, its free border gives attachment to the anterior part of the falx cerebri.

LABYRINTHS

Features

  a. Labyrinth consists of two vertical plates of the bone, one on each side of the perpendicular plate, suspended from the under surface of the cribriform plate.
  b. Each labyrinth encloses number of air cells; they are- Anterior, middle and posterior.

Surfaces

Anterior surface: It articulates with the frontal process of the maxilla to complete the anterior ethmoidal air cells.

Posterior surface: It articulates with the sphenoidal concha to complete the posterior ethmoidal air cells.

Superior surface: It articulates with the orbital plate of frontal bone.

Inferior surface: It articulates with the nasal surface of the maxilla.

  i. Anteriorly, orbital surface of the maxilla,
  ii. Posteriorly, orbital process of the palatine bone.

Medial surface

  i. The medial surface presence superior nasal concha, middle nasal concha, superior meatus lies below the superior concha and middle meatus below the middle concha.
  ii. A rounded swelling projects into the middle meatus called bulla ethmoidalis.

Lateral surface: It forms the medial wall of the orbit.

Perpendicular Plate

Features: It is a thin, quadrilateral piece of bone projects downwards from the inferior surface of cribriform plate forming the upper part of the bony nasal septum.

CLINICAL ANATOMY

CSF rhinorrhea: Fracture of the cribriform plate of ethmoid bone may produce discharge of cerebro spinal fluid (CSF) through the nose.

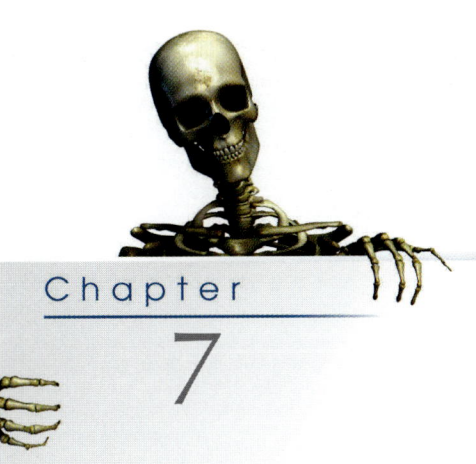

Oral Questions and Answers

Interior of the base of skull (cranial fossae) with foramina and structures transmitting
(Fig. 7.1)

1. **Foramina in the cribriform plate of the ethmoid bone:** Olfactory nerves.

2. **Optic canal:**
   a. Optic nerve
   b. Ophthalmic artery.

3. **Superior orbital fissure:**

   Lateral to the annulus:
   i. From cranial to orbital cavity
      a. Trochlear nerve
      b. Frontal nerve
      c. Lacrimal nerve
      d. Orbital branch of middle meningeal artery
      e. Lacrimal artery
   ii. From orbital to cranial cavity
      a. Superior ophthalmic vein.
      b. Recurrent meningeal branch of lacrimal artery.

   Through the annulus:
   From cranial to orbital cavity
   i. Two divisions of oculomotor nerve
   ii. Nasociliary nerve
   iii. Abducent nerve.

   Medial to annulus:
   i. From orbit to cranium
   ii. Inferior ophthalmic vein.

4. **Inferior orbital fissure:**

Ans. i. Maxillary nerve
   ii. Inferior orbital vessels
   iii. Inferior orbital nerve
   iv. Zygomatic nerve
   v. A few filaments from the pterygopalatine ganglion.

5. **Foramen rotundum:** Maxillary nerve

6. **Foramen ovale:**
   i. Mandibular nerve (motor and sensory roots)
   ii. Accessory meningeal artery
   iii. Occasionally lesser petrosal nerve, an emissary vein and anterior division of middle meningeal sinus.

7. **Foramen spinosum:**
   i. Middle meningeal artery
   ii. Meningeal branch of mandibular nerve (nervus spinosus)
   iii. Posterior division of middle meningeal sinus.

8. **Foramen lacerum:** Internal carotid artery (through the upper opening of the foramen lacerum)

9. **Internal acoustic (auditory) meatus:**
   Entrance
   i. Motor root of facial nerve
   ii. Nervous intermedius
   iii. Internal auditory artery
   iv. A branch from the posterior cerebellar or basilar artery
   Exit
   i. Sensory root of the facial nerve
   ii. The vestibulocochlear (auditory) nerve.
   iii. Internal auditory vein

10. **Jugular foramen:**
    i. **Anterior compartment:** Inferior petrosal sinus
    ii. **Posterior compartment:** Internal jugular vein

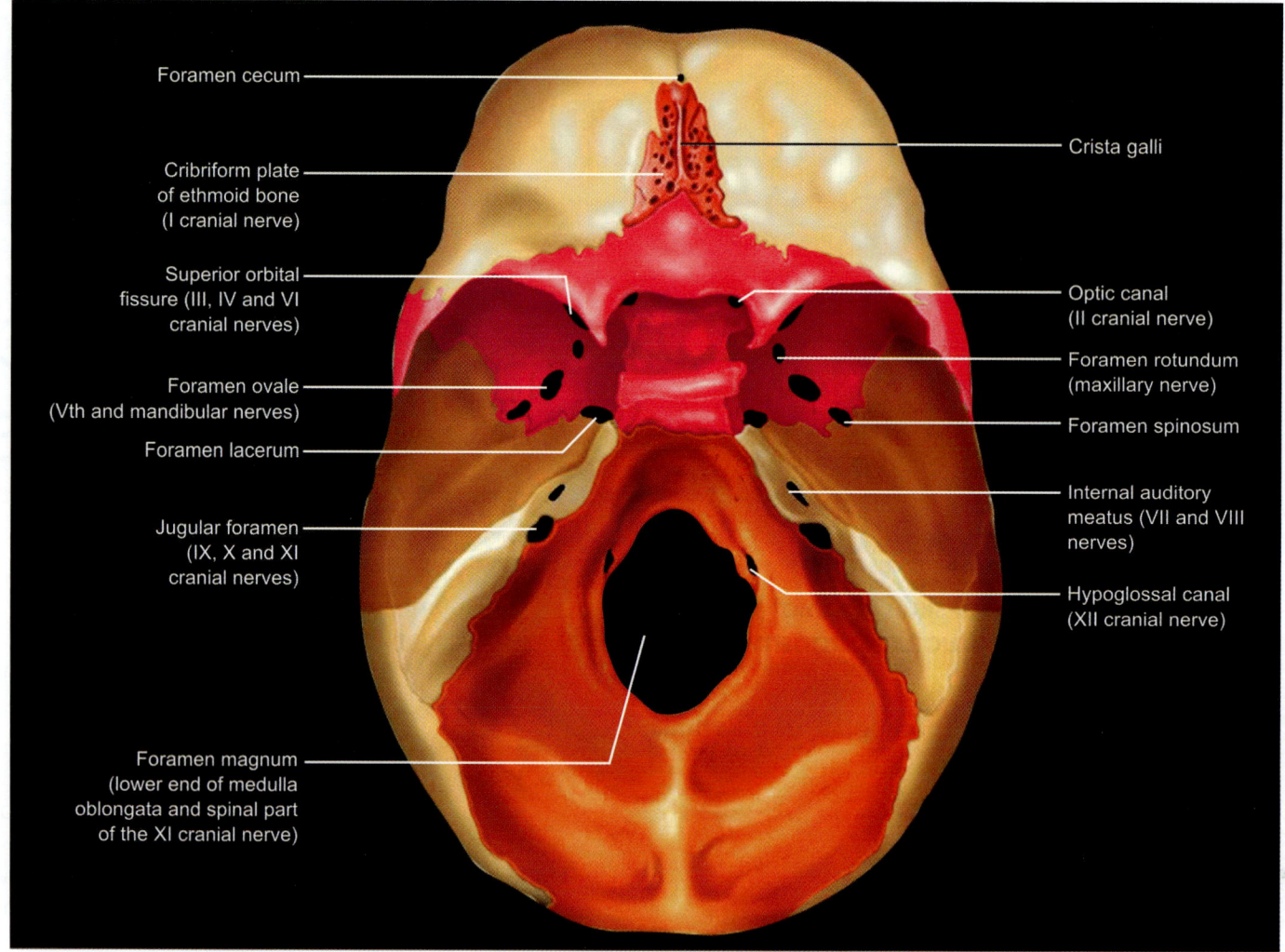

Fig. 7.1: Interior of the base of skull showing its foramina and exit of cranial nerves

iii. **Intermediate compartment:**
    a. Glossopharyngeal nerve
    b. Vagus nerve
    c. Accessory nerve.

11. Hypoglossal (anterior condylar) canal
    i. Hypoglossal nerve
   ii. Meningeal branch of hypoglossal nerve
  iii. Meningeal branch of ascending pharyngeal artery
  iv. Emissary vein

12. Foramen magnum
    i. Structures transmits through the anterior compartment
      a. Apical ligament
      b. The upper band of the cruciate ligament
      c. Odontoid process of axis
      d. Membrana tectoria—it is the continuation of the posterior longitudinal ligament of vertebral column

    ii. Structures pass through the posterior compartment
      • Lower end of the medulla oblongata and its coverings: From outside inwards—
        a. Dura mater
        b. Arachnoid mater
        c. Pia mater.
  iii. Spinal portion of the accessory nerve (ascending)
  iv. Two vertebral arteries with the sympathetic nerve plexus (ascending)
   v. Anterior and posterior spinal arteries (descending).

13. Foramen cecum: An emissary vein connecting the superior sagittal sinus with the veins of the nasal mucosa.

14. Carotid canal: Internal carotid artery with its sympathetic plexus.

15. Stylomastoid foramen: Facial nerve and stylomastoid artery.

16. **Tympanic canaliculus:** Tympanic branch of glossopharyngeal nerve.
17. **Mastoid canaliculus:** Auricular branch of vagus nerve.
18. **Mastoid foramen:** An emissary vein and a small branch of the occipital artery.
19. **Supraorbital canal:** Supraorbital nerve and vessels.
20. **Infraorbital canal:** Infraorbital nerve and vessels.
21. **Supratrochlear foramen or notch:** Supratrochlear nerve and vessels.
22. **Posterior condylar canal:** An emissary vein.

Exterior of the base of skull (norma basalis) with foramina and structures transmitting
(Fig. 7.2)

Anterior part:
1. **Lateral incisive foramen:**
   i. Terminal branches of greater palatine vessels
   ii. Nasopalatine nerve.
2. **Greater palatine foramen:** Greater palatine vessels and nerves.

3. **Lesser palatine foramina:** Lesser palatine vessels and nerves.

Middle part:
4. **Foramen ovale:** *See* page 123.
5. **Foramen spinosum:** *See* page 123.
6. **Foramen lacerum:** Internal carotid artery through the upper opening, but lower part of opening is closed by a plate of cartilage.
   i. **Anterior opening of carotid canal** (present on posterior wall of foramen lacerum)**:** Internal carotid artery and a plexus of sympathetic nerves and veins.
   ii. **Pterygoid canal** (present on anterior wall of foramen lacerum)**:** Pterygoid vessels and nerves.
7. **Lower opening of carotid canal:** Internal carotid artery.

Posterior part:
8. **Foramen magnum:** *See* page 124.
9. **Hypoglossal (anterior condylar) canal:** *See* page 124.
10. **Posterior condylar canal:** *See* above.
11. **Jugular foramen:** *See* page 123.
12. **Stylomastoid foramen:** *See* page 124.

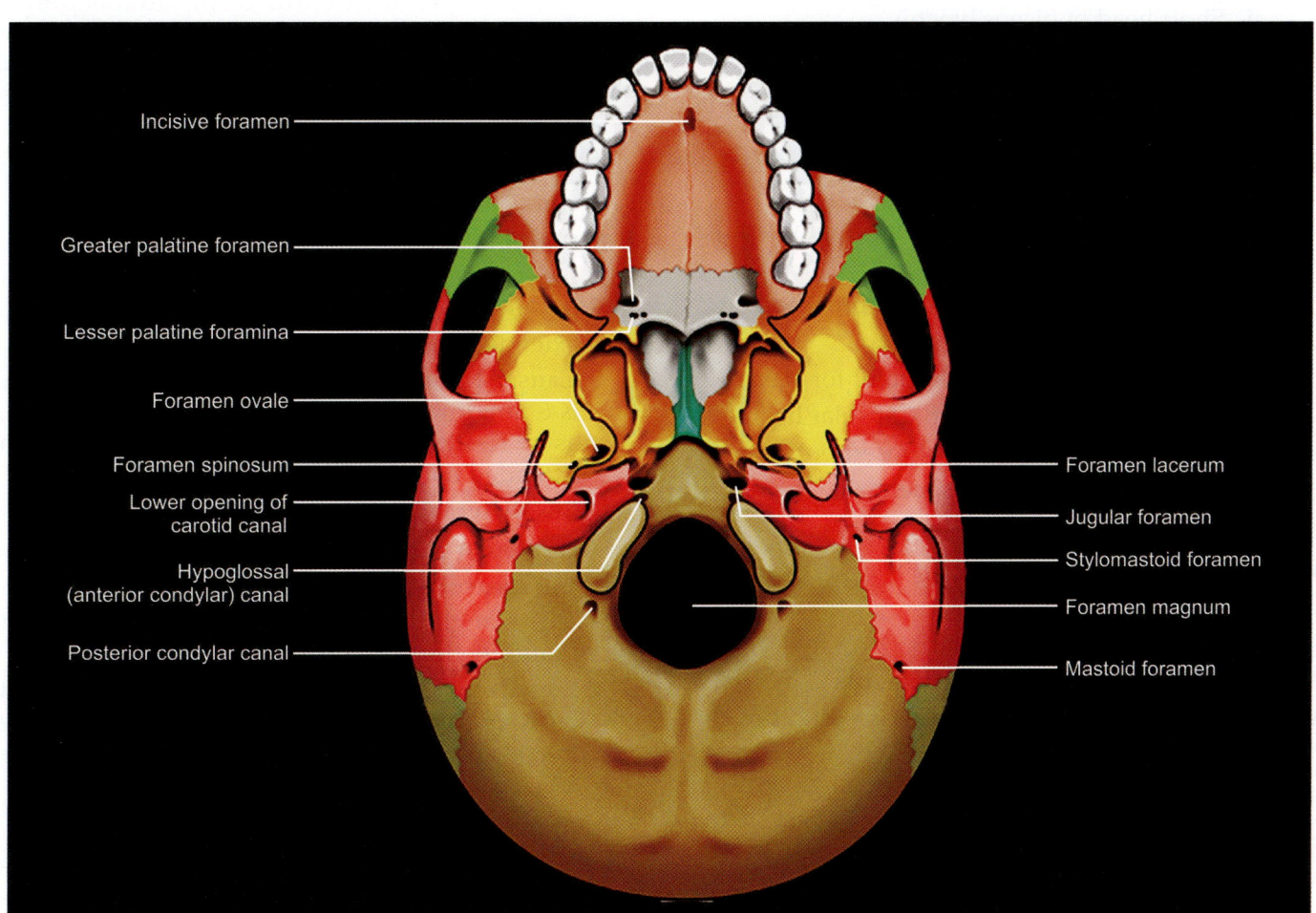

Fig. 7.2: Exterior of the base of skull (norma basalis) showing foramina and structures transmitting

UPPER LIMB

Q. Attachments of medial border of scapula

Ans. Insertion of: On the dorsal aspect

i. Levator scapulae—from superior angle to the upper part of the apex of the spine.

ii. Rhomboideus minor—opposite the apex of the spine.

iii. Rhomboideus major—below the apex of the spine up to the inferior angle.

On the costal surface: Serratus anterior—from whole of the border.

Q. What is the literal meaning of clavicle?

Ans. *"Key".*

Q. What is the literal meaning of scapula?

Ans. "To dig".

Q. What is the meaning of the coracoid process?

Ans. Beak like.

Q. Muscles attached to the coracoid process of scapula.

Ans. i. Coracobrachialis

ii. Short head of biceps brachii

iii. Pectoralis minor.

Q. Structures passing above and below the suprascapular ligament.

Ans. Above the suprascapular ligament: Suprascapular vessels.

Below the suprascapular ligament: Suprascapular nerve.

Q. Structures attached to acromion process.

Ans. i. Lateral border: Deltoid (origin).

ii. Medial margin of articular facet for clavicle.

iii. Margins of articular facet: Capsular ligament.

iv. Medial border: Trapezius (insertion).

v. Tip: Coracoacromial ligament.

Q. What are necks of the humerus?

Ans. i. Anatomical

ii. Surgical

iii. Morphological.

Q. Nerves direct contact with humerus

Ans. i. Axillary *nerve:* At the posterior aspect of the surgical neck.

ii. Radial nerve: At the spiral/radial groove.

iii. Ulnar nerve: At the posterior aspect of the medial epicondyle.

Q. Nerves not contact but related with humerus:

Ans. Nerve to anconeus and musculocutaneous nerve.

Q. Structures related to surgical neck of humerus?

Ans. i. Axillary nerve.

ii. Anterior and posterior circumflex humeral vessels.

Q. Structures passing/lodges through spiral/radial groove.

Ans. i. Radial nerve.

ii. Arteria profunda brachii branch of brachial artery.

Q. Branches of radial nerve in the spiral/radial groove

Ans. i. Muscular branches to—

a. Lateral head of triceps.

b. Nerve to medial head of triceps.

c. Nerve to anconeus.

ii. Cutaneous branches

a. Posterior cutaneous nerve of the forearm.

b. Lower lateral cutaneous nerve of the arm.

Q. Structures related to posterior surface of lower end of radius

Ans. i. Lateral groove—extensor carpi radialis longus laterally and extensor carpi radialis brevis medially

ii. Groove medial to the dorsal tubercle—extensor pollicis longus

iii. Groove more medially—extensor digitorum and more deeply extensor indicis with posterior interosseous nerve.

Q. Carrying angle

Ans. Introduction: It is an angle open laterally between the arm and forearm, when the elbow is fully extended and forearm supinated.

Cause: The medial edge of trochlea of humerus is 6 mm lower than the lateral edge of trochlea., as a result the forearm away from the arm in extended and supinated position.

Sex difference: It is more acute in female.

Degree of angle

i. It measures about 163°.

ii. This angle disappears when the elbow is flexed and the forearm pronated.

Function: The carrying angle prevents contact between the ulnar border of forearm with the lateral surface of the thigh and facilitates to carry a heavy object by the hand.

Q. Angle of humeral torsion

Ans. It is the angle between the axis of head of humerus and with the axis of the lower end of humerus which measures about 164° in adult.

Q. Attachments of greater tubercle of humerus.

Ans. Insertion of muscles:

i. Supraspinatus—to the upper impression

ii. Infraspinatus—to the middle impression

iii. Teres minor—to the lowest impression.

Ligament: Transverse humeral ligament—to the medial margin of the tubercle.

Q. Nerves of the upper limb with their accompanied arteries.

Ans. i. Axillary nerve: Accompanied with posterior circumflex humeral artery branch of axillary artery.

ii. Radial nerve: Accompanied with arteria profunda brachii branch of brachial artery.
Ulnar nerve: Accompanied with superior ulnar collateral artery branch of brachial artery.

iii. Median nerve: Accompanied with arteria nervi mediana branch of anterior interosseous artery.

Q. Structures piercing the clavipectoral fascia.

Ans. **Going out**

i. Thoracoacromial artery

ii. Lateral pectoral nerve

Going in

iii. Cephalic vein

iv. Lymphatics from the breast.

Q. Structures piercing the medial intermuscular septum.

Ans. i. Ulnar nerve

ii. Superior ulnar collateral artery

iii. Posterior branch of inferior ulnar collateral artery.

Q. Structures piercing the lateral intermuscular septum?

Ans. Radial nerve and anterior descending branch of arteria profunda brachii.

Q. Contents of intertubercular sulcus or bicipital groove

Ans. i. Long head of biceps brachii with its synovial sheath,

ii. An ascending branch of anterior circumflex humeral artery.

Q. Attachments of intertubercular sulcus or bicipital groove.

Ans. From lateral to medial insertion of:

i. Lateral lip: Pectoralis major

ii. Floor: Latissimus dorsi

iii. Medial lip: Teres major

Q. Extensor group of forearm muscle but flexor of elbow

Ans. Brachioradialis.

Q. Name two muscles which are flexor of the elbow joint and supplied by the radial nerve

Ans. Brachioradialis and brachialis (only lateral part is supplied by radial nerve).

Q. Name the proximal row of carpal bones.

Ans. Lateral to medial:

i. Scaphoid

ii. Lunate

iii. Triquetral

iv. Pisiform (smallest carpal bone).

Q. Name the carpal bones take part in the formation of wrist joint

Ans. From lateral to medial:

i. Scaphoid,

ii. Lunate,

iii. Triquetral.

Q. Why the pisiform bone does not take part in the formation of wrist joint?

Ans. As the pisiform bone is projected forwards from the anterior aspect of the triquetral bone.

Q. Name the distal row of carpal bones.

Ans. Lateral to medial:

i. Trapezium

ii. Trapezoid

iii. Capitate

iv. Hamate.

Q. Name the smallest and largest carpal bones.

Ans. Smallest—pisiform and largest—capitate.

Q. Which of the carpal bone which is sesamoid and develop in the tendon of flexor carpi ulnaris?

Ans. Pisiform

Q. When does the pisiform bone ossify?

Ans. At the age of 12 years.

Q. Carpal bone starts ossification first

Ans. Capitate

Q. Carpal bone ossified last

Ans. Pisiform

Q. Which is the key carpal bone?

Ans. Capitate.

Q. Which carpal bone commonly fractured on an outstretched hand?

Ans. Scaphoid.

Q. Where do you examine for tenderness in case of scaphoid bone fracture?

Ans. In the anatomical snuffbox.

Q. Bones forming the floor of the anatomical snuffbox

Ans. Proximal to distal:
    i. Styloid process radius
    ii. Scaphoid, trapezium and base of the first metacarpal bone.

Q. Mention importance at the level of insertion of coracobrachialis muscle

Ans.   i. Median nerve crosses the brachial artery from lateral to medial side.
    ii. Upper limit of the medial intermuscular septum.
    iii. Ulnar nerve and the superior ulnar collateral artery pierces the medial intermuscular septum.
    iv. Superior ulnar collateral artery originates.
    v. Radial nerve pierces the lateral intermuscular septum.
    vi. Basilic vein pierces the deep fascia.
    vii. Medial cutaneous nerve of the forearm pierces the deep fascia.
    viii. The upper supratrochlear lymph nodes.
    ix. Deltoid is inserted.

THORAX

Q. What are typical ribs?

Ans. Third to ninth ribs.

Q. What are atypical ribs?

Ans. First, second, tenth, eleventh and twelfth ribs.

Q. Longest rib

Ans. Seventh rib.

Q. Maximum oblique rib

Ans. Ninth rib.

Q. Maximum diameter of thorax

Ans. At the level of eighth rib.

Q. Mention peculiarities of first rib

Ans.   i. It is the most curved rib.
    ii. It has superior and inferior surfaces.
    iii. It is shortest of all the true ribs.
    iv. Head is small and only one facet.
    v. Consists of outer and inner borders.

Q. Structures related to grooves on the superior surface of the first rib

Ans.   i. Anterior groove lodges subclavian vein
    ii. Posterior groove lodges subclavian artery and lower trunk of brachial plexus.

Q. Structures related to neck of the first rib

Ans. From lateral to medial
    i. First thoracic nerve.
    ii. First posterior intercostal vein.
    iii. Superior intercostal artery.
    iv. Sympathetic trunk with the first thoracic ganglion and sometimes stellate ganglion.

Q. Floating ribs

Ans. Eleventh and twelfth ribs.

Q. Structures lodges in the costal groove of typical ribs

Ans. From above downwards:
    i. Intercostal vein.
    ii. Intercostal artery.
    iii. Intercostal nerve.

Q. Ribs producing pump-handle movements

Ans. Second to sixth ribs.

Q. Ribs producing bucket-handle movements

Ans. Seventh to tenth ribs.

Q. What are typical thoracic vertebrae

Ans. These are second to eighth.

Q. What are atypical thoracic vertebrae

Ans. First, ninth, tenth, eleventh and twelfth.

Q. Name the joints between a typical rib and a typical thoracic vertebra.

Ans.   i. **Costovertebral joints:** These are synovial joints between the head of a typical rib articulates with its own vertebra and also with the body of the next higher vertebra.
    ii. **Costotransverse joints:** These are synovial joints between the tubercle of a typical rib articulates with the transverse process of the corresponding vertebra.

Q. Contents of typical intercostal spaces.

Ans. The intercostal spaces are filled by the intercostal muscles and contain the intercostal nerves, vessels and lymphatics.

Q. Name the intercostal muscles.

Ans. From external to internal:
    i. Intercostalis externus
    ii. Intercostalis internus
    iii. Intercostalis intimus.

Q. What is sternal angle or Louis angle mention its importance

Ans. **Introduction:** The sternal angle is the bony angle between the manubrium and body of the sternum.

Situation: It is situated about 5 cm below the suprasternal notch.

Important land marks

i. Termination of arch of aorta into descending thoracic aorta,

ii. End of ascending aorta and beginning of arch of aorta.

iii. Bifurcation of trachea and beginning of the bronchi,

iv. Origin of left recurrent laryngeal nerve,

v. Deep and superficial cardiac plexuses,

vi. Termination of azygos vein into the superior vena cava.

vii. Presence of ligamentum arteriosum,

viii. The site where the pleural sacs meet.

Clinical anatomy: It is an important landmark for counting ribs.

Q. Some important vertebral levels.

Ans. i. Sixth cervical vertebra corresponds to:

a. Cricoid cartilage

b. Terminations of larynx and pharynx

c. Beginning of trachea and esophagus

d. Beginning of second part of vertebral artery

e. Situation of middle cervical sympathetic ganglion

f. Superior belly of omohyoid crossed the front of the common carotid artery

g. Inferior thyroid artery crossed the common carotid artery.

ii. **Second thoracic vertebra corresponds to:** Suprasternal/jugular notch of the manubrium sterni.

iii. **Fourth thoracic vertebra corresponds to**

a. Sternal angle

b. Termination of arch of aorta into descending thoracic aorta

c. End of ascending aorta and beginning of arch of aorta.

d. Bifurcation of trachea and beginning of the bronchi

e. Origin of left recurrent laryngeal nerve

f. Deep and superficial cardiac plexuses

g. Termination of azygos vein into the superior vena cava.

h. Presence of ligamentum arteriosum

i. The site where the pleural sacs meet.

iv. **Eighth and ninth thoracic vertebrae corresponds to**

a. The inferior vena cave (IVC) pierces the diaphragm

b. Ninth thoracic vertebra corresponds to xiphisternal articulation.

ABDOMEN AND PELVIS

Q. Name the typical lumbar vertebrae

Ans. First to fourth.

Q. Name the atypical lumbar vertebra

Ans. Fifth.

Q. Name the five paired processes of lumbar vertebrae.

Ans. i. Transverse processes

ii. Superior articular processes

iii. Inferior articular processes

iv. Mamillary processes

v. Accessory processes.

Q. Structures related to pelvic surface of sacrum.

Ans. i. Sympathetic trunk

ii. Median sacral artery

iii. Rectum

iv. Right and left branches of superior rectal artery

v. Parietal peritoneum.

Q. Which ligament is considered strong in female pelvis?

Ans. Interosseous sacroiliac ligament.

Q. Contents of sacral canal.

Ans. i. Cauda equina

ii. Filum terminale

iii. Spinal meninges with subdural and subarachnoid spaces.

Q. Structures passes through the sacral hiatus.

Ans. i. Filum terminale covered by dura, arachnoid and pia maters

ii. Fifth pair of sacral nerves

iii. Coccygeal nerves.

Q. What is costal element?

Ans. The bar of bone between the pelvic sacral foramina of the same side.

Q. Ala sacralis.

Ans. The non-articular part of the base of the sacrum projects laterally on each side of the articular part as a broad triangular sloping area.

Relations: From medial to lateral

i. Sympathetic trunk

ii. Lumbosacral nerve trunk

iii. Iliolumbar artery

iv. Obturator nerve.

Q. Sacralization of fifth lumbar vertebra.

Ans. The fifth lumbar vertebra or its transverse process may be fused with sacrum and this condition is called sacralization of fifth lumbar vertebra.

Q. What is another name of pelvis and why?

Ans. Pelvis means any basin-shaped structure or cavity. Another name of pelvis is basin which is derived from the Latin word (L., *basin*).

Q. Anatomical position of pelvis:

Ans. i. The anterior superior iliac spine and pubic tubercle are in the same vertical plane
ii. The upper border of symphysis pubis and tip of the coccyx lies on the same level.
Thus in anatomical position of bony pelvis, the dorsal wall looks upwards and ventral wall faces downwards.

Q. Subdivisions of the pelvis.

Ans. The pelvis is subdivided into false or greater pelvis and true or lesser pelvis, by the brim of the pelvis. The brim is formed by the arcuate lines which meet together both in front and behind opposite the median plane.
The arcuate line is formed of each side by the following—sacral promontory, anterior border of the ala sacralis, lower half of medial border of ilium, pectineal line of pubis, pubic crest and the upper border of symphysis pubis.

Q. Boundaries of the pelvic inlet.

Ans. Posteriorly: Sacral promontory and anterior margins of alae of the sacrum.
Laterally: Arcuate and pectineal lines.
Infront: Upper margin of pubic symphysis and pubic crest.

Q. Boundaries of the pelvic outlet.

Ans. Anteriorly: Lower margin of the pubic symphysis.
Anterolaterally: Conjoint ischiopubic ramus on each side.
Laterally: Ischial tuberosity on each side.
Posterolaterally: Sacrotuberous ligament on each side.
Posteriorly: Tip of the coccyx.

Q. Sub-pubic angle in male and female how much?

Ans. In male about 50 to 60° and in female about 80 to 90°.

Q. Boundaries of lumbar (Petit's) triangle and clinical importance

Ans. Boundaries
Anteriorly: By the posterior border of the external obliquus abdominis.
Posteriorly: By the lower part of the lateral border of the latissimus dorsi.

Base: By the crest of the ilium.
Apex: By the union of the external obliquus abdominis and latissimus dorsi muscles.
Floor: By the internal obliquus abdominis.
Clinical importance: Occasionally, it is the site of lumbar hernia.

Q. Important events occurring at L1 vertebra:

Ans. a. Transpyloric plane passes through this level,
b. Superior mesenteric artery arises
c. Pyloric part of stomach lies
d. First part of duodenum lies
e. Superior duodenal flexure lies
f. Coeliac plexus lies
g. Body of pancreas lies
h. Upper part of hilum of right kidney lies
i. Lower part of hilum of left kidney lies.
j. Fundus of gallbladder.
k. Lower end of spinal cord.

Q. Third and fourth lumbar vertebrae correspond to:

Ans. a. Disc between the third and fourth lumbar vertebrae correspond to highest point of iliac crest.
b. Abdominal aorta bifurcates into two common iliac arteries.

LOWER LIMB

Q. Muscles attached to the lesser trochanter of femur.

Ans. Insertion of:
i. Psoas major—on its tip.
ii. Iliacus—to the inferomedial part of its base

Q. Structures related to anterior surface of the lower end of tibia.

Ans. From medial to lateral:
i. Tendon of the tibialis anterior
ii. Tendon of the extensor hallucis longus
iii. Anterior tibial vessels
iv. Deep peroneal nerve
v. Tendon of the extensor digitorum longus
vi. Tendon of the peroneus tertius.

Q. Name the structures related to the posterior surface of the lower end of the tibia.

Ans. From medial to lateral
i. Tendon of the tibialis posterior
ii. Flexor digitorum longus
iii. Posterior tibial vessels
iv. Posterior tibial nerve
v. Tendon of the flexor hallucis longus.

Q. Attachments of iliac tuberosity.

Ans. From before backwards: Iliolumbar ligament, dorsal or posterior sacroiliac and interosseous sacroiliac ligaments.

Q. Name the structures attached to the anterior superior iliac spine.

Ans. i. Lateral end of inguinal ligament
ii. Origin of the sartorius
iii. Origin of tensor fasciae latae and fascia lata
iv. Origin of transversus abdominis
v. Fascia iliaca.

Q. Name the structures attached to the inner lip of iliac crest.

Ans. i. Anterior two-thirds origin of transversus abdominis
ii. Posterior one-third origin of quadratus lumborum.

Q. Name the structures attached to the outer lip of iliac crest.

Ans. i. Fascia lata.
ii. Origin of tensor fasciae latae including ilio-tibial tract.
iii. Insertion of external obliquus abdominis (anterior 1/2 of outer lip).
iv. Origin of latissimus dorsi (posterior 1/3rd of outer lip).

Q. Name the structures attached to the anterior inferior iliac spine.

Ans. i. Upper part: Origin of straight head of rectus femoris.
ii. Lower part: Stem of the iliofemoral ligament (strongest ligament in the body).

Q. Name the structures attached to the pubic tubercle.

Ans. ia. Medial end of the inguinal ligament.
ii. Upper loop of the cremaster muscle.
iii. Anterior layer of rectus sheath.

Q. Name the structures attached to the ischial spine.

Ans. i. Sacrospinous ligament at the tip.
ii. In pelvic surface: Origin of levator ani in front and coccygeus behind.

Q. Why the fracture of neck of femur leads to the necrosis of head?

Ans. Due to interruption of blood supply of the head.

Q. The fracture of tibia at the lower end is slow healing.

Ans. Due to less blood supply.

Q. What will happen if the neck of fibula is fractured?

Ans. Common peroneal nerve is injured.

Q. Structures transmit through the greater sciatic notch:

Ans. The greater sciatic notch is converted into greater sciatic foramen by the sacrotuberous and sacrospinous ligaments.
Further the greater sciatic foramen is divided into upper and lower compartments by the piriformis muscles
i. The upper compartment transmits the following structures:
a. Superior gluteal vessels
b. Superior gluteal nerve.
ii. The lower compartment transmits following structures:
a. Sciatic nerve
b. Posterior femoral cutaneous nerve
c. Internal pudendal vessels
d. Pudendal nerve
e. Nerve to the quadratus femoris
f. Nerve to the obturator internus
g. Inferior gluteal vessels
h. Inferior gluteal nerve.

Q. Name the structures passing through lesser sciatic foramen.

Ans. i. Nerve to the obturator internus
ii. Internal pudendal vessels
iii. Pudendal nerve
iv. Tendon of obturator internus.

Q. Name the structures after exit through the greater sciatic foramen again re-enter through the lesser sciatic foramen.

Ans. i. Internal pudendal vessels.
ii. Pudendal nerve.
iv. Nerve to obturator internus.

Q. What do you mean by symphyseal joint?

Ans. Any joint which occur on the midline of the body.

Q. Name the examples of symphyseal joints.

Ans. Symphysis pubis and sumphysis menti (at birth the two halves of mandible connected at the symphysis menti by fibrous tissue. Bony union takes place during first year of life).

Q. Attachments of linea aspera of femur.

Ans. From medial to lateral
i. Vastus medialis
ii. Medial intermuscular septum
iii. Adductor brevis in the upper part
iv. Adductor longus in the lower part
v. Adductor magnus
vi. Posterior intermuscular septum
vii. Short head of biceps femoris.

viii. Lateral intermuscular septum.

ix. Vastus lateralis.

Q. Name the bone secondary ossification center appears during intrauterine life.

Ans. In the lower end of femur, nine month of intrauterine life.

Q. Attachments intertrochanteric crest.

Ans. Insertion: Quadratus femoris—on the quadrate tubercle (extends to shaft).

Ligament: Capsular ligament—1.3 cm medial to and parallel with the intertrochanteric crest.

Q. Attachments intertrochanteric line.

Ans. Origin:

i. Vastus lateralis—from the upper half of the line.

ii. Vastus medialis—from the lower half of the line.

Ligaments

i. Capsular ligament—attached to its inner part in its whole length.

ii. Lateral and medial bands of iliofemoral ligament attached outside the capsular ligament.

Q. Angle of inclination or neck-shaft angle of femur and its clinical importance

Ans. It is an angle between the long axis of neck and shaft of the femur.

In adults: 127°

In children: 128°

In females: it is less

i. When angle is increased the condition is called coxa valga found in congenital dislocation of hip, which results the adduction of the hip joint is limited.

ii. When angle is decreased the condition is called coxa vara found in fracture in neck of the femur which results in abduction of the hip joint is limited.

Q. Angle of femoral torsion or angle of declination?

Ans. It is an angle between the long axis of neck of femur and transverse axis of the femoral condyles.

Measurements: 14.01°

Q. Which bone is known as knee-cap bone?

Ans. Patella.

Q. What is terrible triad?

Ans. The term used to describe a knee injury involving tears the three most injured structures

i. The tibial (medial) collateral ligament.

ii. The medial meniscus.

iii. The anterior cruciate ligament (ACL).

Q. Smallest and largest tarsal bones

Ans. Smallest is the intermediate cuneiform and largest is the calcaneus.

Q. Muscles attached to the iliotibial tract

Ans. Superficial fibers of the gluteus maximus and tensor fasciae latae.

Lumbar hernia: Boundaries of lumbar (Petit's) triangle and clinical importance

Ans. *See* clinical anatomy of hip bone

Q. Genu varum or bow leg:

The medial angulation of the leg in relation to the thigh, so on standing the knees remain wide apart, commonly seen in children for 1 to 2 years after starting to walk.

Q. Genu valgum or knock knee:

The lateral angulations of the leg in relation to the thigh, so on standing the knees touches together commonly seen in children 2 to 4 years of age.

HEAD NECK AND FACE (HNF)

Q. What are typical cervical vertebrae

Ans. From third to sixth.

Q. What are atypical cervical vertebrae

Ans. First, second and seventh.

Q. Attachments of dens

Ans. Its apex: Apical ligament

Sides: Alar ligament.

Q. Structures transmit through the foramen transversarium of cervical vertebrae (except C7).

Ans. vertebral artery surrounded by plexus of sympathetic nerves and vertebral vein.

Q. Structures transmit through the foramina transversarium of seventh cervical vertebra

Ans. Vertebral vein and sympathetic nerves.

Q. Importance at the level of C6 vertebra

Ans. i. End of larynx and beginning of trachea.

ii. End of pharynx and beginning of esophagus.

iii. Cricoid cartilage.

iv. Beginning of second part of vertebral artery.

v. Position of middle cervical sympathetic ganglion.

vi. Superior belly of omohyoid muscle crossing in front of the common carotid artery.

vii. Crossing of the inferior thyroid artery and common carotid artery.

Q. What is Frankfurt's plane?

Ans. Hold the articulated skull in such a way, that the orbital cavities are directed in front, and the lower margins of the orbits and upper margins of the external acoustic meatuses should lie in the same horizontal plane. Such orbitomeatal position was accepted in an anthropological congress in Frankfurt in 1884; hence this plane is called the Frankfurt plane.

Q. All the joints of skull are fibrous joints only one joint is synovial

Ans. Temporomandibular joint.

Q. Name primary cartilaginous joint and is replaced by bone usually after 25 years

i. First chondrosternal joint

ii. Body of sphenoid unites with basilar part of occipital bone.

Q. Boundaries of orbit

Ans. Roof: It is triangular and concave.

Anteriorly: Orbital plate of the frontal bone.

Posteriorly: Lesser wing of the sphenoid bone.

Floor

i. Mainly by the orbital surface of the maxilla

ii. Orbital surface of the zygomatic bone.

iii. Orbital process of the palatine bone.

Medial wall

i. Frontal process of the maxilla

ii. Anterior lacrimal crest

iii. Lacrimal bone

iv. Orbital plate of the ethmoid bone

v. Small part of the body of the sphenoid bone

vi. Small part of the frontal bone.

Lateral wall

i. Orbital surface of the zygomatic bone

ii. Orbital surface of the greater wing of the sphenoid bone.

Q. Fissures, canals and foramina related to orbit

Ans. i. Superior orbital fissure

ii. Inferior orbital fissure

iii. Optic canal

iv. Infraorbital groove

v. Supraorbital notch

v. Anterior and posterior ethmoidal foramina

vii. Nasolacrima canal.

Q. Attachments of the mastoid part including mastoid process of temporal bone

Ans. i. Origin of

a. Auricularis posterior.

b. Occipital belly of occipitofrontalis

c. Posterior belly of digastric (from the mastoid notch).

ii. Insertion of: Above downwards and forwards

a. Sternocleidomastoid

b. Splenius capitis

c. Longissimus capitis

Q. Structures attached to the lower border of the hyoid bone.

Ans. i. Sternohyoid

ii. Omohyoid

iii. Thyrohyoid

iv. Pretracheal fascia.

Q. Structures attached to external occipital protuberance.

Ans. Highest point of the ligamentum nuchae.

Q. Structures attached to styloid process of temporal bone.

Ans. i. Styloglossus muscle

ii. Stylohyoid muscle

iii. Stylopharyngeus muscle

iv. Stylohyoid ligament

v. Stylomandibular ligament.

Q. Structures passing through mental foramen.

Ans. i. Mental artery: Branch of inferior alveolar artery

ii. Mental nerve: Branch of inferior alveolar nerve.

Q. Muscles attached to genial tubercle.

Ans. i. Upper genial tubercle: Genioglossus muscle.

ii. Lower genial tubercle: Geniohyoid muscle.

Q. Ligaments attached to mandible.

Ans. i. Capsular ligament with synovial membrane.

ii. Lateral temporomandibular ligament

iii. Stylomandibular ligament

iv. Sphenomandibular ligament

v. Pterygomandibular ligament.

Q. Muscles of mastication attached to mandible.

Ans. i. Medial pterygoid

ii. Lateral pterygoid

iii. Temporalis

iv. Masseter

v. Buccinator (accessory).

Q. Name the largest muscle of mastication? And how is it identified?

Ans. Masseter. Ask the patient to bite his teeth, this muscle become prominenet on both sides.

Q. Name the main muscle for opening the mouth

Ans. Lateral pterygoid.

Q. Name the main muscle for closing the mouth

Ans. Medial pterygoid

Q. Arteries related to mandible.

Ans. **Arteries:**
i. Maxillary artery (first part)
ii. Inferior alveolar artery
iii. Facial artery
iv. Masseteric, mylohyoid and mental arteries.

Q. Salivary glands related to mandible:
i. *Parotid gland* with the posterior border and upper posterior smooth part of the external surface of the ramus.
ii. *Submandibular gland* in the submandibular fossa.
iii. *Sublingual gland* in the sublingual fossa.

Q. Nerves closely related to mandible:
i. **Inferior alveolar (dental) nerve:** Branch of mandibular nerve—passes through the mandibular canal.
ii. **Lingual nerve branch of mandibular nerve:** Behind the posterior end of mylohyoid line.
iii. **Masseteric nerve:** Branch of mandibular nerve, pass through the mandibular notch.
iv. **Auriculotemporal nerve branch mandibular nerve:** Medial side of the neck of the mandible.
v. **Mylohyoid nerve branch of inferior alveolar nerve:** In the mylohyoid groove.
vi. **Mental nerve branch of inferior alveolar nerve:** Outer surface of the body of the mandible passes through the mandibular foramen.
vii. **Marginal mandibular branch of facial nerve:** On the outer surface of the body at the anteroinferior angle of masseter muscle.

Q. Venous sinuses related to occipital bone.

Ans. i. **Superior sagittal sinus:** At the sagittal sulcus.
ii. **Transverse sinus:** At the transverse sulcus.
i. **Confluence of sinuses:** At the point of union between the right transverse sinus with the superior sagittal sinus and the occipital and straight sinuses continuous with left transverse sinus.
iv. **Occipital sinus:** At the internal occipital crest.
v. **Inferior petrosal sinus:** At the basilar part of occipital bone.
vi. **Basilar plexus or sinus:** At the basilar part of occipital bone.
vii. **Sigmoid sinus:** At the jugular process of occipital bone.

Q. Venous sinuses related to temporal bone.

Ans. i. **Inferior petrosal sinus:** At the petrous part of temporal bone
ii. **Superior petrosal sinus:** At the groove on the superior part of the petrous part of temporal bone.
iii. **Sigmoid sinus:** At the mastoid part of temporal bone.

Q. Confluence of sinuses, its situation and formation:

Ans. **Situation:** At the area internal occipital protuberance of occipital bone.

Formation: Superior sagittal sinus is continuous with the right transverse (larger than left) sinus and the occipital and straight sinuses continuous with left transverse sinus.

Q. Pterion and its clinical importance:

Ans. i. In articulated skull it meets with four bones and the area is known as pterion.
The four bones are:
a. Frontal
b. Parietal
c. Greater wing of sphenoid
d. Squamous part of temporal bone.
ii. Center of pterion: About 4 cm above the zygomatic arch and 3.5 cm behind the frontozygomatic suture.
iii. Relations:
a. Anterior division of middle meningeal vessels
b. Stem of lateral sulcus of cerebrum (Sylvian point).

Clinical importance of pterion
It is very thin and weakest part of the skull, therefore, blows or ingury to the side of the skull may fracture the pterion and rupture of the anterior division of middle meningeal vessels and produce extradural hemorrhage.

Q. Asterion:

Ans. i. It corresponds to the asterion or meeting points of three bones on the skull.
ii. The three bones are:
a. Posteroinferior angle of parietal bone
b. Lateral angle of occipital bone
c. Mastoid part of temporal bone.

Q. Most fragile bone of the skull:

Ans. Ethmoid

Q. Name the unpaired facial bones:

Ans. Mandible, vomer and ethmoid.

Q. Cephalic index:

Ans. It is calculated as follows:
Maximum breadth/maximum length × 100.

Q. Maximum cranical length:

Ans. It is measured from glabella to the furthest point at the occipital bone.

Q. Maximum cranical breath:

Ans. It is measured at right angle to the sagittal plane opposite the parietal tubers.

Q. Maximum cranial hight:

Ans. It is measured from the basion (median point on the anterior margin of the foramen magnum to the bregma)

Q. Cranial capacity:

Ans. An average of 1350 to 1400 cc

Q. What is craniometry:

Ans. Craniometry is the study of skulls of different races and species, to take various measurements of the skull.

MISCELLANEOUS

Bones and Joints

1. **Growing ends of long bones in upper and lower limbs**

Ans. The growing ends are opposite the direction of the nutrient foramen.

Upper limb: Upper end of humerus and lower ends of radius and ulna.

Lower limb: Lower end of femur and upper end of tibia.

2. **Direction of nutrient foramen of bones of upper and lower limbs**

For upper limb: Towards the elbow.

For lower limb: Flee (run away) from knee.

3. **Name the longest bone:** Femur.

4. **Name the smallest bone:** Stapes.

5. **Movable bone of skull:** Mandible.

6. **Ring like bone:** Atlas

7. **'U'-shaped bone:** Hyoid.

8. **First bone to start ossification:** Clavicle.

9. **Last bone to complete ossification:** Clavicle.

10. **Bone develops after birth:** Sesamoid bones (e.g. patella).

11. **Key bone of the ankle:** Talus

12. **Two halves of bone unites after birth:** Mandible.

13. **Bone having no muscle attachment:** Talus

14. **Which bone is called key bone of tarsus?**

Ans. Talus.

15. **Which bone is called donor's bone? and why?**

Ans. Fibula, because it does not transmit body weight. So if part of the fibula is removed a person can walk, run, and jump normally.

16. **Why fibula does not transmit body weight?**

Ans. Because fibula does not articulate with the femur.

17. **Why fibula does not part of knee joint?**

Ans. Because fibula does not articulate with the femur.

18. **In which bone secondary center of ossification appears before birth**

Ans. Lower end of femur (nine month of intrauterine life).

19. **Which bone is called rider's (heterotopic) bone:**

Ans. Horse riders develop this bone in their thighs (in the tendon of adductor longus) due to straining the muscles that adduct the thighs.

20. **Functions of interosseous membrane?**

i. Holds the radius and ulna together in forearm and tibia and fibula in leg.

ii. Provides attachments to muscles.

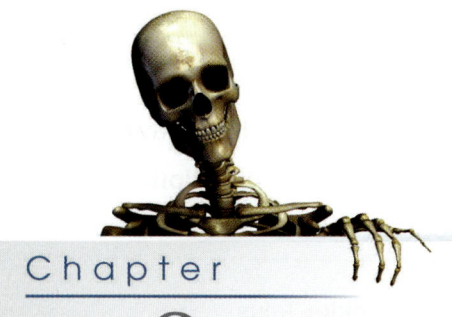
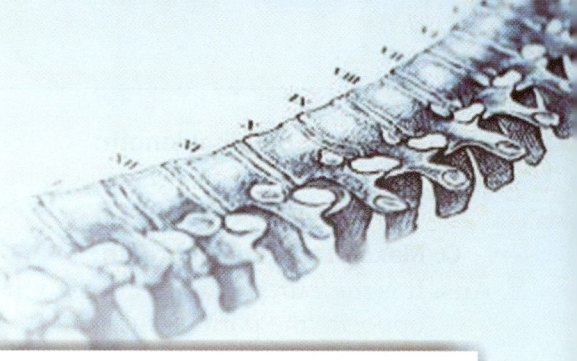

Muscles of Whole Body

The chapter of 'myology' contains the different muscles of the whole body in a nutshell, in relation to origin, insertion, nerve supply, actions and clinical anatomy. Which will be helpful to the students of anatomy for their examinations and also they can easily understood from this schematic representation of myology.

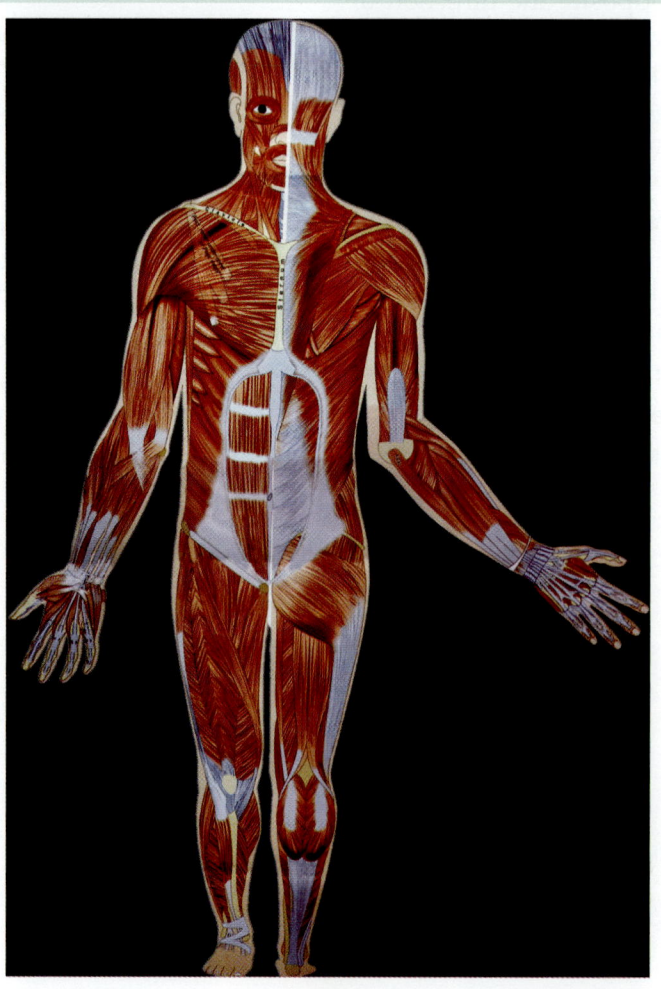

Table 8.1 | Muscles connecting upper limb to vertebral column

Muscles	Origin	Insertion	Nerve supply	Actions/Functions	Clinical anatomy
1. **Trapezius**	i. External occipital protuberance ii. Superior nuchal line (medial 1/3rd) of occipital bone iii. Ligamentum nuchae iv. Spine of C7 to T12 vertebrae v. Supraspinal ligaments	i. Upper fibers—posterior border of lateral 1/3rd of clavicle ii. Middle fibers—medial margin of acromion process of scapula iii. Lower fibers—upper lip of the crest of the spine of scapula	Spinal root of the accessory nerve and branches from the C3 and C4 spinal nerves	i. Upper fibers: Elevates scapula and point of shoulder ii. Middle fibers: Draws the scapula towards mid line. iii. Draw the head and neck backwards and to the same side	**Triangle of auscultation and its importance:** Above: Lateral border of the trapezius Below: Upper border of the latissimus dorsi Laterally: Medial border of the scapula Floor: 7th rib and 6th and 7th intercostal spaces Importance: i. Ausculation of the swallowed liquids is obtained over this triangle ii. It is a suitable site for the auscultation of the lungs on the back
2. **Latissimus dorsi** (climber's/ swimmer's muscle)	i. From posterior 1/3rd of outer lip of ventral 2/3rd of illiac crest ii. Posterior lamella of lumbar fascia iii. Spines of lower 6 thoracic, all lumbar and sacral spines iv. Lower 3 or 4 ribs v. Dorsal aspect of the inferior angle of scapula	Floor of intertubercular sulcus of humerus between pectoralis major and teres major	Thoraco-dorsal nerves (C6,C7,C8) or nerve to latissimus dorsi	i. Draws the humerus backwards, adductors and medial rotator of the shoulder. ii. Raises body upwards and forwards during climbing iii. Helps in forceful expiration and violent exp. efforts like coughing, sneezing.	
3. **Levator scapulae**	i. Posterior tubercles of transverse processes of C3 and C4 vertebrae ii. Transverse processes of C1 and C2 vertebrae	Superior part of medial border of scapula from the superior angle to the apex of spine	Dorsal sca-pular (C5) and directly from cervical (C3, C4) nerves	i. Elevates the scapula ii. Depresses the point point of shoulder	
4. **Rhomboid minor and major**	**Minor:** Ligamentum nuchae, spinous processes of C7 and T1 vertebrae **Major:** Spinous processes and supraspinal ligaments of T2 to T5 vertebrae	Medial border of scapula opposite the apex of the spine Medial border of scapula below the apex of spine	Dorsal scapular (C5) nerve or nerve to rhomboids	i. Draws the scapula back-wards and depresses the point of shoulder ii. Fixes scapula to thoracic wall	

| **Table 8.2** | **Muscles of pectoral region** | | | | |

Muscles	Origin	Insertion	Nerve supply	Actions/Functions	Clinical anatomy
1. **Pectoralis major**	i. Anterior surface of the medial half of the clavicle ii. Half of the breadth of the sternum downs the level of 6th costal cartilage iii. 2nd to 6th costal cartilages iv. Aponeurosis of external obliquus abdominis	At the lateral lip of the intertubercular sulcus of humerus as trilaminar tendon	Medial (C8, T1) and lateral (C5, C6 and C7) pectoral nerves	i. Flexion, adduction and medial rotation of shoulder joint ii. Draws the arm forwards and medially iii. It draws the trunk upwards and forwards during climbing iv. Adduction and medial rotation of the humerus against resistance v. An inspiratory muscle during deep forcible inspiration	i. **Test the function of pectoralis major:** Abducts the arms about 60° then flexes the elbows now person attempts to bring the arms together. The examiner follows the prominence the anterior axillary folds ii. **Poland anomaly:** It is congenital absence of pectoralis major which causes anterior axillary fold is absent
2. **Pectoralis minor**	i. From the outer surfaces of the 3rd, 4th and 5th ribs close to their costal cartilages ii. Fascia covering the external intercostal muscle	Medial border and upper surface of the coracoid process of scapula	Medial (C8, T1) and lateral (C5, C6 and C7) pectoral nerves	i. Depresses the point of shoulder ii. Elevates the upper ribs	It is the key muscle for surgical landmark to identify axillary lymph nodes in diagnosis and surgical treatment of breast cancer
3. **Serratus anterior** (Boxer's muscle)	It arises by eight or nine digitations from the outer surfaces and upper borders of the upper eight ribs close to the anterior angle and from the aponeurotic fascia of the intercostal muscles. The first digitation arises from the first and second ribs, whereas all other digitations from their corresponding ribs	It is inserted into the costal surface of the medial border of the scapula	Long thoracic nerve or nerve to serratus anterior (C5, C6 and C7)	i. It draws the scapula forwards for pushing and punching movements ii. It keeps the medial border of scapula in contact with the chest wall iii. Its lower four or five digitations pulls the inferior angle of scapula forwards around the thorax	**Winging of the scapula:** Paralysis of the serratus anterior results following effects i. The inferior angle and medial border of scapula become unduly prominent ii. Unable to perform pushing, punching and raise the arm fully
4. **Subclavius**	Upper surface of the 1st rib and the adjoining 1st costal cartilage	Subclavian groove on the inferior surface of the middle 2/3rd of the clavicle	Nerve to subclavius (C5, C6)	Depresses the clavicle and steadies the sternoclavicular joint	

Table 8.3 — Muslces of shoulder region

Muscles	Origin	Insertion	Nerve supply	Actions/Functions	Clinical anatomy
1. Deltoid (multipennate muscle)	i. Anterior border of lateral 1/3rd of clavicle (anterior fiber) ii. Lateral border of acromion process of scapula (middle fiber) iii. Lower lip of spine of scapula (posteropr fibers)	Deltoid tuberosity of humerus	Axilliary nerve (C5, C6) from the posterior cord of brachial plexus	i. Anterior fibres along with clavicular head of pectoralis major flexes and medially rotates the arm ii. Middle fibers along with supraspinatus abduct the arm iii. Posterior fibers along with latissimus dorsi and teres major extend and laterally rotate the arm	i. Fracture of surgical neck of humerus due to injury of axillary nerve results in paralysis of deltoid and loss of abduction of arm ii. Paralysis of deltoid results into atrophy of it and loss of rounded contour of shoulder
2. Subscapularis	i. Medial 2/3rd of the subscapular fossa ii. Bony ridges in subscapular fossa	Lesser tubercle of humerus	Upper and lower subscapular nerves (C5, C6, C7) from the posterior cord of brachial plexus	i. Medially rotates the humerus ii. Helps to hold humeral head in glenoid cavity	
3. Supraspinatus	i. Medial 2/3rd of supraspinous fossa of scapula ii. Upper surface of spine of scapula	Superior facet on greater tubercle of humerus	Suprascapular nerve (C5, C6)	i. Helps deltoid to abduct the arm ii. Hepls in stabilising the head of the humerus	Degeneration of the supraspinatus tendon occurs from the age of 40 and above. Hence rupture, inflammation and calcium deposition are very common. Supraspinatus tendinitis producing painful abduction from 60 to 120°
4. Infraspinatus	i. Infraspinous fossa of scapula ii. Infraspinous fascia	Middle facet on greater tubercle of humerus	Suprascapular nerves (C5, C6)	i. Laterally rotates the arm ii. Hepls in stabilising the head of the humerus	
5. Teres minor	Superior part of lateral border of scapula	Inferior facet on greater tubercle of humerus	Axilliary nerve (C5, C6) posterior division	i. Lateral rotator and abductor of the arm. ii. Stabilising the head of humerus in the glenoid cavity	
6. Teres major	Dorsal surface of inferior angle of scapula and adjoining its lateral border	Medial lip of bicipital groove of humerus	Lower subscapular nerve (C5, C6, C7)	i. Adduction of the arm ii. Stabilising the head of humerus in the glenoid cavity	

Table 8.4 — Rotator Cuff/musculotendinous cuff

Muscles	Origin	Insertion	Nerve supply	Actions/Functions	Clinical anatomy
1. **Subscapularis** 2. **Supraspinatus** 3. **Infraspinatus** 4. **Teres minor**		These are rotator cuff muscles Descibed in Table 8.3			As cuff is deficient below, dislocation of shoulder joint commonly occur inferiorly

Table 8.5 — Anterior arm mucles

Muscles	Origin	Insertion	Nerve supply	Actions/Functions	Clinical anatomy
1. **Biceps brachii**	**Short head:** Tip of coracoid process of scapula **Long head:** Supraglenoid tubercle of scapula	i. Posterior part of radial tuberosity of the radius ii. Bicipital aponeurosis fuses with infront of deep fascia of forearm	Musculocutaneous nerve (C5, C6)	i. Flexion of elbow joint ii. Supination of forearm iii. Long head helps in retaining the head of humerus in glenoid cavity	
2. **Brachialis**	i. Lower 1/2 of anterolateral and anteromedial surfaces of humerus ii. Medial and lateral intermuscular septa	i. Tuberosity of ulna. ii. Anterior surface of coronoid process of ulna	i. Musculocutaneous nerve (C5, C6) ii. Radial nerve supply the small lateral part	Flexes the elbow joint	
3. **Coraco-brachialis**	i. Tip of coracoid process of scapula ii. Medial aspect of upper part of the common tendinous origin	Middle of the medial border of shaft of humerus	**Musculocutaneous** nerve (C5, C6)	Helps in flexion and adduction of shoulder joint	

Table 8.6 — Posterior arm muscles

Muscles	Origin	Insertion	Nerve supply	Actions/Functions	Clinical anatomy
Triceps brachii	**Long head:** Infraglenoid tubercle of scapula **Lateral head** i. Ridge on the posterior surface of the shaft of the humerus above the spiral groove ii. Lateral intermuscular septum **Medial head** i. Posterior surface of the shaft of humerus below the spiral groove ii. Lateral and medial intermuscular septa	i. Posterior part of the upper surface of olecranon process of ulna ii. Capsule of the elbow joint iii. Antebrachial fascia	Radial nerve (C5, C6 C7, C8, T1)	i. Strong extensor of the elbow joint ii. Long head adducts the shoulder joint	

Table 8.7   Anterior forearm muscles

Superficial layer

Muscles	Origin	Insertion	Nerve supply	Actions/Functions	Clinical anatomy
1. Pronator teres	**Humeral head** i. From the medial epicondyle of the humerus ii. From the intermuscular septum **Ulnar head:** Medial margin of the coronoid process of ulna	Middle part of lateral surface of radial shaft	Median nerve (C5, C6, C7, C8, T1)	i. Pronation of the forearm. ii. Helps in flexion of elbow joint.	
2. Flexor carpi radialis	i. Medial epicondyle of the humerus ii. Antebrachial fascia	Palmar surface of the bases of second and third metacarpal bones	Median nerve (C5, C6, C7, C8, T1)	Flexion and abduction of the wrist	
3. Palmaris longus	From the medial epicondyle of the humerus	i. Palmar aponeurosis ii. Flexor retinaculum of hand	Median nerve (C5, C6, C7, C8, T1)	i. Flexion of wrist. ii. Tightens the palmar aponeurosis as an anchor for skin and fasciae of the hand	
4. Flexor carpi ulnaris	**Humeral head** • Medial epicondyle of humerus **Ulnar head** i. Medial margin of the olecranon process and the proximal two-thirds of the posterior border of the ulna ii. From the intermuscular septum	Pisiform, hamate, flexor retinaculum and fifth metacarpal bones	Ulnar nerve (C7, C8, T1)	i. Flexion of the wrist joint. ii. Adducts the wrist.	
5. Flexor digitorum superficialis	**Humeral head** i. Medial epicondyle of the humerus ii. Ulnar collateral ligament iii. Medial margin of the coronoid process of ulna iv. Intermuscular septum **Radial head** Oblique line of the anterior border of shaft of the radius	Sides of the middle phalanges of medial 4 fingers by dividing into 4 slips	Median nerve (C5, C6, C7, C8, T1)	Flexes the middle and proximal phalanges and the wrist joint	

Contd.

Table 8.8 — Anterior forearm muscles (Contd.)

Deep layer

Muscles	Origin	Insertion	Nerve supply	Actions/Functions	Clinical anatomy
1. **Pronator quadratus**	Oblique ridge on the lower 1/4th of the anterior surface of the shaft of the ulna and area medial to it	Distal one-fourth of anterior border and surface of radius and triangular area above the ulnar notch of the radius	Anterior interosseous branch of median nerve (C5, C6, C7, C8, T1)	i. Pronation of forearm (principal pronator) ii. Deep fibers bind radius and ulna together	
2. **Flexor digitorum profundus**	i. Upper 3/4th of medial and anterior surfaces of the ulnar shaft ii. Upper three-fourths of the posterior border of the ulna iii. Medial half of the upper 3/4th of the interosseous membrane iv. Medial surface of the olecranon process of the ulna	Palmar surfaces of the bases of distal phalanges of medial 4 digits by dividing into 4 tendons	i. Medial half by the ulnar nerve (C7, C8, T1). ii. Lateral half by the median nerve (C5, C6, C7, C8, T1)	i. Flexes distal interphalangeal joints of medial 4 fingers ii. Strong gripping muscle when wrist is extended	
3. **Flexor pollicis longus**	i. Upper 3/4th of the anterior surface of shaft of the radius ii. Adjacent interosseous membrane iii. Medial margin of the coronoid process of ulna	Palmar surface of base of distal phalanx of thumb	Anterior interosseous branch of median nerve (C5, C6, C7, C8, T1)	i. Flexes the distal phalanx of thumb ii. Flex the metacarpophalangeal and wrist joints	

Table 8.9 — Posterior forearm muscles

Superficial layer

Muscles	Origin	Insertion	Nerve supply	Actions/Functions	Clinical anatomy
1. **Anconeus**	Posterior surface of the lateral epicondyle of humerus	Lateral surface of olecranon preocess and superior part of posterior surface of the shaft of the ulna	Radial nerve (C5, C6, C7, C8, T1)	Helps triceps in extending the elbow	
2. **Brachioradialis**	i. Proximal two-thirds of the lateral supracondylar line of the humerus ii. Lateral intermuscular septum	Base of the styloid process of the radius	Radial nerve (C5, C6, C7, C8, T1)	i. Flexes the elbow joint ii. Helps pronating from supine to mid position of forearm iii. Helps supinating from prone to mid position of forearm	

Contd.

Table 8.9	Posterior forearm muscles (Contd.)				
Muscles	Origin	Insertion	Nerve supply	Actions/Functions	Clinical anatomy
3. Extensor carpi radialis longus	i. Distal one-third of lateral supracondylar ridge of humerus ii. From lateral intermuscular septum iii. Lateral epicondyle of the humerus	Dorsal surface of base of 2nd meta-carpal bone	Radial nerve (C5, C6, C7, C8, T1)	i. Extension of wrist joint ii. Abduction of wrist joint	
4. Extensor carpi radialis brevis	i. Lateral epicondyle of humerus ii. Adjacent intermuscular septum iii. Radial collateral ligament of elbow joint	Dorsal surface of base of 3rd metacarpal bone	Posterior interosseous nerve	i. Extension of wrist joint ii. Abduction of wrist joint	
5. Extensor digitorum	i. Lateral epicondyle of the humerus ii. Lateral intermuscular septum iii. Antebrachial fascia	Inserted by three slips i. Intermediate slip back of the middle phalanx ii. Two collateral slips soon reunite to be inserted back of the distal phalanx	Posterior interosseous nerve	i. Extends the digits at proximal and distal interphalangeal joints of medial 4 digitis ii. Extends the wrist joint	
6. Extensor carpi ulnaris	i. Lateral epicondyle of the humerus ii. Posterior border of ulna iii. Antebrachial fascia	Tubercle on the medial side of the base of 5th metacarpal bone	Posterior interosseous nerve	i. Extension of wrist joint ii. Adduction of wrist joint	
7. Extensor digiti minimi	i. Lateral epicondyle of the humerus ii. Interosseous membrane	Dorsal aspect of the base of the proximal phlanax of 5th digit	Posterior interosseous nerve	Extends proximal phalanx of the little finger	
Deep layer					
1. Supinator	i. Lateral epicondyle of humerus ii. Radial collateral ligament of elbow joint iii. Supinator crest of the ulna	Lateral surface of upper one-third of the radius	Posterior interosseous nerve	i. Supination of the forearm ii. Rotates the radius to turn the palm anteriorly	
2. Abductor pollicis longus	i. Posterior surface of the shaft of the radius ii. Upper part of the lateral area on the posterior surface of the ulna iii. Interosseous membrane	Radial side of the base of the 1st metacarpal bone	Posterior interosseous nerve	i. Abducts the thumb ii. Extends the thumb	

Contd.

Table 8.9 — Posterior forearm muscles (Contd.)

Deep layer

Muscles	Origin	Insertion	Nerve supply	Actions/Functions	Clinical anatomy
3. Extensor pollicis brevis	i. Posterior surface of radius ii. Interosseous membrane	Dorsal aspect of the base of proximal phalanx of the thumb	Posterior interosseous nerve	Extends and abducts the proximal phalanx of the thumb	
4. Extensor pollicis longus	i. Lateral part of the posterior surface of the shaft of the ulna ii. Interosseous membrane	Dorsal aspect of the base of distal phalanx of thumb	Posterior interosseous nerve	Extends the metacarpo-phalangeal and carpo-metacarpal joints and extends the distal phalanx of the thumb	
5. Extensor indicis	i. Posterior surface of ulna distal to the extensor pollicis longus ii. Interosseous membrane	Extensor expansion of index finger	Posterior interosseous nerve	i. Extends the proximal phalanx of the index finger ii. Assist in extension of wrist	

Table 8.10 — Intrinsic muscles of hand

Muscles of thenar eminence and adductor pollicis

Muscles	Origin	Insertion	Nerve supply	Actions/Functions	Clinical anatomy
1. Abductor pollicis brevis	i. Flexor retinaculum ii. Tubercles of the scaphoid and trapezium bones iii. From the tendon of the abductor pollicis longus	i. Tubercle on the lateral margin of the base of proximal phalanx of thumb ii. Lateral margin of the extensor pollicis longus	Median nerve (C5, C6, C7, C8, T1)	i. Abduction of thumb. ii. Flexes the metacarpo-phalangeal joint of thumb	
2. Flexor pollicis brevis	**Superficial head** i. Distal border of flexor retinaculum ii. Crest of the trapezium **Deep head** i. From the trapezoid and capitate bones	The two heads unite and inserted to the lateral side of base of proximal phalanx of thumb	**Superficial Head** Median nerve (C5, C6, C7, C8, T1) **Deep head** Ulnar nerves (C7, C8, T1)	i. Abduction of thumb ii. Flexes the metacarpo-phalangeal joint of thumb.	
3. Opponens pollicis	i. Flexor retinaculum ii. From the tubercle (crest) of the trapezium	Lateral border and anterolateral surface of the first metacarpal bone	Median nerve (C5, C6, C7, C8, T1)	If flexes and medially rotates the thumb	
4. Adductor pollicis	**Oblique head:** Bases of 2nd and 3rd metacarpal bones **Transverse head:** Ridge on the anterior aspect of the third metacarpal bone	Medial side of base of proximal phalanx of thumb with a sesamoid bone intervening	Deep branch of ulnar nerve (C7, C8, T1)	i. Adducts the thumb which helps in gripping ii. Week flexor of the distal phalanx of the thumb	

Contd.

Table 8.10	Intrinsic muscles of hand (Contd.)

Muscles of hypothenar eminence and palmaris brevis

Muscles	Origin	Insertion	Nerve supply	Actions/Functions	Clinical anatomy
1. **Abductor digiti minimi**	Pisiform bone	Palmar aspect of the base of the proximal phalanx of little finger	Deep branch of ulnar nerve (C7, C8, T1)	Abducts the little finger	
2. **Opponens digiti minimi**	i. Hook of hamate ii. Flexor retinaculum	Medial aspect of 5th metacarpal bone	Deep branch of ulnar nerve (C7, C8, T1)	i. Flexes the 5th metacarpal bone ii. Adductor of the little finger	
3. **Flexor digiti minimi**	i. Hook of hamate ii. Flexor retinaculum	Palmar aspect and the ulnar side of the proximal phalanx of little finger	Deep branch of the ulnar nerve (C7, C8,T1)	Flexes the proximal phalanx of littel finger	
4. **Palmaris brevis**	i. Flexor retinaculum ii. Medial border of the central part of the palmar aponeurosis	To the skin along the ulnar border of the hand	Superficial branch of the ulnar nerve (C7, C8, T1)	i. Wrinkles the skin on the ulnar side of the palm of the hand ii. Deepens the hollow of the palm iii. Helps in palmar gripping	

Lumbrical muscles

1. **1st and 2nd lumbricals** (unipennate muscles)	All arising from tendon of flexor digitorum profundus for the index and middle fingers	All the lumbricals Via the dorsal digital expansion of the dorsum of bases of distal phalanx of the 2nd to 5th digits	1st and 2nd lumbricals by the median nerve (C5, C6, C7, C8, T1)	All the lumbricals flex the digits at the metacarpophalangeal joints and extend interphalangeal joints of 2nd to 5th digits	
2. **3rd and 4th lumbricals** (bipennate muscles)	3rd arising from the adjacent sides of the tendons of the middle and ring fingers and 4th from the adjacent sides of the ring and little fingers		3rd and 4th by the deep branch of the ulnar nerve (C7, C8, T1)		

Interossei mucles

1. **Palmar interossei muscles**	**1st:** From the medial side of the base of the 1st metacarpal bone	**1st:** Medial side of the base of proximal phalanx of thumb	All palmar interossei supplied by the deep branch of the	i. Adduct the fingers towards the middle finger	

Contd.

Table 8.10 Intrinsic muscles of hand (Contd.)

Interossei muscles

Muscles	Origin	Insertion	Nerve supply	Actions/Functions	Clinical anatomy
(unipennate muscles) four in number	**2nd:** Medial side of the shaft of the 2nd metacarpal bone **3rd:** Lateral side of the shaft of the 4th metacarpal bone **4th:** Lateral side of the shaft of the 5th metacarpal bone	Via extensor expansion into dorsum of bases of distal phalanges of 2nd, 4th and 5th digits	ulnar nerve (C7, C8, T1)	ii. Flexion of the meta-carpophalangeal joints and extension of the inter-phalangeal joints	
2. **Dorsal interossei muscles** (bipennate muscles) four in number	**1st:** From the adjacent sides of the shaft of the 1st and 2nd metacarpal bones **2nd:** From the adjacent sides of the shaft of the 2nd and 3rd metacarpal bones **3rd:** From the adjacent sides of the shaft of the 3rd and 4th metacarpal bones **4th:** From the adjacent sides of the shaft of the 4th and 5th metacarpal bones	Via extensor expansion of the dorsum of bases of distal phalanges of 2nd, 3rd, 4th and 5th digits	All dorsal interossei supplied by the deep branch of the ulnar nerve (C7, C8, T1)	i. Flexion of the meta carpophalangeal joints ii. Extension of the interphalangeal joints of 2nd to 5th digits	

Table 8.11 Muscles of lower limb

Anterior thigh muscles

Muscles	Origin	Insertion	Nerve supply	Actions/Functions	Clinical anatomy
1. **Quadriceps femoris muscles:** i. **Rectus femoris**	**Straight head:** From the anterior inferior iliac spine **Reflected head:** Groove just above the margin of acetabulum of the hip bone	Base of the patella	By the posterior division of the femoral nerve (L2, L3 and L4)	i. Extension of the knee joint ii. Flexion of the hip joint is done by rectus femoris iii. Vastus medialis prevents the lateral dislocation of patella iv. Maintain the posture and locomotion	i. This muscle may rupture due to sudden and violent extension of the knee joint ii. Fracture of the patella may occur due to sudden forceful contraction of the rectus femoris

Contd.

Table 8.11   Muscles of lower limb (Contd.)

Anterior thigh muscles

Muscles	Origin	Insertion	Nerve supply	Actions/Functions	Clinical anatomy
ii. Vastus lateralis	i. Upper part of the inter-trochanteric line ii. Anterior and inferior aspects of the greater trochanter of femur iii. Lateral lip of gluteal tuberosity iv. Upper half of the lateral lip of linea aspera v. Lateral intermuscular septum	To the base and lateral border of patella, to the capsule of the knee joint and to the lateral condyle of the tibia	By the posterior division of the femoral nerve (L2, L3, and L4)	Same as rectus femoris	
iii. Vastus medialis	i. Lower part of intertrochanteric line ii. Spiral line of femur iii. Medial lip of linea aspera iv. Upper two-thirds of the medial supracondylar line v. Medial intermuscular septum vi. Tendon of adductor magnus	i. Medial border of patella and quad-riceps tendon ii. Medial condyle of tibia	By the posterior division of the femoral nerve (L2, L3, and L4)	Same as rectus femoris	
iv. Vastus intermedius	i. Upper two-thirds of the anterior and lateral surfaces of femoral shaft ii. Lateral intermuscular septum	Deep surface of the tendon of rectus femoris and upper part of the patella	By the posterior division of the femoral nerve (L2, L3 and L4)	Same as rectus femoris	
2. Sartorius (longest muscle in the body and it is also known as Tailor's muscles)	i. Anterior superior iliac spine of hip bone ii. Upper half of notch inferior to anterior superior iliac spine of hip bone	Superior part of medial surface of shaft of tibia	Anterior division of femoral nerve (L2, L3, L4)	i. Abduct and laterally rotate the thigh ii. Flexions of the knee and hip joints	
3. Articularis genu	Anterior surface of lower part of shaft of femur	Into the suprapatellar bursa	From nerve to vastus imter-medius	It pulls the suprapatellar bursa upwards during extension of the knee joint	

Table 8.12   Hamstring muscles

Muscles	Origin	Insertion	Nerve supply	Actions/Functions	Clinical anatomy
1. **Semitendinosus**	From the lower and medial part of ischial tuberosity in common tendon with long head of biceps femoris	Upper part of the medial surface of the shaft of the tibia	Tibial division of the sciatic nerve (L4, L5, S1, S2, S3)	i. Flexion of the knee ii. Extension of the hip iii. Medial roation of the leg and the hip joint	**Hamstring muscles pulled or torn:** It is most commonly occur among the athletes, football players, etc.
2. **Semimem-branosus**	From upper lateral area of upper quadrilateral part of ischial tuberosity	In the groove behind the medial condyle of the tibia	Tibial division of sciatic nerve (L4, L5, S1, S2, S3)	Same as of semitendinosus	
3. **Biceps femoris** (long head)	From the lower and medial part of the ischial tuberosity in common tendon with semitendinosus	i. Upper and lateral side of the head of the fibula ii. Adjoining part of the lateral condyle of tibia	Tibial division of sciatic nerve (L4, L5, S1, S2, S3)	i. Flexor of the knee ii. In semiflexed knee acts as lateral rotator of knee iii. Weak extensor of the hip	
Biceps femoris (short head)	i. Lower part of the lateral lip of the linea aspera of femur ii. Upper two-thirds of the lateral supracondylar line of femur	Same as long head	Common peroneal division of the sciatic nerve (L4, L5, S1, S2, S3)	Same as long head	
4. **Adductor magnus** (Ischial fibers of the adductor magnus)	See muscles of the medial aspect of the thigh				

Table 8.13   Adductor muscles

Muscles	Origin	Insertion	Nerve supply	Actions/Functions	Clinical anatomy
1. **Gracilis** (donor's muscle)	i. Anterior aspect of body and inferior ramus of the pubis ii. Anterior aspect of the ramus of the ischium	At the upper part of the medial surface of the shaft of the tibia just below the medial condyle	By the anterior division of obturator nerve (L2, L3, L4)	i. Adduction of the hip. ii. Flexion and medial rotation of the leg iii. Week flexion of the knee	**Transplantation of the gracilis:** This muscle as a whole or part of the muscle is used for transplantation
2. **Pectineus** (hybrid muscle)	Pectineal line and adjoining pectineal surface of the superior ramus of pubis	Line extends from lesser trochanter to the linea aspera of femur	i. Femoral nerve (L2, L3, L4) ii. Branch of obturator nerve (L2, L3, L4)	Flexor and adductor of hip and lateral rotator of thigh	In horse back riders, adductor longus muscle may strain and
3. **Adductor longus**	From anterior surface of the body of the pubis	By an aponeurosis into the linea aspera of femur	Anterior division of obturator nerve (L2, L3, L4)	a. Adducts the thigh b. Medially rotates the thigh c. Flexes the thigh	

Contd.

Table 8.13 — Adductor muscles (Contd.)

Muscles	Origin	Insertion	Nerve supply	Actions/Functions	Clinical anatomy
					sometimes ossification may occur in the tendon of the muscle. The ossified tendon sometimes called **rider's** bones
4. Adductor magnus (hybrid muscle)	i. From the infero-lateral aspect of the ischial tuberosity (Hamstring part). ii. From the external surface of ramus of the ischium iii. A small part of the inferior ramus of the pubis	i. Pubic fibers: Medial margin of the gluteal tuberosity of the femur ii. Fibers from the ischial ramus: Linea aspera and upper part of the medial supracondylar line of the femur iii. Fibers from the "ischial tuberosity: Into the adductor tubercle of the femur	i. Obturator nerve (L2, L3, L4) ii. Tibial division of the sciatic nerve (L4, L5, S1, S2, S3)	i. Adductor of the thigh ii. Extensor of the thigh iii. Medial rotator of the thigh iv. It controls the posture	
5. Adductor brevis	Femoral surface of the body and the inferior ramus of pubis	Along a line from lesser trochanter to linea aspera of femur	Obturator nerve (L2, L3, L4)	i. Adducts the thigh. ii. Assist in flexion of thigh iii. Lateral rotation of hip joint	

Table 8.14 — Muscles of gluteal region

Muscles	Origin	Insertion	Nerve supply	Actions/Functions	Clinical anatomy
1. Gluteus maximus	i. Outer sloping area of the dorsal segment of the iliac crest ii. Area above and behind the posterior gluteal line of hip bone iii. Aponeurosis of erector spinae iv. Gluteal aponeurosis v. Sides of the last two segments of the sacrum and 1st three segments of the coccyx vi. Sacrotuberous ligament	i. Superficial fibers at the iliotibial tract ii. Deep fibers at the gluteal tuberosity of femur	Inferior gluteal nerve (L5, S1 and S2)	i. Extension, flexion and lateral rotation of thigh ii. Powerful abduction of thigh. iii. Raises the body from stooping position. iv. Cycling, walking and climbing v. It is the tensor of the fascia lata.	i. This muscle is a common site for itramuscular injection of drugs ii. Injection is always made above the line joining the posterior superior ilia spine to the greater trochanter of femur

Contd.

Table 8.14 Muscles of gluteal region (Contd.)

Muscles	Origin	Insertion	Nerve supply	Actions/Functions	Clinical anatomy
2. Gluteus medius	i. Outer surface of the ilium between the posterior and anterior gluteal lines ii. Strong fascia that covers this muscle	Oblique ridge on lateral surface of greater trochanter of femur	Superior gluteal nerve (L4, L5, S1)	i. Abducts and medially rotates the thigh during flexion and rotates laterally during extension ii. Maintain the trunk erect when the foot of the opposite side is raised from the ground during walking and running	**Trendelenburg's sign:** When gluteus medius and minimus of one side are paralyzed due to injury of the superior gluteal nerve The pelvis sinks on the healthy side. If that foot is of the ground. The affected person walks with a Lurching gait
3. Gluteus minimus	External surface of ilium between anterior and inferior gluteal lines	i. Anterior surface of the greater trochanter of femur ii. Capsule of the hip joint	Superior gluteal nerve (L4, L5, S1).	Same as gluteus medius	
4. Piriformis	i. Anterior surface of the sacrum by three digits ii. Upper border of the greater sciatic notch iii. Sacrotuberous ligament	Superior border of greater trochanter of femur	Ventral rami of S1 and S2 nerves	Rotates the thigh laterally	
5. Gemellus superior *(twin muscles)*	Upper part of lesser sciatic notch	Into medial surface of greater trochanter of femur	Nerve to obturator internus	Lateral rotation and abduction of thigh	
6. Gemellus inferior	Lower part of lesser sciatic notch	Into medial surface of greater trochanter of femur	Nerve to quadratus femoris	Lateral rotation and abduction of thigh	
7. Obturator internus	i. Pelvic surface of obturator membrane ii. Pelvic surface of the body of ischium, ischio-pubic rami and ilium below the pelvic brim	Medial surface of the greater trochanter of femur	Posterior branch of the obturator nerve (L2, L3, L4)	Lateral rotation of thigh	
8. Obturator externus	i. Outer surface of obturator membrane ii. Outer surface of the margins of obturator foramen	Inserted into the trochanteric fossa	Posterior branch of the obturator nerve (L2, L3, L4)	Lateral rotation of thigh	
9. Quadratus femoris	Upper part of the outer border of the ischial tuberosity	Quadrate tubercle and the area below it	Nerve to quadratus femoris (L4, L5, S1)	Lateral rotation of thigh	
10. Tensor fasciae latae	Anterior 5 cm of the outer lip of the iliac crest up to the tubercle of the iliac crest	Iliotibial tract 3–5 cm below the level of greater trochanter	Superior gluteal nerve (L4, L5 and S1)	i. Abduction and medial rotation of thigh ii. Extensor of knee joint	

Table 8.15 — Calf muscles (Triceps of lower limb or triceps surae)

Muscles	Origin	Insertion	Nerve supply	Actions/Functions	Clinical anatomy
1. **Gastrocnemius** (lateral and medial heads)	i. **Lateral head:** Lateral surface of lateral condyle of femur and the lateral supracondylar line of femur and capsule of the knee joint ii. **Medial head** a. Upper and posterior part of the medial condyle of the femur b. Popliteal surface of femur and capsule of the knee joint	The tendon of this muscle fuses with the tendion of the soleus to from tendocalcaneus or Achilles, which is inserted in to the middle 1/3rd of the posterior surface of the calceneus	Tibial nerve (L4, L5, S1, S2, S3)	i. Raises the heel during walking, running, etc. ii. Acts as plantar flexor of the foot iii. Flexes the knee joint	**Calf pump:** Venous plexus lies deep to the calf muscles help in venous return from the leg when the calf muscles actively contract
2. **Soleus** (peripheral heart)	i. Posterior aspect of head and proximal one-fourth of the shaft of the fibula ii. Soleal line of the tibia iii. Middle one-third of the medial border of tibial shaft iv. From a fibrous band between the tibia and fibula	The fibers of the muscle become thick and narrower and join with the gastrocnemius to form the tendocalcaneus.	Tibial nerve (L4, L5, S1, S2, S3)	i. Act as a plantar flexor of the foot at the ankle joint ii. Steading the leg on the foot in standing, walking, running, etc.	**Peripheral heart:** The soleus muscle contains larger sinusoids filled with blood. So when this muscle contracts the blood pumps into the deep veins but when the muscle relaxes blood from the superficial veins enter into the sinusoids for this reason the soleus muscle is explained as peripheral heart

Table 8.16 — Muscles of sole

Muscles of first layer of sole

Muscles	Origin	Insertion	Nerve supply	Actions/Functions	Clinical anatomy
1. **Abductor hallucis**	i. Medial calcaneal tubercle of the calcaneus ii. Flexor retinaculum iii. Plantar aponeurosis iv. Medial intermuscular septum	Medial side of the base of the proximal phalanx of the great toe (hallux).	Midial plantar nerve (S1 and S2)	Abduction and flexion of the proximal phalanx of the great toe	
2. **Flexor digitorum brevis**	i. Medial calcaneal tubercle of the calcaneus ii. Lateral and medial intermuscular septa iii. Central part of the plantar aponeurosis	It divides into four tendons. Each tendon divides into two slips that are inserted on either sides of the shaft of the middle phalanges of lateral four toes	Midial plantar nerve (S1 and S2)	Flexes lateral four toes at the proximal interphalangeal joints	

Contd.

Table 8.16   Muscles of sole *(Contd.)*

Muscles of first layer of sole

Muscles	Origin	Insertion	Nerve supply	Actions/Functions	Clinical anatomy
3. Abductor digiti minimi	i. Medial and lateral tubercles of the calcaneus ii. Lateral intermuscular septum iii. Deep fascia covering it	At the lateral side of base of proximal phalanx of little toe	Lateral plantar nerve (S2 and S3)	i. Abduction of the little toe ii. Flexion of the little toe	

Muscles of second layer of sole (with two extrinsic tendons)

Muscles	Origin	Insertion	Nerve supply	Actions/Functions	Clinical anatomy
1. Flexor digitorum accessorius	**Medial head:** Medial surface of the calcaneus **Lateral head:** Distal to the lateral tubercle of the calcaneus	To the lateral side of the tendon of flexor digitorum longus	Lateral plantar nerve (S1, S2 and S3)	Plantar flexor of lateral four toes	
2. Lumbricals (1st—unipennate and 2nd to 4th—bipennate)	i. 1st Medial border of the first tendon of the flexor digitorum longus ii. Rest of lumbricals: From the adjacent sides of the tendons of the flexor digitorum longus	Digital expansions of lateral four toes.	i. 1st: Medial plantar nerve ii. Rest: Deep branch of the lateral plantar nerve	Extension of the digits at the interphalangeal joints of the lateral four toes	
3. Flexor digitorum longus	From upper 2/3rd of the medial part of the posterior surface of tibial shaft below the soleal line	The muscle divides into four tendons. Each is inserted to the plantar surface of distal phalanges of 2nd to 5th digit	Tibial nerve	i. Plantar flexion of lateral four toes ii. Plantar flexion of ankle iii. Maintains medial longitudinal arch	
4. Flexor hallucis longus	Lower 3/4th of the posterior surface of fibula expect lowest 2.5 cm and adjoining interosseous membrane	Plantar surface of the base of the distal phalanx of the great toe	Tibial nerve	Plantar flexor of the great toe, plantar flexor of ankle joint, maintains medial longitudinal arch	

Mucles of third layer of sole

Muscles	Origin	Insertion	Nerve supply	Actions/Functions	Clinical anatomy
1. Flexor hallucis brevis	**Lateral limb** i. Lateral cuneiform bone ii. Plantar surface of cuboid bone **Medial limb** Continuation of tendon of tibialis posterior	Sides of the base of proximal phalanx of great toe by dividing into medial and lateral parts	Medial plantar nerve (S1 and S2)	Flexes the proximal phalanx of the great toe	

Contd.

Table 8.16   Muscles of sole (Contd.)

Mucles of third layer of sole

Muscles	Origin	Insertion	Nerve supply	Actions/Functions	Clinical anatomy
2. Adductor hallucis	i. *Oblique head:* Bases of 2nd to 4th metatarsal bones and fibrous sheath of peroneus longus tendon ii. *Transverse head:* Plantar metatarsophalangeal ligaments of 3rd to 5th toes and deep transverse ligament of the foot	Lateral side of the base of the proximal phalanx of the great toe	Deep branch of lateral plantar nerve (S2, S3)	i. Adductor of great toe towards the 2nd toe. ii. Maintains transverse arch of the foot	
3. Flexor digiti minimi brevis	i. Plantar surface of the base of the fifth metatarsal bone ii. Sheath of peroneus longus tendon	Lateral side of the base of proximal phalanx of little toe	Superficial branch of lateral plantar nerve (S2, S3)	Flexes metatarsophalangeal joint of the little toe	

Muscles of fourth layer of sole (with two extrinsic tendons)

Muscles	Origin	Insertion	Nerve supply	Actions/Functions	Clinical anatomy
1. Plantar interossei (3 in no and unipennate muscles)	Bases and medial sides of matatarsal bones from third to fifth	Medial sides of bases of proximal phalanges of extensor expansions of third to fifth toes	1st and 2nd: Lateral plantar nerve (deep branch) 3rd: Lateral plantar nerve (superficial branch)	i. Adducts third to fifth toes ii. Flexes the metatarso-phalangeal and extend the interphalangeal joints	
2. Dorsal interossei (4 in no and Bipennate muscles)	Ajacent sides of matatarsal bones (first to fifth)	At the bases of proximal phalanges and dorsal digital expansions **First**-medial side of second toe Second, third and fourth lateral sides of second, third and fourth toes.	1st, 2nd and 3rd by: Lateral plantar nerve (deep branch). 4th: dorsal inter-osseous branch of lateral plantar nerve	i. Abductors of toes. ii. 1st and 2nd causes medial and lateral abductors of 2nd toe. 3rd and 4th for abduction of 3rd and 4th toes	
3. Tibialis posterior	i. Upper 2/3 of lateral part of posterior surface of tibia below the soleal line ii. Posterior surface of fibula in front of the medial crest iii. Posterior surface of the interosseous membrane	i. Principal insertion to the tuberosity of the navicular bone ii. Planter aspects of all tarsal bones except talus iii. 2nd to 4th metatarsal bones at their bases	Tibial nerve	i. Plantar flexor of ankle joint. ii. Main invertor of foot iii. Supports the medial longitudinal arch of foot	
4. Peroneus longus	i. Head of the fibula ii. Upper 2/3rd of lateral surface of shaft of fibula iii. Deep surface of the fascia cruris	Lateral side of the first metatarsal bone and the adjoining part of the medial cuneiform bone	Superficial peroneal nerve	i. Evertor of the foot ii. Maintain the lateral longitudinal arch and transverse arch of foot	

Table 8.17   Musles of mastication

Muscle	Origin	Insertion	Nerve supply	Actions/Functions	Clinical anatomy
1. Temporalis	Temporal fossa of the temporal bone and temporal fascia	Anterior border of the ramus, margins and deep surface of coronoid process of the mandible	Deep temporal nerves branches of anterior division of mandibular nerve	i. Elevates the mandible ii. Retracts the mandible iii. Side-to-side grinding movements	**Testing of masseter and temporalis muscles:** Ask the patient to bite his teeth, the temporalis and masseter muscles should equal prominence on both sides. This can be better checked by palpation over the muscle, in case if there is paralysis. The muscles on that side will fail to become prominent
2. Masseter	i. **Superficial layer:** Anterior twothirds of the inferior border of the zygomatic arch and adjoining zygomatic process of maxilla. ii. **Deep layer:** Deep surface of the zygomatic arch iii. **Middle layer:** Lower border of posterior 1/3rd of zygomatic arch	i. **Superficial layer:** Angle and lower part of lateral surface of the mandibular ramus ii. **Deep layer:** Rest part of the mandibular ramus iii. Central part of the mandibular ramus	Masseteric branch of the anterior division of mandibular nerve	i. Elevates the mandible to close the mouth. ii. Exerts force of compression between mandibular and maxillary teeth. iii. Side-to-side movements, and protrusion of mandible	
3. Lateral pterygoid	**Upper head:** From infratemporal surface and crest of the greater wing of sphenoid bone **Lower head:** Lateral surface of the lateral pterygoid plate of sphenoid bone	i. Articular capsule and disk of the temporomandibular joint ii. Anterior surface of neck of mandible	Branch from the anterior division of the mandibular nerve	i. It depresses the mandible to open the mouth. ii. Helps in chewing by upper head iii. Protrudes the mandible forwards. iv. Right lateral pterygoid turns the chin to left side.	**Testing:** The patient is asked to open the mouth widely gainst gentle resistance. If the chin deviates to one side, it indicates the paralysis of lateral pterygoid of the same side
4. Medial pterygoid	**Deep head** i. Medial surface of the lateral pterygoid plate of the sphenoid bone ii. Pyramidal process of the palatine bone **Superficial head:** Lateral surface of the pyramidal process of palatine bone and maxillary tuberosity	Medial surface of the ramus and angle of the mandible	Nerve to medial pterygoid branch of trunk of mandibular nerve	i. It elevates the mandible ii. Moves the mandible from side-to-side iii. Protrudes the mandible forwards	
5. Buccinator (accessory of muscle of mastication)	i. Outer surface of the alveolar processes of the maxilla and the mandible opposite the three molar teeth ii. Pterygomandibular ligament	i. Upper fibers pass to lower lip ii. Lower fibers pass to upper lip iii. Middle fibers intersect at the angle of mouth	Lower buccal branch of facial nerve	i. Compress the cheek against the gum and teeth ii. Helps whistling, sucking and blowing	Paralysis of buccinator muscle occurs in facial palsy, causes the food accumulates between cheek and gum during mastication

Table 8.18   Muscle of the Side of neck

Muscle	Origin	Insertion	Nerve supply	Actions/Functions	Clinical anatomy
1. Sterno-cleido-mastoid	i. **Sternal head:** Superolateral part of the anterior surface of manubrium sterni ii. **Clavicular head:** Superior surface of the medial one-third of clavicle	i. Lateral surface of the mastoid process of temporal bone ii. Lateral half of superior nuchal line of occipital bone	i. Spinal accessory nerve ii. Branches from the ventral rami of C2 and C3 (sometimes C4) nerves	i. Draws the head and neck towards the adjacent shoulder and towards opposite side ii. It raises the head from recumbent to sitting posture iii. Rotation of head and draws the head forwards iv. It helps the muscles of forced inspiration v. Extension and flexion of neck	**Wryneck or torticollis** i. In this deformity the head is bent to the affected side while the face turns to the opposite side. ii. It is caused by difficult labor which results in hemorrhage occurs in the muscle

Index